Public Health in the 21st Century

Caregivers

Challenges, Practices and Cultural Influences

PUBLIC HEALTH IN THE 21ST CENTURY

Additional books in this series can be found on Nova's website under the Series tab.

Additional e-books in this series can be found on Nova's website under the e-book tab.

PUBLIC HEALTH IN THE 21ST CENTURY

CAREGIVERS

CHALLENGES, PRACTICES AND CULTURAL INFLUENCES

ADRIANNA THURGOOD
AND
KASHA SCHULDT
EDITORS

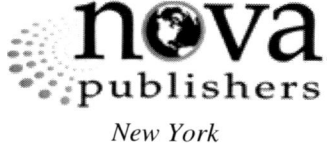

New York

Copyright © 2013 by Nova Science Publishers, Inc.

All rights reserved. No part of this book may be reproduced, stored in a retrieval system or transmitted in any form or by any means: electronic, electrostatic, magnetic, tape, mechanical photocopying, recording or otherwise without the written permission of the Publisher.

For permission to use material from this book please contact us:
Telephone 631-231-7269; Fax 631-231-8175
Web Site: http://www.novapublishers.com

NOTICE TO THE READER

The Publisher has taken reasonable care in the preparation of this book, but makes no expressed or implied warranty of any kind and assumes no responsibility for any errors or omissions. No liability is assumed for incidental or consequential damages in connection with or arising out of information contained in this book. The Publisher shall not be liable for any special, consequential, or exemplary damages resulting, in whole or in part, from the readers' use of, or reliance upon, this material. Any parts of this book based on government reports are so indicated and copyright is claimed for those parts to the extent applicable to compilations of such works.

Independent verification should be sought for any data, advice or recommendations contained in this book. In addition, no responsibility is assumed by the publisher for any injury and/or damage to persons or property arising from any methods, products, instructions, ideas or otherwise contained in this publication.

This publication is designed to provide accurate and authoritative information with regard to the subject matter covered herein. It is sold with the clear understanding that the Publisher is not engaged in rendering legal or any other professional services. If legal or any other expert assistance is required, the services of a competent person should be sought. FROM A DECLARATION OF PARTICIPANTS JOINTLY ADOPTED BY A COMMITTEE OF THE AMERICAN BAR ASSOCIATION AND A COMMITTEE OF PUBLISHERS.

Additional color graphics may be available in the e-book version of this book.

Library of Congress Cataloging-in-Publication Data

ISBN: 978-1-62618-030-7

Library of Congress Control Number: 2013931034

Published by Nova Science Publishers, Inc. † New York

CONTENTS

Preface		vii
Chapter 1	A Lifespan Developmental Approach to Assessing and Addressing Neurodevelopmental Disorders: A Comprehensive Guide to Meeting Individual and Caregiver Needs *Rebecca H. Foster, Elliott W. Simon, Elizabeth B. B. Lee, LaNaya Shackelford and Sarah H. Elsea*	1
Chapter 2	The Family Caregivers of Patients with Cancer: Roles and Challenges *Sabrina Cipolletta*	57
Chapter 3	Zooming (In) – Zooming (Out): From Feeling Exclusively like a Caregiver to Integrating Caregiving in Daily Life. Understanding Sudden Informal Caregivers' Paths *Helder Rocha Pereira*	77
Chapter 4	Parental and Educators´ Judgments and Attitudes toward Life Challenges of people with Intellectual Disabilities: Functional Measurement Contributions to Special Education from a Cognitive Algebra Approach *Guadalupe Elizabeth Morales, Ernesto Octavio Lopez, David Jose Charles, Claudia Castro Campos and Martha Patricia Sanchez*	97
Chapter 5	The Experience of Caregiving across Myths and Cultures *Camilla Pietrantonio, Francesco Pagnini, Paolo Banfi, Gianluca Castelnuovo and Enrico Molinari*	119
Chapter 6	Resilience in Caregivers *Violeta Fernández-Lansac and María Crespo*	137
Chapter 7	Caregiver Burden in a Hong Kong Chinese Population: Risk Factors, Consequences and Remedies *P. H. Chau, T. Kwok and J. Woo*	157
Chapter 8	Managing Compassion Fatigue among Professional Cancer Caregivers: Understanding the Problem and Possible Treatment Strategies *Amanda C. Kracen and Teresa L. Deshields*	171

Chapter 9	Caregiving in Clinical Oncology *Carola Locatelli, Marcella Cicerchia and Lazzaro Repetto*	**183**
Chapter 10	Caregiver Burden of Older Adults: A Southeast Asian Aspect *Panita Limpawattana and Jarin Chindaprasirt*	**195**
Chapter 11	Community-Based Education Concerning Palliative Care for the Elderly in Japan *Yoshihisa Hirakawa and Kazumasa Uemura*	**207**
Chapter 12	Does Caregiver Perception Reflect Oral Health in Cerebral Palsy Children? *Renata Oliveira Guaré, Daniel Cividanis Gomes Nogueira Fernandes and Maria Teresa Botti Rodrigues Santos*	**217**
Chapter 13	Role of Assistive Technologies for Person-Centered Dementia Care: An Exploratory Case Study in Japan *Taro Sugihara and Tsutomu Fujinami*	**225**
Index		**243**

PREFACE

In this book, the authors discuss the challenges, practices and cultural influences of caregiving. Topics include caregiving for individuals with neurodevelopmental disorders and intellectual disabilities; family caregivers for patients with cancer; elder caregiving in South Asian families in the U.S. and India; study of caregiver's resilience; caregiver burden in a Hong Kong Chinese population; managing compassion fatigue among professional cancer caregivers; community-based education for palliative care for the elderly in Japan; caregiver perception and oral health in cerebral palsy children; and the role of assistive technologies for person-centered dementia care in Japan.

Chapter 1 - Individuals living with neurodevelopmental disorders (NDs) require substantial specialized supports and resources across the lifespan. Parents and siblings are typically at the forefront of caring for these individuals and ensuring that individualized medical and psychosocial needs are met. Within their roles as primary caregivers, numerous benefits and challenges are often encountered while working to promote the best quality of life possible for the entire family unit. Using a lifespan developmental approach, this chapter highlights the experiences of those caring for individuals diagnosed with NDs, with an emphasis on the unique needs of those acting as caregivers for individuals diagnosed with Smith-Magenis, Williams, or Down syndrome. Challenges associated with each predominant developmental period are explored, including methods of assessing specific challenges via psychological or neuropsychological evaluation. Example recommendations made to address these challenges are provided, and how primary caregivers can seek out resources aimed at addressing challenges is discussed. Advocating within educational systems, independent living and vocational planning, and overall family-oriented quality of life are emphasized. Given that siblings are frequently called upon to assume caregiver roles and financial responsibility as they age, distinct challenges within this relationship dynamic are considered. Legal concerns regarding guardianships and alternatives to guardianships are also highlighted.

Chapter 2 - Assisting a loved one with cancer implies assuming a role that may fit or contrast with the person's previous role, thereby allowing the person to adjust to the new role or provoking suffering. In order to explore the constraints and challenges this situation may pose, a research project was developed at the University of Padua (Italy). A first study explored if it was possible to identify different profiles of caregivers on the basis of their different ways of giving and receiving help. Fifty Italian family caregivers of patients with cancer completed the Beck Anxiety Inventory, the Beck Depression Inventory-II and Kelly's

Dependency Grids. Cluster analysis was conducted on the indices derived from the three instruments. Three profiles emerged and were described on the basis of the balance/imbalance between the usual and present role of the caregiver. If there was congruence between the situation of giving help that the caregivers experienced and their personal role, then anxiety and depression decreased, otherwise they increased. The implications of the balance /imbalance between the usual and present role depended also on the typicality of the caregivers' experience, as related to their caring role. A subsequent study, was aimed at investigating in depth the meaning and impact of cancer in patients and caregivers' lives and relationships. Semi-structured interviews were carried out with eight patients admitted to a hospice in northern Italy and their family caregivers using interpretative phenomeno-logical analysis to analyze the interview transcripts. This discovered a complex relationship between patients and caregivers' narrations, also influenced by their relationship with health professionals. These results suggest that personalized support to family caregivers may empower them, allowing them to find new ways to play their helping role.

Chapter 3 - What are the experiences faced by informal caregivers that suddenly and unexpectedly are forced to begin such a role? What are the stages of their unexpected paths? What experiences do they consider most relevant? What works or does not work for them in their interactions with professionals whose mission is to give them support in their new role?

The experiences of informal caregivers of loved ones are a widely studied topic, both in terms of assessing the caregivers' needs, of support programs available and of the implications that the responsibility of giving care (*burden*) represents to caregivers' health and well-being, amongst other things.

Nevertheless, when the unforseen focus is placed on the informal caregiver, who did not anticipate seeing him/herself as such, the available evidence is still scarce and reveals gaps that need to be addressed.

This chapter is based in the results of a phenomenological hermeneutical study (N=14 sudden informal caregivers), as well as on the integration of those results with published narratives of personal experiences of informal caregiving and relevant knowledge in this area, enabling a better understanding of the phenomenon.

The focus of this chapter is to globally understand the non linear path between two distinct poles, which are characterized by unstable points of balance. There are two extremes: seeing oneself as exclusively a caregiver (Zooming (in) in the caregiver situation) and integrating caregiving in one's life (Zooming(out).

In truth, for sudden caregivers, the experience in developing their role is that of an "attack/theft" on/of their previous life. The main focus in the sudden caregiver's life becomes that of being a caregiver (giving care, worrying, feeling insecure, having to be constantly present, as well as many other aspects). Taking on that role quickly consumes the caregiver's whole life. Their focus becomes almost exclusively to develop that new role.

The unexpected, urgent and "unprepared" nature of such a situation results in focusing solely on caregiving. As time goes by and and reflecting upon the situation, the caregiver realizes that he/she cannot be committed to a situation that limits or affects his/her wellbeing, freedom, social contacts, mental health and other responsibilities in the remaining facets of his/her life. In order to regain a sense of normality, the caregiver must detach his/herself from his/her situation and allow the role of caregiving to be harmoniously integrated along with other roles and competing needs emerging from their daily lives (Zooming (out).

This chapter (i) explores those processes based upon the experiences reported by the study participants, (ii) recalls relevant knowledge to broaden professionals' understanding of the phenomenon (for example: the transitions theory, the caregivers' career or the need of respite care) and (iii) presents a group of high clinical value indicators, identified in the research process, that may help professionals to better understand and monitor new caregivers' paths in this process of adapting themselves to suddenly becoming a caregiver.

Chapter 4 - For a long time, a person with an intellectual disability (ID) was ignored as a human being. Their interests, aspirations and needs were not contemplated as a priority. Fortunately, in many societies this inappropriate and deep-rooted vision seems to be changing. New efforts coming from parents, teachers and carriers to promote the human rights of this population have had a direct effect on improving the quality of their lives. For example, nowadays a more open attitude can be identified. ID individuals may be included in regular school and work. Their right to exercise a sexual life is considered. In this chapter, the authors argue that comprehending the cognitive nature of parents and caregivers´ beliefs, attitudes and judgments toward persons with ID, will provide significant life improvements in this population. Specifically, the Information Integration Theory (IIT) research approach will be introduced. It allows scientific scrutiny about how contextual and human factors of a society are integrated into systematic thinking (cognitive algebra). The authors discuss how the IIT approach can be used whenever improvement of life conditions of people with ID is considered.

Chapter 5 - The person who gives care, the caregiver, must be aware of the disease, should be taught by qualified staff about strategies and optimal techniques to be applied on behalf of the care receiver to deal with the difficulties of everyday life.

The vast literature on the subject has now shown that caregiving cannot be reduced to a simple phenomenon that is attuned only to the fulfillment of a patient's needs. The question of assistance is very complex because it involves many aspects of health and the level of support necessary to the individual in need, but also to the organization of social care, to the policies that manage and ensure its delivery. The notion of assistance regards all those cultural elements and values that relate to field of ethics, justice and social equality, individual well-being and community.

Culture gives meaning to the events that occur in our lives, by ascribing to each one different values and emotions so the importance of cultural influences is essential in caregiving too. A broad range of literature has investigated the relationship among the characteristics of caregivers' culture, the role of the emotions and the mode of action of caregivers.

In the present and, even more so, in the future, it appears that daily confrontation with illness, disability, non-self-sufficiency will be a continuing challenge to our civilization, social welfare systems and health systems so a new vision of the "economy of care" is warranted.

Chapter 6 – Caring for a dependent relative is a major source of stress and it is common to consequently suffer emotional issues, such as depression or anxiety symptoms. However, a large number of caregivers perceive their situation as a positive experience, and feel uplifts or satisfaction at times. Hence, why do some caregivers adapt to this situation while others do not? This study of resilience aims to answer this question.

Resilience in caregivers refers to the overall capacity of individuals to face caregiving without having their mental health severely compromised, or their usual functioning altered.

This capacity comprises a number of resources and individual skills, among which the following can be found: competence, tenacity, trust in one's instincts, tolerance to negative affect, strengthening effects, positive acceptance to change, secure relationships, control, and spiritual influences. Research has shown that the sum of these subcapacities acts as an important protective factor that attenuates the impact of objective stressors on mental health. Elucidating the variables that determine the development of caregivers' resilience is therefore a major step forward to identify how individuals overcome chronic stress situations.

Bearing this in mind, the study at hand has been conducted with a sample of 111 Spanish non-professional caregivers of elderly relatives. Its aim was to analyze the connection between resilience, as a mediator factor, with different variables regarding: care context, primary and secondary stressors, appraisals, other mediator variables (social support, intrapsychic resources and personality characteristics), together with the emotional status of caregivers. The outcomes of this study will be integrated into a conceptual model of caregivers' resilience. The implications of this work in clinical practice will be discussed in this chapter.

Chapter 7 – To achieve the goal of ageing-in-place, informal family caregivers who look after older people at home are of crucial importance. In Hong Kong, over half of all elderly people, who receive informal care, are cared for by their children. Despite traditional Chinese beliefs concerned with filial piety, these caregivers, particularly if they have to deal with dementia or stroke patients, often face very heavy burdens, which may in turn lead to higher risk of institutionalization, and in some extreme cases abuse of the elderly. Deterioration in functional and cognitive status of the care recipient produces two of the main factors adding to the caregiver burden, while assistance from domestic helpers and a sense of self-efficacy may reduce it. Some initiatives, such as training programs for caregivers, which may ameliorate their situation have been established. In this chapter, existing and new evidence is presented on the risk factors and consequences of caregiver burden among the Hong Kong Chinese population, and strategies to tackle such burdens are discussed.

Chapter 8 – Professional cancer caregivers work with patients who are ill and vulnerable. Caregivers have opportunities to support and care for patients, and hopefully, to offer comfort and healing. However, as a result of the empathy and personal involvement they bring to their jobs, compassion fatigue (CF) is a common professional challenge. Recognizing that CF negatively affects many caregivers, as well as their colleagues and patients, this chapter provides an overview of recent research into CF in professional cancer caregivers. Specifically, the chapter defines CF and related constructs, reviews the prevalence and effects of CF, highlights why CF is a concern in oncology, and provides an overview of evidence-based interventions and personal coping strategies to ameliorate symptoms and enhance resiliency among caregivers.

Chapter 9 – More often, family play a central role in providing support to the complex needs of cancer patients; there are 4.6 million Americans who care for someone with cancer at home.

Informal caring may involve considerable physical, psychological and economic stresses. Several recent studies have examined the effect of caregiving on the health and well-being of cancer caregivers. These studies indicate that stress and demands associated with caregiving can cause problems and changes for caregivers in areas such as their psychological, physical, and financial well-being. This impairment has an important impact not only on the caregiver but also on the patient. We have to consider that caregivers who had high emotional distress in the course of illness had a significant negative effect on the adjustment of patients with cancer. Although many studies are set up to determine the link between the stressors in caregiving and the impact on the family caregiver and/or on the patient's outcomes, the results remained inconclusive. A range of supportive programmes for caregivers is being developed including psychological support and practical assistance. A recent (2011) and systematic review has detected an encouraging growth in the number of intervention studies that aim to improve outcomes for caregiver in cancer and palliative care and an improvement in the study designs used. However, this activity needs to continue to focus on mechanisms of intervention, powerful designs and a plurality of models and target populations/settings.

There is an urgent need for health care providers and policy makers to recognize the pivotal role of family caregivers in patients' care and a need to view them as care partners establishing tailored training programs. These intervention programs should give to caregivers the knowledge and skills to manage the patients' changing needs, also should grant tax credits or compensation for the care they provide and for the financial damages they make. A concerted effort is needed to train health professionals about the needs of caregivers and the importance of assessing them as part of routine cancer care. Training programs should ensure that clinicians are prepared to work with caregivers, to understand their needs, and to recognize the range of responsibilities being asked of them. For the caregivers training should incorporate strategies that would help caregivers to develop positive lifestyle behaviors, effective coping skills, and ways to access resources. Improved patient outcomes, including early detection or better management of adverse effects, increased adherence to oral medication, would result in reduced health care use and costs.

In respect to this topic the authors are performing a study aimed to demonstrate the mutuality of psychological distress in both cancer patients and their caregivers, by validation of a new assessment tool able to identify the risk factors to develop mental disorders in the caregivers' population.

We need to integrate a different point of view beginning to consider the patient-caregiver dyad as a unit of care. If the patient-caregiver dyad is treated as the unit of care, we can promote important synergies that can increase the well-being of both patients and caregivers.

Chapter 10 – Disability is common among the elderly; it worsens with age and erodes the well-being of the caregiver(s). Caregivers of the elderly with chronic illness (eg. dementia and stroke) will likely experience personal life strain, social isolation, financial burden, and lack of intrinsic reward. The perception of burden varies based on socioeconomic and cultural backgrounds. From a Southeast Asian perspective, a considerable burden for the care of older persons with disability is based on informal care by family members. It, however, varies considerably even within the region and data are limited. Developing a better understanding of the caregiving process—include all of the factors contributing to the caregiver's burden among these populations—would help allied-health workers provide support in dealing with the various stressors more effectively. Intervention(s) to lessen the caregivers' burden would include (a) assessment of the associated portions by focusing on acknowledged specific concerns (b) evaluating of caregivers' perspective regarding patients' illness and (c) management of a care plan with family members.

Chapter 11 – Japan is confronted with shifting preferences of elderly patients and their families regarding their care. Namely, an increasing number of elderly people are now opting to spend their last few years of life in community settings such as long-term care facilities or in their own home. The community is therefore expected to assume a growing responsibility in caring for the dying elderly. Improving the quality and quantity of palliative care provision at home or at long-term care facilities has become an urgent priority in Japan. We believe that community-based palliative care education is one of the most important aspects of palliative care for the elderly.

Although a number of palliative care educational intervention programs have reportedly been implemented, many of these programs were formulated for university education rather than for community-based education.

In this chapter, the authors described the current situation of community-based education concerning palliative care for the elderly in Japan. They also explained the details of community-based education programs concerning palliative care for the elderly, with special focus on community staff education.

Chapter 12 – *Purpose:* This study is aimed to evaluate the quality of life of children with CP concerning oral health/dental caries and their caregivers' perception.

Methods: Forty-three children with CP, aged 1-15 years-old (8.7 ±3.7) were evaluated regarding dental caries experience (DMF Index; WHO 1997) and grouped as Group I (GI, n=20; carie-free; DMFT=0), and Group II (GII, n=23; with caries, DMFT≥1). Caregivers completed the questionnaire Early Childhood Oral Health Impact Scale (B_ECOHIS) composed of 13 questions with frequency scores ranging from 0 to 4, such that the higher the score, the greater the impact on the child, the family and the overall value. Comparison between the groups was performed by the Fisher Exact and Mann-Whitney tests, with the significance level set at 5%.

Results: Significant differences were observed between the group impact scores for child (GI 0.95 ±1.67 and GII 3.00 ±3.93, p=0.044), family (GI 0.05 ±0.22 and GII 1.13 ± 1.84, p=0.007) and overall (GI 1.00 ±1.78 and GII 4.14 ±4.82, p=0.004), with higher values for Group II.

Conclusion: Caregiver perception does not reflect the real condition of the child's oral health and caries increase the impact and diminish the quality of life in children with CP.

Chapter 13 – This chapter discusses the potential role of assistive technologies for dementia care. Despite urgent needs for person-centered care, it is difficult for care houses in Japan to achieve it because of a lack of resources and fatigue caused by the shortage of funds and caregivers. Assistive technologies for dementia care are fruitful in helping care work. However, little attention has been focused on the influence of these technologies on person-centered care. To investigate effects of assistive technologies on the care house, the authors installed a video monitoring system for caregivers in three homes and observed the effects of applying the system to caregiving by interviews and video observations.

As results, the video monitoring system enabled caregivers to optimize their work and helped them concentrate on their tasks at hand, reducing both mental and physical stresses. Finally, the authors established the concept of a triage support environment, which can augment dementia care.

In: Caregivers: Challenges, Practices and Cultural Influences
Editors: Adrianna Thurgood and Kasha Schuldt
ISBN: 978-1-62618-030-7
© 2013 Nova Science Publishers, Inc.

Chapter 1

A LIFESPAN DEVELOPMENTAL APPROACH TO ASSESSING AND ADDRESSING NEURODEVELOPMENTAL DISORDERS: A COMPREHENSIVE GUIDE TO MEETING INDIVIDUAL AND CAREGIVER NEEDS

Rebecca H. Foster[1,2]*****, *Elliott W. Simon*[3],
Elizabeth B. B. Lee[4], *LaNaya Shackelford*[1]
and Sarah H. Elsea[5]

[1]Department of Psychology, Winona State University, Winona, Minnesota, US
[2]Gundersen Lutheran Medical Center, La Crosse, Wisconsin, US
[3]Research and Health Services, Elwyn, Elwyn, Pennsylvania, US
[4]Department of Psychology, St. Jude Children's Research Hospital, Memphis, Tennessee, US
[5]Department of Molecular and Human Genetics, Baylor College of Medicine, Houston, Texas, US

ABSTRACT

Individuals living with neurodevelopmental disorders (NDs) require substantial specialized supports and resources across the lifespan. Parents and siblings are typically at the forefront of caring for these individuals and ensuring that individualized medical and psychosocial needs are met. Within their roles as primary caregivers, numerous benefits and challenges are often encountered while working to promote the best quality of life possible for the entire family unit. Using a lifespan developmental approach, this chapter highlights the experiences of those caring for individuals diagnosed with NDs, with an emphasis on the unique needs of those acting as caregivers for individuals diagnosed with Smith-Magenis, Williams, or Down syndrome. Challenges associated

---

***** Correspondence should be addressed to: Rebecca H. Foster, Ph.D., Dept. of Psychology, Winona State University, Winona, MN 55987 USA, Phone: 507-457-5543, Fax: 507-457-2327, Email: rfoster@winona.edu

with each predominant developmental period are explored, including methods of assessing specific challenges via psychological or neuropsychological evaluation. Example recommendations made to address these challenges are provided, and how primary caregivers can seek out resources aimed at addressing challenges is discussed. Advocating within educational systems, independent living and vocational planning, and overall family-oriented quality of life are emphasized. Given that siblings are frequently called upon to assume caregiver roles and financial responsibility as they age, distinct challenges within this relationship dynamic are considered. Legal concerns regarding guardianships and alternatives to guardianships are also highlighted.

Keywords: Neurdevelopmental disorders, Smith-Magenis syndrome, Williams syndrome, Down syndrome, caregivers, siblings

INTRODUCTION

"[Having a sibling with a neurodevelopmental disorder] has taught me to respect life the way it is made."

12 year-old sibling of 5.5 year-old diagnosed with Down syndrome

Promoting the best quality of life possible for individuals with neurodevelopmental disorders (NDs) and their families requires significant time and attention to both individual- and family-based needs. For many of these families, substantial specialized care and resources are needed across the lifespan of the diagnosed individual. Parents and siblings are typically at the forefront of providing supportive care and ensuring that individualized medical and psychosocial needs are met. Within their roles as primary caregivers[1], numerous benefits and challenges are often encountered. Primary caregivers must learn to cope with these challenges in such a way that meets the child's specific needs while also preserving the well-being of the entire family unit. Therefore, this chapter investigates the experiences of those caring for individuals diagnosed with NDs, with an emphasis on the unique lifelong needs of those acting as caregivers for individuals diagnosed with Smith-Magenis syndrome (SMS), Williams syndrome (WS), or Down syndrome (DS). Challenges associated with each predominant developmental period are explored, including those encountered during infancy, early childhood, middle childhood, adolescence, and adulthood. Methods of assessing specific individual and family needs via developmental, psychological, neuropsychological, and vocational evaluation will be discussed within the context of each developmental period. Example recommendations made to address identified challenges are presented, along with examples of how caregivers can seek out resources aimed at addressing those identified needs. Approaches to coping with developmental and behavioral concerns are highlighted. Common challenges related to educational systems, independent living, vocational planning, and overall family-oriented quality of life are emphasized. Given that siblings are frequently called upon to assume supportive roles and financial responsibility as they age, distinct challenges within this relationship dynamic are considered. Legal concerns regarding guardianship and alternatives to guardianships are also discussed.

---

[1] For the purposes of this chapter, the term "primary caregivers" or "caregivers" generally refers to parents and/or other legal guardians.

WHAT ARE NEURODEVELOPMENTAL DISORDERS?

"My daughter was just diagnosed today. It has been 32 years of trying to find out if there was some unifying reason for all of her differentnesses."

Parent of 32 year-old diagnosed with SMS

By definition, neurodevelopmental disorders (NDs) are a classification of disabilities that predominately affect the development and functioning of the nervous system (Reynolds and Goldstein, 1999). Multiple disorders have been classified as NDs, including intellectual disability, learning disorders, autism spectrum disorders (ASD), and attention-deficit /hyperactivity disorder (ADHD). Those diagnosed with NDs experience a variety of challenges, such as problems with speech and language, motor function, adaptive behaviors, emotional expression, memory, and age-appropriate learning. Although specific problem areas and needs often change across the lifespan, the majority of children who are diagnosed with a ND will continue to experience challenges as they age. Addressing these ever-changing needs can be quite difficult, and day-to-day management typically requires intensive time and commitment in the form of home- and school-based interventions, community-based therapies, and medication management. As expected, the totality of these stressors can place tremendous demands on primary caregivers and siblings.

HOW ARE NEURODEVELOPMENTAL AND GENETIC DISORDERS RELATED?

"Children with SMS require lots and lots of patience and understanding. They have mental disabilities that cause major behavior meltdowns and delayed learning."

Parent of a child diagnosed with SMS

"Now that I know that there is a legitimate medical reason for her delays, I am not so anxious for my daughter to "catch up" to an appropriate stage of development for her age. I am more relaxed knowing that she has her own timetable, and that she will grow and progress eventually."

Parent of a child diagnosed with SMS

In the United States (U.S.), approximately 12-13% of children between the ages of 3 and 17 are diagnosed with one or more NDs (Pastor and Reuben, 2009). Both medical communities and educators have observed what appears to be a genuine increase in the prevalence of children with NDs (Grupp-Phelan, Harman, and Kelleher, 2007; Kelleher, McInerny, Gardner, Childs, and Wasserman, 2000; U.S. Department of Education, 2007). Recent research suggests that the percentage of children diagnosed with such a disability will continue to rise, in part due to increased public awareness and modifications in diagnostic criteria (Froehlich, Lanphear, Epstein, Barbaresi, Katusic, and Kahn, 2007; Grandjean and

Landrigan, 2006; Newschaffer, Falb, and Gurney, 2005; Prior, 2003; Rutter, 2005; Visser, Bitsko, Danielson, Perou, and Blumberg, 2010).

Genetics likely plays a salient role in the etiology of NDs, and children diagnosed with genetic disorders are often found to have some type of ND as an expression of the genetic condition. Throughout the world, more than 7.6 million children are born with some type of severe genetic condition annually (World Health Organization, 2005), resulting in a large number of families who must learn to cope with related stressors, including medical problems, developmental delays, and/or intellectual impairments.

Approximately half of intellectual disabilities have a known genetic basis (Emery and Rimoin, 1990), with the expression of the disability typically being attributed to both genetic and environmental factors (Dykens, Hodapp, and Finucane, 2000). Based on the current DSM-IV-TR (American Psychiatric Association (APA), 2000) diagnostic criteria, an individual can be diagnosed with an intellectual disability if there is evidence of impaired intellectual functioning prior to age 18 and if they also demonstrate deficits in adaptive functioning. Impaired intellectual functioning is typically defined as having an intelligence quotient (IQ) of approximately 70 or less, based on a standardized, well-validated intelligence assessment. Adaptive functioning refers to daily living skills, such as communication, self-care behaviors, independent living, or social/interpersonal skills (American Association of Intellectual and Developmental Disabilities, 2012; Schroeder, 2000). The DSM-IV-TR further categorizes intellectual disabilities into four sub-groups, including 1) mild (i.e., intellectual quotient of 50-55 to approximately 70), 2) moderate (i.e., IQ of 35-40 to 50-55), 3) severe (i.e., IQ of 20-25 to 35-40), or 4) profound impairment (i.e., IQ below 20-25; Greenberg et al., 1996; Martens, Wilson, and Reutens, 2008; Meyer-Lindenberg, Mervis, and Berman, 2006). The majority of individuals with Smith-Magenis, Williams, or Down syndromes, the primary foci of this chapter, will have IQs falling in the range of mild to moderate intellectual impairment.

Of note, the term "intellectual disability" is the preferred term utilized among disability sectors when describing intellectual impairments. However, the term "mental retardation" continues to be utilized, most often in law and public policy sectors. It is anticipated that the term "mental retardation" will be largely replaced with "intellectual disability" or "intellectual developmental disorder" when the DSM-5 is released in 2013 (Comer, 2013). In addition, "mental retardation," which is now categorized in the grouping of "Disorders Usually First Diagnosed in Infancy, Childhood, or Adolescence" will be listed in a new grouping called "Neurodevelopmental Disorders" along with ADHD, learning disorders, communication disorders, coordination disorders, and autism spectrum disorders. Other commonalities among both neurodevelopmental and genetic disorders, such as problems with learning and attention, will be discussed elsewhere in this chapter.

DIAGNOSING SMITH-MAGENIS, WILLIAMS, AND DOWN SYNDROMES

This chapter provides a broad overview of individual, primary caregiver, and family needs among those coping with NDs. Discussion topics will include challenges that often emerge across specific developmental periods, perceived family benefits that result from the disorder, and available resources and services aimed at assisting individuals and families coping with NDs. In addition to this broad overview, special attention will be paid regarding the needs of those living with and supporting individuals diagnosed with Smith-Magenis syndrome (SMS), Williams syndrome (WS), and Down syndrome (DS).

Smith-Magenis Syndrome

> "I feel so very blessed to have my brother in my life. His bright spirit and his sweetness - even in the face of overwhelming obstacles he faces daily - are a constant inspiration to me. My relationship with him has made me a better person - a more loving, patient, kind and happy person. My relationship with my developmentally-typical siblings is closer because of the bond that we share in having a brother with special needs. My brother is an essential part of my family and of my life. And while there certainly have been challenges (I don't think I slept a full night once during my high school years), I can honestly say that I wouldn't trade my experience of being his sister for anything in the world."
>
> 26 year-old sibling of 13 year-old with SMS

Smith-Magenis syndrome (SMS) is a chromosomal disorder caused by either a deletion of a portion of chromosome 17 or a mutation of the *RAI1* gene, which lies within the SMS chromosome 17p11.2 region (Elsea and Girirajan, 2008; Smith et al., 2006). This syndrome affects approximately 1 out of 15,000 to 1 out of 25,000 live births worldwide and is typically a sporadic syndrome that is not inherited from a parent. Individuals are affected equally across genders and racial groups. The syndrome is characterized by physical, developmental, and behavioral features (Smith et al., 2006). Common features among those diagnosed with SMS include craniofacial anomalies, a hoarse voice, feeding problems in infancy, low muscle tone, developmental delays, including early speech and language problems, intellectual disability, decreased pain sensitivity, chronic sleep disturbances, hyperactivity, arm hugging, hand squeezing, attention problems, emotional lability, and self-injurious behaviors that include skin picking and nail yanking (Elsea and Girirajan, 2008; Slosky, Foster, and Elsea, 2012; Smith et al., 2006). Intellectual functioning typically falls within the mild to moderate range of intellectual disability, with a mean full scale IQ score of 47 (range: 20 to 78, Greenberg et al., 1996). Specific intellectual weaknesses are often seen on sequential processing tasks; however, relative strengths are observed in areas of acquired knowledge and reading (Dykens, Finucane, and Gayley, 1997). Medical problems also commonly exist, including congenital heart defects, seizure disorders, peripheral neuropathy, scoliosis, vision problems, and urinary tract anomalies (Edelman et al., 2007; Smith et al., 2006).

SMS was first documented in the literature in the early 1980s (Smith, McGavran, Waldstein, and Robinson, 1982). Diagnostically, SMS may first be suspected based on phenotypic appearance and behaviors. The small chromosomal deletion indicative of diagnosis was often overlooked until fluorescent in situ hybridization (FISH) became more readily accessible (Dykens et al., 2000). Comparative genomic hybridization (CGH) microarray is now commonly utilized to verify a suspected SMS diagnosis.

Williams Syndrome

"It is a privilege to live with someone that has Williams syndrome because you grow a new-found respect for all the different people we live with day to day."

14 year-old sibling of 7 year-old with WS

Williams syndrome (WS) is a rare ND caused by a hemizygous contiguous gene deletion of the 7q11.23 region of chromosome 7 (Peoples et al., 2000). This region of chromosome 7 spans approximately 28 genes, including the elastin gene (*ELN*), which is deleted in over 95% of individuals with WS (Schubert, 2009). This syndrome affects 1 in 7,500 to 1 in 20,000 people worldwide, with equal rates across genders and racial groups. As with SMS, it is a sporadic syndrome typically not inherited from a parent (Schubert, 2009; Stromme, Bjomstad, and Ramstad, 2002). WS can be conceptualized as a multi-system disorder with distinct physical, developmental, and social features and medical complications. Common features include intellectual disability and learning difficulties, developmental delays, craniofacial anomalies, low birth weight, and feeding problems (Burn, 1986). Physically, people with WS have a distinct appearance with a wide mouth, full lips, full cheeks, short upturned noses, periorbital fullness, broad brows and foreheads, and curly hair (Martens, Wilson, and Reutens, 2008). Common medical concerns include supravalvular aortic stenosis, hypertension, hypercalcemia, vision, hearing, and dental problems, glucose intolerance, subclinical hypothyroidism, early onset puberty, gastrointestinal problems, and genitourinary tract problems (Burns, 1986; Cambiaso et al., 2007; Pober, 2010; Stagi et al., 2005; Wessel et al., 2004). Socially, WS is characterized by a unique interpersonal demeanor, and individuals are often described as having a "cocktail party" personality, defined as being overly friendly, highly sociable, and displaying high degrees of empathy (Schubert, 2009). Despite being exceedingly friendly and empathetic, those with WS also demonstrate a poor understanding of social relationships and boundaries, making it difficult to develop and maintain friendships. Cognitively, individuals with WS show a broad range of intellectual ability, with an average IQ of 50-60 (range: 40 to 100), in the range of mild to moderate intellectual disability (Martens et al., 2008; Meyer-Lindenberg et al., 2006). Verbal abilities tend to be strong, but weaknesses exist with respect to visuospatial processing and reasoning (Martens et al., 2008). People with WS often show a strong affinity towards music, display strong emotional reactions towards music, and are noted to display creativity in their musical abilities (Martens et al., 2008). Children with WS are usually first identified by their characteristic facial appearance (Burns, 1986). FISH testing can be utilized to verify the diagnosis, as the chromosome deletion is usually too small to visualize on karyotype (Borg, Delhanty, and Baraitser, 1995; Elcioglu, Mackie-Ogilvie, Daker, and Berry, 1998). However, testing may also be done by CGH microarray, which is the current recommended methodology.

Down Syndrome

"If only the world was as simple in their perspective and as pure as a kid with Down syndrome, the world would be a better place. We could learn a lot from them all."

15 year-old sibling of 10 year-old with Down syndrome

Down syndrome (DS), or trisomy 21, is a chromosomal condition caused by an extra copy of chromosome 21. In 94% of cases of DS, there is full trisomy; 2.4% of cases are mosaic trisomy, and in 3.3% of cases there is a translocation involving chromosome 21 (Jones, 2006). The syndrome affects approximately 1 in 800 births worldwide, with a slightly increased incidence of DS in males as compared to females, with the ratio being 1.15 to 1 (Canfield et al., 2006). Individuals with DS show distinct physical, developmental, and social features. Cognitively, people with DS have an IQ in the range of 35 to 70, or the mild to moderate range of intellectual disability (Jones, 2006). Overall, people with DS have a good rhythm and enjoy music. Although delayed, social functioning tends to be approximately three years more advanced than mental age (e.g., if intellectual functioning is at a 6 year-old level, social functioning is at an approximately 9 year-old age level). Physical features of individuals with DS may include short stature, epicanthal folds, hypotonia (i.e., poor muscle tone), single transverse palmar crease, protruding tongue, small ears, and a short appearing neck. Around 50% of children with DS are born with a congenital heart defect. People with DS may experience gastrointestinal problems such as Hirschsprung disease, which can cause chronic constipation, and urinary tract abnormalities (Jones, 2006). Persons with DS experience accelerated aging with initial signs of aging typically beginning in the fourth decade of life; 60 to 75% of individuals with DS will eventually develop Alzheimer disease. Leukemia is also more common in individuals with DS (Wiseman et al., 2009).

DS is typically identified at birth based upon physical appearance. A standard peripheral blood karyotype will identify the trisomy 21, including translocations and other variants involving chromosome 21 that may be associated with DS. Many individuals may be identified prenatally. Parental screening tests, including ultrasound and maternal serum screening, may lead to diagnostic testing, such as chorionic villus sampling (CVS) or amniocentesis, which identify DS through karyotypic analysis of cells from the placenta or fetus.

Comparison and Summary of Syndromes

Individuals with SMS, WS, and DS all demonstrate unique physical, developmental, and social traits. However, the extent to which individuals will be affected by the specific features of their syndromes varies both across and within the diagnoses. For example, in comparison to SMS, individuals with WS or DS tend to have a good-natured disposition and demonstrate fewer behavioral concerns. However, individuals with WS and DS tend to have more medical complications than individuals with SMS. In addition to medical concerns, individuals with WS display high incidences of psychiatric conditions, including anxiety and depression. These psychiatric problems often progress with age (Schubert, 2009) and are not seen as frequently among those with SMS or DS. One unique psychiatric concern seen in individuals with WS is auditory allodynia, which is a substantial aversion to, or fear of, certain sounds that are not typically found aversive (Levitin, Cole, Lincoln, and Bellugi, 2005). With respect to cognitive functioning, individuals with SMS, WS, and DS all function within the mild to moderate range of intellectual disability. The specific pattern of cognitive strengths and weaknesses may vary by diagnosis.

Regardless of the specific syndrome, the complexity of these medical, developmental, intellectual, and social concerns, as well as the varied presentation, requires significant medical and psychosocial management by an integrated multidisciplinary team of highly trained professionals. While these teams include physicians and other medical professionals, families coping with NDs such as SMS, WS, and DS, benefit from psychosocial support teams, including case managers, psychologists, social workers, and educational advocates, as well as other ancillary providers such as physical, occupational, and speech/language therapists. The services required vary depending upon specific individual and family needs, which often change across the developmental lifespan.

CHALLENGES, ASSESSMENTS, AND INTERVENTIONS: INFANCY AND EARLY CHILDHOOD

"It has given us a greater appreciation for the value of the lives of those who society may not see as perfect. We have all grown in patience, love, understanding, and compassion, and we wouldn't trade it, as challenging as it is."

Parent of a 7 year-old without WS and a 4 year-old with WS

"I feel very ill equipped to handle the aggressive and impulsive behaviors of our son with WS. And these behaviors cause me consistent and extreme stress. We have yet to find professionals (doctors, therapists, teachers, psychologists, etc.) that are able to truly provide us with ways to help our son in these critical areas. It is quite discouraging as a caregiver to realize that the "professionals" are at a loss as to how actually help my child and they are supposed to be the ones with the education, experience, expertise, etc. I can explain the behaviors to my spouse, my friends, medical professionals, etc. but when it is you dealing with the same stuff every day from this little person who does not seem to be improving, it is a heavy weight to carry daily."

Parent of a child diagnosed with WS

Developmental Challenges

Children with NDs often face numerous challenges that emerge as early as infancy and/or early childhood. Common concerns in this developmental period include problems related to sleep and feeding, maladaptive behavior, poor motor development, and delays in speech and language development.

Sleep, Feeding, and Behavioral Concerns

Sleep-related concerns can be tremendous barriers to wellness among families coping with NDs. This is especially true among individuals and families coping with SMS. Those with SMS usually experience nocturnal wakefulness and persistent daytime hypersomnia, shortened sleep cycles, problems falling asleep, and reduced periods of rapid eye movement (REM) sleep (Smith, Dykens, and Greenberg, 1998b). Research has demonstrated that these sleep problems are highly detrimental to caregiver and family well-being (Hodapp, Fidler, and Smith, 1998). Moreover, families report a greater number and intensity of maladaptive behaviors when sleep disturbances increase (Dykens and Smith, 1998). Sleep problems are also present among individuals with WS. Specific problems often include significant bedtime resistance and periods of wakefulness throughout the night (Annaz et al., 2010).

Feeding problems are also not uncommon among individuals diagnosed with NDs. For example, children with WS often experience both reflux and constipation in addition to atypical weight gain and abdominal pain of unknown etiology (Pober, 2010). They are also at risk for hypercalcemia, which can lead to decreased feeding, irritability, and colic (Cooper-Brown et al., 2008). Similar feeding and digestive problems are observed in children with SMS and DS (Smith et al., 2012). For example, infants with DS often experience oral motor and dental problems (Cooper-Brown et al., 2008). These problems collectively contribute to feeding difficulties, which may include aversions to certain food textures, chewing and swallowing difficulties, choking, hypotonia, and poor motor coordination, which can limit self-feeding behaviors. The severity of feeding problems may lead children with these disorders to be labeled as failure to thrive (FTT), and the chronicity of these problems may not resolve without intensive feeding interventions (e.g., feeding clinics, modified feeding schedules, feeding tubes).

Significant maladaptive behaviors, which are observed somewhat frequently among individuals with NDs, can create high levels of stress among caregivers and families, which, in turn, can negatively impact both individual and family functioning. Individuals with SMS typically display more maladaptive behaviors than those with WS or DS. Among individuals with SMS, these maladaptive behaviors often include problems with aggression and self-injury, including self-biting and nail-pulling (Colley, Leversha, Voullaire, and Rogers, 1990; Stratton et al., 1986). Disobedience, tantrums, stubbornness, destruction of property, enuresis, and encopresis are also common problems (Dykens and Smith, 1998). A study of 19 children with SMS found that, on average, the children displayed 13 different stereotypic behaviors, including self-hugging, teeth grinding, hand flapping, and repetitive rocking (Martin, Wolters, and Smith, 2006). Based on parent report, the children also displayed an average of five self-injurious behaviors such as self-hitting and/or self-biting, headbanging, skin picking, and insertion of fingers or objects into body orifices other than the mouth.

Motor Development and Speech and Language Concerns

Problems with motor and/or speech and language development are also common among children with NDs, including those with SMS, WS, or DS; however, the etiology and expression of these difficulties vary by diagnosis. For example, a study of 11 children with SMS, ages 5 to 34 months, found moderate to severe delays in both motor functioning and expressive language acquisition (Wolters et al., 2009); however, receptive language was less severely affected (Smith et al., 2012). Results showed that toddlers (ages 24 to 34 months) demonstrated more significant deficits than infants in these domains, suggesting that these delays become more apparent over time. Problems with motor and speech and language development have been attributed to generalized cognitive deficits, as well as to hypotonia, oral-motor abnormalities, and middle ear dysfunction. Neuropathies in the upper and lower extremities may also play a role in the motor delays experienced by children with SMS, as well as contributing to self-injury.

Children with WS have delays in both fine and gross motor development, due to problems with musculoskeletal development (Burns, 1986; Udwin and Yule, 1991). One study assessing psychomotor development in young children with WS (less than 42 months of age) found severe delays in motor functioning in the majority of children as compared to typically developing children, prompting researchers to recommend occupational and physical therapies (Tsai, Wu, Liou, and Shu, 2008). Visuospatial deficits have also been reported among children with WS, which further contribute to problems with tasks requiring fine motor coordination (Nakamura et al., 2009). Language acquisition can be significantly delayed as well, with expressive language skills developing at approximately three years of age (Mervis et al., 2000).

Children with DS are also at risk for motor and/or speech and language delays as a function of impaired cognitive functioning, hypotonia, and craniofacial abnormalities that often include a protruding tongue (Canfield et al., 2006; Jones, 2006). Language deficits tend to be more significant than general cognitive, motor, or social deficits, although deficits often exist in all of these domains (Clibbens, 2001; Fowler, 1990; Miller, 1992; Rondal and Comblain, 1996; Tager-Flusberg, 1999). In terms of language development, specific problems with morphology and syntax have been identified, with related deficits present well into adulthood. However, research results have varied widely when exploring language development among children with DS. Specifically, some research findings suggest that nonverbal cognitive functioning and receptive language development tend to be more advanced than expressive language development (Miller, 1999). Others have found no differences between nonverbal and verbal cognitive ability, while further research has shown delays in both receptive and expressive language.

Early Child Interventions Programs and Developmental Assessments

Fortunately, a number of interventions are available to help children and families meet the wide range of developmental needs that are present in SMS, WS, and DS. Identification of specific areas of strength and weakness is important when designing individually tailored interventions. This process typically begins with a developmental assessment, which can be utilized to evaluate children from birth through ages 5 to 6. Most children with complex genetic disorders, who are known to be at risk of significant neurodevelopmental delays, will qualify for such an assessment. Developmental assessments are usually conducted by a psychologist, psychological examiner, or neuropsychologist, although additional aspects of developmental assessments may be completed by developmental pediatricians, speech and language pathologists, occupational therapists, or physical therapists. It is becoming more common for developmental assessments to be completed in interdisciplinary care clinics that include some or all of these specialty services, and they are often completed through state-run early intervention programs, in hospitals, and in other community-based settings. Primary caregivers who bring their children to a developmental assessment can expect to participate in an intake interview, during which they will be asked to provide background information about their child's medical and developmental history, and to discuss their ongoing concerns. Clinicians will typically make note of behavioral observations while engaging the child in a formal, standardized assessment of their development in the areas of early cognitive ability, receptive and expressive language, fine and gross motor functioning, and social skills.. Depending on the primary presenting concerns and the age of the child, the evaluation may also include assessments of pre-academic skills, behavioral and emotional functioning, and/or attention and impulsivity. Each child's performance on these measures will be compared to what would be expected given the child's age, based on normative data. Once the assessment is complete, a report will be written and provided to the caregiver(s). A typical report will consist of an overview of the child's medical, developmental, family, and social history, a detailed description of the assessment results, a summary of results with any associated diagnoses, and a list of recommendations and resources aimed at helping the primary caregiver(s) meet both the child and family's needs.

Examples of Recommendations Found in a Developmental Assessment

Clinicians are able to provide a variety of recommendations following the completion of a developmental assessment, and these are typically listed within the report that caregivers receive. These recommendations should be specific to each child's age, developmental needs, cultural and language background, and make note of available services and resources in the community. Although not an exhaustive list, below are examples of recommendations that may be provided for an infant who is found to have cognitive and/or neurodevelopmental delays:

Referral for Early Intervention Services
1) The child's parent(s) are encouraged to share the results of this assessment with Early Intervention Services. Early Intervention Services can assist in setting up appropriate local services and therapies for children under the age of 3 years.

Recommendation to Participate in Occupational Therapy, Physical Therapy and/or Speech and Language Therapy
2) It is strongly recommended that the child (and family) participate in occupational therapy, physical therapy, and speech and language therapy. Referrals for each of these services can be provided if desired by the family. For children in bilingual families, it is further recommended that these services be completed with a bilingual therapist.

Recommendations to Address Fine and Gross Motor Delays
3) The following recommendations are provided to the child's parent(s) to address his/her delays in motor development. These activities can be incorporated into the child's play activities within the home environment.
   a. Engage the child in activities that require him/her to sit independently.
   b. Encourage the child to play on the floor in a prone position (i.e., on his/her stomach) so that he/she builds strength in his/her arms and legs. This position with also encourage neck strength, fine motor control as he/she reaches for toys, and gross motor control, which will help him/her learn to crawl.
   c. Encourage the child to stand and bounce while holding onto furniture or adults for support. This will help him/her develop leg strength and balance.
   d. Play hide-and-seek games that encourage the child to find toys hidden under washcloths or cups to develop fine motor control.
   e. While reading stories together, encourage the child to turn the pages of the books.

    f.   Fine motor skills can be practiced in conjunction with self-care behaviors, such as feeding himself/herself. In addition to allowing the child to hold his/her own bottle, practice using sippy cups. He/she can also practice using a pincer grasp to pick up cereal or grasping a spoon while eating rice cereal or other table foods.

Recommendations to Address Speech and Language Delays

4) The following recommendations are provided to the child's parent(s) to promote language development. The parents are encouraged to consistently integrate these activities into the child's daily routine.
   a. Encourage the child to mimic words and word sounds in his/her environment.
   b. Begin to teach the child the words for common objects in his/her environment, as well as the names for colors and body parts. He/she will learn how to understand these words first and then learn how to say the words as he/she ages.
   c. Use songs to practice words, numbers, and counting.
   d. Pair nonverbal gestures with words in the child's environment. For example, point to objects when talking about them so that he/she learns to associate words with the objects.
   e. Spend time reading to the child. Infants enjoy brightly colored books that include simple language and nursery rhymes. Cloth books and "touch and feel" books are also recommended.
   f. Although television time should be limited, allowing the child to utilize television programs for learning activities can help promote his/her language development. His/her parent is encouraged to work with him/her to understand and express words when watching television.
   g. Once the child has mastered the naming of common objects, encourage his/her use of words when making requests. Require the child to attempt to use words before providing him/her with the desired object, and praise him/her for effort.
   h. For children with severe problems mastering spoken language, sign language, picture exchange programs (e.g., Picture Exchange Communication Systems), and/or augmentative assistive language devices should be utilized. There are a number of such devices available, including many low cost iPad and tablet applications that can be downloaded. Utilization of these resources can facilitate adaptive verbal and non-verbal communication and decrease the frequency of behavioral outbursts and self-harming behaviors.

Recommendations to Address Feeding Problems

5) For picky eaters and infants who are reluctant to try new foods, take things slowly and be patient, choose feeding times when the child is feeling well, happy, and not too hungry, expect messes and distractibility, keep mealtimes fun, and focus on the positive while feeding the child. When an infant or young child refuses a new food, wait a few weeks before trying it again and consider mixing it with a preferred food.

Recommendations for a pre-school aged child who is found to have cognitive and/or neurodevelopmental delays *may* include some or all of the following:

Implementation of 504 Plan or Individualized Education Plan (IEP[2])
1) The child's parents are encouraged to share the results of the current evaluation with appropriate school personnel so that they may be considered in the development of a 504 Plan or an Individualized Education Plan (IEP). Results of this evaluation indicate that the child is exhibiting deficits that will require classroom accommodations and curriculum modifications to be successful in school.

Recommendations for Therapy Services to Address Behavioral Concerns
2) The child and family would benefit from participating in outpatient and/or home-based individual/family-based therapy to help address communication difficulties, oppositional behaviors, aggression, and self-injurious behaviors. Applied behavior analysis, parent-child interaction therapy, and other evidence-based parenting strategies may be especially helpful in addressing these concerns. An in-home therapist may be especially beneficial in setting up consistent expectations for the child within the home and helping to create cohesive behavioral expectations between home and school.

Recommendations for Address Behavioral Concerns in the Home
3) Specific behavioral interventions can be applied in the home to promote the child's social and emotional well-being. The following strategies and techniques are recommended:
   a. Maintain predictable classroom and home routines; keep the daily schedule as consistent as possible. A schedule builds a sense of safety, reduces anxiety, sets reasonable expectations, and breaks things down into manageable components. Keeping the child on a routine will help him/her manage his/her behaviors and give him/her the best chance to succeed. Create visual schedules for the child so that he/she may be reminded of "what comes next" throughout the day.
   b. Activities that require the child to sit still should not be more than 15 to 20 minutes in length. After 15 to 20 minutes, allow the child to get up and move around before returning to the task he/she needs to complete.
   c. Before addressing the child, speak his/her name and make eye contact; keep oral directions short and uncomplicated. Ask him/her to repeat the directions or demonstrate that he/she understands what is required.
   d. Actively ignore minor, undesired behaviors that are not harmful to oneself or others. Parents often unintentionally provide children with attention for inappropriate behavior, which can inadvertently increase the likelihood that the child will engage in that same inappropriate behavior in the future. Therefore, it is important to ignore, minor negative behaviors, while at the same time, providing specific praise and attention when the child engages in appropriate, positive behavior.
   e. When agitated, have the child move to a separate area away from peers and siblings (in a different room close by if possible). Many children are able to calm themselves if given the opportunity and materials. Allowing the child to engage in

---

[2] See the section entitled *Advocacy, Psychoeducational Assessments, and Academic Accommodations* for more information on IEPs and 504 Plans.

activities that require organization and repetition may help the child calm down. Doing puzzles, counting, singing, listening to music or a story, or writing letters and shapes repetitively may help facilitate this process. These strategies should only be used when the child has become overwhelmed or upset, and not when the child has misbehaved.

f. Try to identify the child's strengths that can be publicly announced or praised. When praising the child, label specific aspects of what is being done well, and use brief statements. For example, rather than saying, "Great job!" say "I really like it when you sit nicely and eat your lunch!" or "Good job saying 'thank you'!"

g. Try to offer immediate reinforcement for appropriate behavior (i.e. stickers for chart, free-time, etc.). Waiting too long for rewards may lose the desired effect.

h. When the child is having a tantrum, ensure that he/she is safe (e.g., move him/her away from hard floors, walls, or any dangerous objects), but do not engage with him/her in any other way (e.g., do not talk to him/her or provide other forms of attention). He/she is likely using self-injurious behaviors as a form of communication and control. Engaging with him/her while he/she is participating in such behaviors will only prolong the behaviors. As the child begins to understand that tantrums and self-injury no long produce their desired outcomes, the behaviors will reduce in frequency and severity.

i. When the child is aggressive with others or property belonging to others, remove him/her from the situation whenever possible. Follow through with consequences such as time-outs or removal of fun activities. Do not interact with him/her while he/she is in time-out. If he/she gets up from his/her time out location, simply bring him/her back without speaking to him/her. When the time out is over, give him/her a one sentence explanation of why he/she was punished and have him/her repeat the explanation to ensure that he/she understands. If a time-out is assigned due to the child's oppositional or defiant behavior, have the child follow the original instruction and assign a second time-out if he/she again fails to comply.

Recommendations to Address Fine Motor Delays

4) The following recommendations are provided to the child's parent(s) to address his/her fine motor difficulties. These activities should be incorporated into the child's play activities within the home environment.

   a. Provide the child with a variety of writing materials (e.g. pencils, colored pencils, crayons, paint brushes) to strengthen his/her basic writing skills.

   b. Model the appropriate technique for gripping a pencil and how to position the paper when writing.

   c. Provide the child with supplies that will aid him/her in appropriately gripping his/her pencil (e.g., oversized pencils, pencil grips).

   d. Engage the child in fine motor play that includes tracing, coloring within the lines, stringing beads, lacing cards, building objects with blocks or Legos, putting puzzles together, and forming objects with play dough.

   e. Encourage the child to correct or rewrite poorly formed letters; monitor his/her practice to ensure letters are formed correctly.

   f. For some children, fine motor deficits may be severe. In such cases, expecting the child to engage in traditional written communication may not be realistic.

Continuing to insist that the child participate in challenging fine motor tasks may result in significant frustration, tantrums, and other aggressive behaviors. In such cases, it is recommended that the child be encouraged to utilize tablets or other assistive devices. These skills can promote learning, decrease disruptive behaviors, and improve overall quality of life. Typing can also be introduced as the child ages.
  g. Reinforce his/her successful efforts when engaging in traditional writing activities and/or utilization of technology-based assistive devices to participate in written communication. Provide corrective feedback as needed.

Recommendations to Address Gross Motor Delays

5) The following recommendations are provided to the child's parent(s) to address his/her gross motor difficulties. These activities can be incorporated into the child's play activities within the home environment.
   a. Ride tricycles or scooters. Be sure to have the child wear a helmet and other protective pads to protect the child and teach good self-care behaviors.
   b. Practice kicking and throwing balls, pushing carts, and pulling wagons.
   c. Participate in obstacle courses and relay races.
   d. Walk across balance beams, jump on trampolines, and climb and swing on playground equipment.
   e. Dig in the dirt and plant gardens.

Recommendations to Address Speech and Language Delays

6) It is recommended that the child's family and school personnel actively work on his/her conversational skills to increase the likelihood of communication success and competence. Given the child's sporadic use of phrases and sentences to obtain items and activities, and his/her limited ability to echo the speech of others, it is recommended that his/her family members learn skills to improve his/her independent speech. The most effective method for teaching independent speech is by teaching a child to request desired items. There are several steps in the progression toward independent requesting.
   a. First, a parent must know the items and activities that are desired by the child. These may include edible items such as chips, juice, cookies, peanuts, or crackers. These may also include items or access to activities such as watching a cartoon, playing with a musical toy, mom singing, or throwing a ball back and forth. Anything that your child enjoys can be used to teach requesting. The more items and activities that are available, the more opportunities to teach requesting there are.
   b. The next step is to restrict access to the most desirable items. This does not mean putting all of the child's toys away. It simply means putting his/her favorite toys out of reach so that it creates a motivation for the child to ask for the item. If the child is able to go and get desired items by himself/herself, he/she has no reason to communicate with you. However, if he/she needs the parent to get things for him/her, he/she is more likely to communicate verbally. Favorite toys, videos, snacks, and other items should be put out of reach but in sight.

c. Once the child is unable to get things on his/her own, the parent should follow the child until he/she indicates that he wants something. The child may indicate by pointing, pulling you to the item, crying, or glancing at the item. If the parent knows what the child wants, he/she should say the name of the item and pause for the child to repeat it. If the child does not repeat the name, say the name once more and then deliver the item anyway. Do not withhold items for too long or the child may become frustrated and learn that talking is too difficult. The goal is for the child to learn that talking is a good way to get his/her needs met. With snack items, the parent should give the child only a small portion. By giving only a small amount, the child will need to come back to ask for more and so there is another opportunity to teach the child to ask. If the parent gives the child a full glass of juice instead of only a few sips, then he/she may become full and not want anymore. Therefore, only give small portions to increase the number of opportunities to teach.
d. With activities, only allow a small amount of time with the items. Try not to take things away, but when the child puts a toy down, the parent should pick it up. Then, when he/she wants it again, the parent has it, and there is another opportunity to teach him/her to ask. Always say the name of the item and pause to see if he/she will repeat what the parent said before giving the item or snack. Requesting items and activities is best done in the context of playtime.
e. Games can also be played that promote language acquisition.
   i. Sing songs using preschool tapes or videos.
   ii. Play "what is it?" games by putting objects in a bucket and labeling the objects as they are pulled from the bucket.
   iii. Play games such as I Spy, Pictionary, or acting games that require verbalization.

Recommendations to Address Sleep Concerns

7) The child's parents are encouraged to speak to a pediatrician concerning his/her sleep difficulties, as there may be behavioral interventions that can help him/her to fall asleep. It will be important to implement a consistent sleep routine (e.g., bath, then story, then lights out at 8:30 every night). Suggestions for establishment of this routine include slowly weaning his/her daily naptime, along with waking him/her up earlier in the morning. As much as possible, allow the child to help determine a plan that will make him/her more comfortable at night and set up a consistent, calming sleep environment (e.g. getting a soft blanket, putting pictures of the family beside his/her bed, selecting soothing music to listed to before bed, etc.).

8) Encourage the child to fall asleep independently by putting him/her to bed when drowsy, but still awake. If the child avoids bedtime, set consistent limits, and if the child gets out of bed during the night, matter of factly walk him/her back to his/her bed.

9) Specific sleep concerns related to SMS should be addressed with a pediatrician and sleep specialist. Sleep phase shift programs may be successful in creating and sustaining a more normative sleep schedule. Medications such as melatonin and other modifications such as bright light therapy may be required to sufficiently address sleep concerns in this population.

Recommendations to Address Feeding Problems

10) For young children who exhibit behavioral problems during mealtimes, try to conceptualize the mealtime as an opportunity to teach the child appropriate behaviors and manners. Establish a routine that includes sit-down, family style meals, and keep the television turned off. Set reasonable time limits for meals and provide only small portions of preferred foods to encourage the child to expand his/her diet. Avoid "clean your plate" rules that may lead children to develop unhealthy eating habits, and include the child in conversation and social interaction during the meal to make it enjoyable.

11) Establish a set of mealtime rules, starting with only 2 or 3. Remind the child of the rules before each meal and provide specific praise for appropriate mealtime behavior. Have the child practice the correct behavior the first two times he/she breaks a rule and reserve time-out for the third time the rule is broken. Avoid providing the child with snacks in between meals if he/she did not eat appropriately at mealtime.

Recommendations to Address Development of Self-Care Behaviors

12) The following recommendations are provided to the child's parent(s) to promote development of self-care behaviors. They are encouraged to consistently integrate these activities into the child's daily routine.
   a. Encourage the child to practice self-care behaviors such as getting dressed and putting on his/her own shoes. Be patient with him/her as these activities will likely take a significant amount of time at first.
   b. Practice allowing the child to button his/her own buttons and zip his/her own zippers. This will help improve fine motor skills as well.
   c. Assist the child in learning appropriate bathroom hygiene, such as washing his/her own hair, brushing his/her own teeth, and taking care of his/her own toileting behaviors. To ensure cleanliness, it may be helpful to allow the child to attempt these behaviors independently at first and then assist him/her as necessary.
   d. Set expectations for the child to complete simple household chores such as putting away his/her own toys, putting his/her jacket in the closet, helping set the dinner table, or putting his/her laundry in the hamper. Setting these expectations now will help the child develop independent living skills as he/she ages.
   e. Use positive reinforcement (e.g., praise, small rewards) to encourage the child to engage in self-care behaviors.

Promoting Social Skill Development

13) The following recommendations are being made to promote the child's social skill attainment.
   a. Model the appropriate use of manners (e.g., saying please and thank you, refraining from interrupting others during conversations, sharing toys and games, raising his/her hand to ask a question in class).
   b. The child may also benefit from learning simple scripts for initiating play, such as "That looks like fun. Can I play too?" or "Would you like to play with these blocks with me?" Such scripts could be practiced at home and school, and the

child should be prompted to use these phrases when he/she is around other children.
   c. Play activities should include activities that require turn-taking and one-on-one interactions. Examples include throwing a ball back and forth or playing games such as Candyland or Chutes and Ladders that have simple rules and require at least two people to play. Other activities may include racing cars side by side, playing with puppets, or building or making something with manipulatives.
   d. Model and practice pretend play with the child. This could include any number of activities such as playing dress-up or house, pretend cooking, playing pirates or dinosaurs, or pretending to be superheroes.

Recommendations to Promote Toilet Training

14) The following recommendations are provided to the child's parent(s) to promote toilet training.
   a. Determine whether the child is ready to be toilet trained. The child must achieve bladder control prior to initiating toilet training. Signs of bladder control include remaining dry during short (i.e., 30 minute) naps, urinating all at once rather than "dribbling" throughout the day, and engaging in facial expressions suggesting that the child needs to urinate or is urinating.
   b. Recognize that toilet training is a multi-step process that is more manageable if broken down into smaller steps. Focusing on mastering one step at a time will increase the child's chances of success.
   c. The child is more likely to eliminate on the toilet once he/she feels comfortable sitting on the toilet to potty chair. The child will feel more comfortable if this activity is perceived as being enjoyable. Reading stories or singing toileting songs that are only accessible when sitting on the toilet or potty chair can reinforce the child's desire to use the toilet. Use praise or small rewards such as stickers, hugs, or M&M's to encourage these behaviors.
   d. After the child is comfortable sitting on the toilet or potty chair, setting up a "sitting schedule" can increase the chances of successful elimination. Set up the schedule around the times that the child is most likely to naturally want to eliminate such as immediately after waking, 30 minutes after a meal, shortly after active play, and/or after bathing. On days when the primary caregiver is home with the child, the caregiver is encouraged to provide the child with a favorite beverage to help ensure the need to eliminate during scheduled times. When the child successfully eliminates on the toilet or potty chair, be sure to use lots of praise. Other small rewards may also help reinforce this behavior.
   e. Teach the child to ask to utilize the toilet or potty chair by requiring that the child ask permission prior to going into the bathroom. The parent can prompt the child to do one of the following: 1.) make the sign for potty 2.) Say "potty," or 3.) Say, "I need to go to the potty." Praise the child for asking, and then immediately take him/her to the toilet or potty chair.
   f. If the child continues to demonstrate difficulties transitioning out of diapers, it may be helpful to have the child wear underpants under the diaper. This will help the child sense when he/she is wet, thus increasing discomfort and the chance that the child will want to eliminate on the toilet or potty chair.

Recommendations to Promote Pre-Academic Skill Development

15) The following recommendations are provided to the child's parent(s) to strengthen pre-academic skills development. They are encouraged to use these techniques at home, perhaps incorporating them into play.
    a. Practice identifying numbers and shapes using age appropriate games and books.
    b. Integrate learning opportunities into daily activities. For example, have the child count objects in the grocery store, identify common road signs while driving, identify left and right turns while driving, or identify letters and numbers in the home environment.
    c. Use songs to practice learning letters or counting.
    d. Use matching games to identify objects, associative pairs, quantities, and upper and lowercase letters.
    e. Engage the child in sorting activities to arrange toys/objects by color, size, functions, features, or categories.
    f. Use blocks or alphabet and number magnets to help the child learn sequencing skills.
    g. Spend time reading to the child. While reading, help him/her identify letters and matching initial words sounds to pictures within the stories (e.g., "c" goes with "cat"). Consider choosing books that provide examples of how to behave appropriately in social situations, that are reassuring and foster development of healthy self-esteem, and that are imaginative, humorous, and silly.
    h. Utilize repetition to learn how to write letters, especially those in the child's name. Repetition or songs can be used to help the child learn his/her address and phone number as well.
    i. Although videogame/computer and television time should be limited, allowing the child to utilize these tools for learning activities can help promote his/her pre-academic skills. His/her parents are encouraged to work with him/her to learn skills when playing on the computer or watching television.

Addressing Safety Concerns

16) The following recommendations are provided to help the family address safety concerns.
    a. Teach appropriate social boundaries such as remaining in close proximity to caregivers, how to refrain from speaking to unfamiliar others, and asking permission to go places with peers or other adults.
    b. For particularly active children, who enjoy exploring their environment and have difficulty remaining within arm's reach of their caregivers when outside or in public places, use of a child tracking device may be helpful. Several companies produce GPS systems that include a tracking bracelet worn by the child and a parent monitor that both sounds an alarm when children wander off too far, and that also can be used to determine the location of the child.
    c. Practice teaching the child how to cross the street safely.
    d. If the child has a tendency to leave the house without permission, it may be beneficial to place locks on doors that are out of the child's reach and/or install alarms on doors and windows. Door alarms may be particularly helpful for

caregivers of children who have a tendency to get out of bed at night and roam the house.

Many developmental assessment reports will also include some type of recommendation for when the child should return to complete a follow-up assessment.

Early Developmental Resources for Families

As stated in the preceding section, developmental assessment results may include recommendations for occupational, physical, and/or speech and language therapies, feeding clinics, and/or behavioral interventions, depending on the individualized needs of the child and family. The following sections offer brief descriptions of what these resources are and the benefits of each for families coping with SMS, WS, or DS.

Occupational and Physical Therapy
Evaluations for occupational and/or physical therapy may be conducted as part of a larger developmental assessment, as described in the preceding section, or may be conducted independently. Occupational therapy evaluations can be helpful in assessing a variety of potential concerns including visual-motor and visual-perceptual skills (e.g., handwriting, cutting with scissors), upper extremity utilization (e.g., range of motion, bilateral hand coordination, strength), gross motor control, and activities of daily living (e.g., hygiene, dressing, feeding; Children's Healthcare of Atlanta, 2012). The content of a physical therapy evaluation can vary as well. However, broadly speaking, caregivers can expect that the initial evaluation will include an objective assessment of posture, joint functioning, skeletal alignment, movement analysis, strength and flexibility, reflexes, pain, and sensory processing (Physician Therapyworks, 2012). Most hospital systems offer occupational and physical therapy services. Larger cities may also have community-based rehabilitation clinics offering these services. Public educational systems should provide these services for qualifying children; however, caregivers may want to inquire as to how frequently the services can be offered, as services may be limited depending upon the school system's resources.

Speech and Language Therapy
Speech and language evaluations are typically conducted by speech and language pathologists but may be conducted as part of larger development evaluations as well. The age-based evaluation will likely include an assessment of receptive and expressive language, verbal fluency, voice and resonance, oral motor skills, articulation, and hearing ability. If deficits exist, ongoing speech and language therapy will be recommended. In addition to the services offered through hospitals and pediatric rehabilitation centers, speech and language therapy should be available through the child's public school system.

Sign language, in combination with other augmentative and alternative communication systems, has been shown to be useful in promoting language acquisition and generalized communication skills among individuals with NDs (Clibbens, 2001). These interventions can also reduce frustrations and maladaptive behaviors among children with communication difficulties. New technologies, such as such as iPads or the DynaVox®, have been shown to be especially helpful. For many children with NDs, the utilization of sign language or other alternatives to spoken language can be phased out as speech improves; however, for some, these speech and language alternatives may continue to be beneficial throughout the individual's life.

Feeding Clinics

Feeding clinics are available to help families with children and adolescents who experience challenges with feeding behaviors. Such clinics may comprise a number of pediatric specialty services; however, most of these clinics are run by speech and language pathologists, psychologists, nutritionists, or a combination of these services. Feeding clinics can be found at most children's hospitals and/or pediatric rehabilitation centers that offer speech and language therapy. When caregivers bring their child to a feeding clinic, they can expect an evaluation that will consist of an intake assessment of feeding behaviors, medical concerns, and developmental delays. Problems with chewing and swallowing, food and texture aversions, and mealtime anxiety will be explored. The child's anatomy and behaviors related to drinking and eating will be explored to the extent that the child may be observed engaging in these activities. It may also be necessary to conduct a swallowing study, in which a videofluoroscopy is utilized to assess whether food and liquids can move through the mouth and throat safety and effectively.

As stated previously, children with SMS, WS, and DS are likely to experience significant problems with feeding behaviors, requiring ongoing supports beyond the initial feeding clinic evaluation. Thus, these families are encouraged to request a referral from their pediatrician to participate in intensive feeding therapy or seek out such services on their own. In addition to feeding therapy, the pervasive feeding and gastrointestinal problems seen among these children may also require ongoing care from a pediatric gastroenterologist, especially if feeding problems are severe enough to require feeding tubes. Moreover, kidney problems, enuresis, and frequent urinary tract infections are often reported, which may require additional assistance from pediatric nephrologists and/or urologists (Pober, 2010). The family's pediatrician can assist with making these referrals as well.

Behavioral Therapy

Maladaptive behaviors can be among the most challenging issues faced by caregivers. While behavioral concerns can exist among most children (and adults) with NDs, extreme and persistent maladaptive behaviors are more often reported among those with SMS as compared to those with WS or DS (Elsea and Girirajan, 2008; Slosky, Foster, and Elsea, 2012; Smith et al., 2006). It is important to remember that for individuals with SMS, WS, or DS, the etiology of these behaviors is typically both genetic and environmental. This suggests that although standard behavioral interventions can be very helpful in reducing and effectively managing maladaptive behaviors, knowledge of the specific syndrome can aid in developing a behavioral support plan that takes into consideration a specific syndrome's medical, cognitive, and behavioral profile. Therefore, in addition to ongoing behavioral therapy, psychoeducation can be a highly important first step in helping caregivers better understand the behaviors they are most likely to encounter. This educational process needs to be initiated immediately following diagnosis so that caregivers can preemptively prepare for potential concerns before they develop and/or become severe. For example, if caregivers are aware that self-injurious behaviors are likely to develop, they can actively spend time prompting or helping the child participate in more adaptive methods of coping with frustration (i.e., playing outside, squeezing silly putty or play dough, taking a bath) from the time the child is very young. As stated in a previous section, language delays or deficits can lead to significant frustration and behavioral problems. If caregivers are aware that speech and language problems are likely, they can teach sign language or the use of assistive devices before delays are apparent. Finding professionals who are specially trained to understand the complexity of these severe maladaptive behaviors can be difficult. However, more children's hospitals or larger pediatric medical clinics will have pediatric psychologists or developmental specialists who are familiar with addressing behavioral concerns among children with NDs. Early intervention programs also employ psychologists and certified behavior analysts who are trained in assessing the function of specific behaviors. Knowledge of syndromic profiles can greatly aid these professionals in conducting functional behavioral assessments that take etiology into account.

CHALLENGES, ASSESSMENTS, AND INTERVENTIONS: THE MIDDLE CHILDHOOD YEARS

"I am very happy to have my brother. I cannot imagine him being anything but himself, my little brother with Down syndrome. He can get on my nerves, but mostly I like having him around and wish that I could take him to school and show him off - plus teach some of the bullies how he is not different from them. He CAN read and do all things, and I would love to show them my brother and have him with me at my school. They don't let him go to my school because he has Down syndrome, and this school system separates them in other classes and my school does not have those classes. He has to go to a different elementary than this one. I think my brother should be able to go to the same school that I go to."

14 year-old sibling of 8-year-old diagnosed with DS

"The hardest part in raising him and for our other two children was the school years. Everything was a battle from getting services to finding teachers who wanted him in their class to IEP wording to appropriate assignments to friendships in school. I look back on those years and wonder how I retained any sanity at all. I wish we could have done those years better for everyone's sake."

Parent of 24 year-old with DS and 22 year-old sibling without DS

Developmental Challenges

New and ongoing developmental challenges exist during the middle childhood years (i.e., ages 6 to 11, approximately), particularly for children with NDs. Previously established home-, school-, and community-based interventions often need to continue throughout the elementary and middle school years. In addition to already implemented interventions, new developmental needs and milestones specific to this period need to be considered. Common concerns include problems with social relationships, learning, inattention, hyperactivity, and impulsivity.

Peer Relationships and Bullying

Peer relationships become increasingly important as children enter the middle childhood years. Regardless of whether NDs exist, the significance of friendships in promoting quality of life and relationship development has been well-established (e.g., Bagwell, Schmidt, Newcomb, and Bukowski, 2001; Bierman, 2004). Irrespective of disability status, children desire similar characteristics in friendships, such as shared social interactions and experiences, empathy, and trust (Heiman, 2000; Turnbull, Blue-Banning, and Pereira, 2000). Inadequate social skills, poor self-esteem, and previous peer rejection tend to predict a lack of friendships (Bierman, 2004; Odom et al., 2006). Given that children with severe NDs are likely to experience problems with social skills, making and maintaining friendships can be especially challenging (Shokoohi-Yekta and Hendrickson, 2010). Children with NDs have commonly expressed feelings of loneliness due to their struggles to make friends (Solish, Perry, and Minnes, 2010). Additionally, when a child is perceived as being different or less socially competent, he/she can become a target of bullying.

In general, children without NDs participate in significantly more social activities than children with NDs (Solish et al., 2010). Additionally, children with NDs typically encounter most of their friend and peer interactions at school as compared to home environments (Shokoohi-Yekta and Hendrickson, 2010). Geisthardt, Brotherson, and Cook (2002) found that children with physical disabilities are more likely to experience friendships within the home environment than children with behavioral problems or intellectual disability. While this study did not explicitly address social concerns among children with SMS, WS, or DS, the results suggest that children with these disorders may experience significant problems making friends based on the cognitive and behavioral deficits displayed. Living in a secluded area further prevents children with NDs from having friendships outside of school, although living near other children does not guarantee interactions with peers (Geisthardt et al., 2002).

Based on this literature, social concerns and potential problems with peer relationships are important considerations for children with SMS, WS, and DS. However, for children with WS, these problems are particularly salient. Individuals with WS display a significant lack of stranger anxiety, which is often described as having a "cocktail party personality" (Pober, 2010, p. 245). Being highly sociable and empathetic may be perceived as a good character trait; however, this hyper-sociability can also cause problems and lead to significant concerns among primary caregivers. Studies have found that children with WS often fail to recognize threatening facial cues and do not understand social boundaries, which may lead them to associate with people who may cause them harm (Schumann, Bauman, and Amarai, 2010). While this leads to a need for increased monitoring around unfamiliar adults, social skills deficits and difficulty understanding social cues can also cause problems with peer relationships, as these children may be easily manipulated into engaging in undesired activities. Despite possessing hyper-sociability, children with WS also report feeling socially isolated and experiencing anticipatory anxiety in social situations (Dykens, 2003). Children with WS have been described as demonstrating problems with obsessive thinking and being overly attentive (Davies, Udwin, and Howlin, 1998). With respect to socialization, such behaviors may translate into poor boundaries, which may lead potential friends to become overwhelmed and shy away from ongoing social interactions.

Learning Disorders

It is not uncommon for children with genetic disorders such as SMS, WS, and DS to experience problems with learning. These difficulties may be the direct result of intellectual disability, a specific learning disorder, attention problems, or a combination of the all three. Although problems with learning may be identified prior to school entry, specific learning disorders, which are a type of NDs in and of themselves, are most commonly identified during the primary and/or secondary school years. The DSM-IV-TR (APA, 2000) provides diagnostic criteria for three types of learning disorders. These include mathematics disorder, reading disorder, and disorder of written expression. All three learning disorder diagnoses require a level of achievement in reading, mathematics, or written expression that is significantly lower than would be expected given a child's age, IQ, and education level. The soon-to-be published DSM-5 (Comer, 2013) will place learning disorders within a new grouping called "neurodevelopmental disorders." It is anticipated that mathematics disorder will be renamed as dyscalculia, and reading disorder will be renamed dyslexia.

Given these diagnostic criteria, while children with SMS, WS, and DS are likely to experience problems with learning, they may be unlikely to meet full criteria for diagnosis of a learning disorder, given their intellectual disability. At the same time, they may benefit from interventions that are designed for children with specific learning disabilities.

Inattention and Hyperactivity

Like intellectual disability and learning disorders, children with genetic disorders such as SMS, WS, and DS often display problems with inattention, impulsivity, and hyperactivity. Depending upon the intensity and number of symptoms, a child demonstrating problems in these domains may meet DSM-IV-TR diagnostic criteria for attention-deficit/hyperactivity disorder (APA, 2000). An ADHD diagnosis requires that a child display ongoing symptoms of inattention and/or hyperactivity and impulsivity in multiple settings (e.g., school and home) for a period of no less than six consecutive months with symptoms beginning prior to age 7. For example, children with ADHD may demonstrate significant difficulties completing chores or homework, paying attention in class, or following directions. They may seem forgetful, be easily distracted, or avoid tasks that require sustained attention. Children with ADHD may also have significant problems sitting still to the extent that they are constantly fidgeting, climbing on furniture or other objects at inappropriate times, and/or talking excessively. They may have difficulties with peer interactions because it is hard for them to take turns or engage in play activities for age-appropriate lengths of time. Three different categories of ADHD diagnoses currently exist. If symptoms are primarily inattentive in nature, the diagnosis is ADHD, Predominantly Inattentive Type. If symptoms are primarily hyperactive-impulsive in nature, the diagnosis is ADHD, Predominantly Hyperactive-Impulsive Type. Most children display a combination of inattentive and hyperactive-impulsive symptoms, which is diagnosed as ADHD, Combined Type. Although currently classified within the DSM-IV-TR as a "disruptive behavior disorder," the DSM-5 (Comer, 2013) will re-categorize ADHD as a "neurodevelopmental disorder."

Problems with inattention, hyperactivity, and impulsivity have been documented among children diagnosed with DS, SMS and WS (Colley, Leversha, Voullaire, and Rogers, 1990; Stratton et al., 1986). Among those with WS, one study found that more than 80% of children meet diagnostic criteria for ADHD, an anxiety disorder, or both disorders (Leyfer, Woodruff-Borden, Klein-Tasman, Fricke, and Mervis, 2006), while a recent study on ADHD among those with DS revealed a prevalence of approximately 44% (Ekstein, Glick, Weill, Kay, and Berger, 2011). Pharmacological intervention to treat ADHD and other psychiatric disorders in individuals with genetic syndromes often does not show adequate success (Laje, Bernert, Morse, Pao, and Smith, 2010). Of note, pharmacologic intervention should be considered on an individual basis with careful monitoring and the recognition that some medications may exacerbate existing sleep or behavioral problems and may cause undesired weight loss (Smith et al., 2012).

Advocacy, Psychoeducational Assessments, and Academic Accommodations

Regardless of the child's diagnosis or the severity of delays or deficits, most families want their child to engage in age-appropriate activities, such as attending school, reaching his/her learning potential, building relationships with teachers and peers, and participating in extracurricular activities. For children with NDs, meeting academic needs requires a continuous partnership among the school system, family, and child's medical and psychosocial teams. An important initial step for caregivers is to work with the child's school to help personnel better understand the child's genetic syndrome diagnosis. Such psychoeducation on the child's diagnosis needs to begin as soon as the child enters school and should continue each time the child encounters new educators and support staff. Given the wide variety of complex diagnoses and needs that children have in educational settings, primary caregivers cannot expect that schools will be knowledgeable about specific diagnoses prior to their child entering the school system. Proper education and training often needs to be provided, and for rare diagnoses, such as SMS or WS, the caregivers and/or child's hospital-based team may be called upon the help with such training. Although this can be frustrating and time consuming, it also offers them an opportunity to advocate for the child. In-services between families and school personnel can not only provide disorder-specific education, but they can also help form partnerships that are designed to best serve the child as he/she ages. Such interactions can also help the child learn to feel more comfortable advocating for himself/herself.

Schools in the United States are expected to educate children within the least restrictive environment (LRE), which means that many children with NDs will spend at least a portion of the school day with typically developing children (National Center for Learning Disabilities, 2012). As such, it can be helpful for schools to address children's perceptions of individuals with NDs and offer in-services or interventions to educate the child's classmates on their diagnosis as well (Staub, 1998; Vignes et al., 2009). Offering classmates an opportunity to ask questions about the syndrome or disorder and its associated features can be very important in helping to promote a supportive environment for the child (Rillotta and Nettelbeck, 2007). These interactions can also help to alleviate caregivers' concerns about peer relationships and potential bullying. The child's peers may benefit from being provided with the opportunity to ask questions about the physical manifestations of the disorder or syndrome, such as facial features, as well as medical concerns (Rillotta and Nettelbeck, 2007). Allowing classmates to ask questions about the child's learning needs, classroom assistance, maladaptive behaviors, and social concerns can foster compassion, minimize stereotyping, promote normalization, and improve the likelihood that the child with a ND will be able to develop adaptive and meaningful friendships as he/she moves through the educational system (Hemmeter, 2000; Rillotta and Nettelbeck, 2007).

In addition to the benefit of in-services aimed at educating teachers and classmates, children with NDs are eligible to receive specialized school-based accommodations through the Individuals with Disabilities Education Act (IDEA) or Section 504 of the Rehabilitation Act (National Center for Learning Disabilities, 2012). IDEA is a federal statute that was developed to provide free and appropriate education to children between the ages of 3 and 21, who have specific disabilities that adversely impact their educational attainment. Children qualifying under IDEA receive federally mandated and funded supplemental services and/or supports in excess of those provided within the general curricula. These accommodations are provided free of charge to the family and may include assistance with learning disorders, developmental delays, intellectual deficits, social and emotional difficulties, behavioral concerns, and managing complex medical issues. In addition to the IDEA, Section 504 is a broad civil rights law that protects the rights of those with a physical or mental disability in a way that enables the individual to participate in education with his/her peers. The law requires that schools eliminate barriers that may prevent the individual from fully participating in his/her education.

In order to obtain and ensure that educational accommodations are provided through IDEA and Section 504, a formal educational plan needs to be written, either in the form of an Individualized Education Plan (IEP) or 504 Plan. Children with diagnosed intellectual deficits, learning disorders, and/or other NDs, including those with SMS, WS, or DS should qualify for an IEP, and it is recommended that a plan be put in place as soon as the child enters the public school system (i.e., as young as age 3). Of note, private school systems are not obligated to implement an IEP or 504 Plan, but they may be open to establishing such a plan or implementing similar accommodations upon request. Once a referral is made by the parent, school, or other entity, a meeting will be held to determine what types of accommodations are needed. These meetings, which are held at least annually once a plan has been established, are important opportunities for family and others providing support to build partnerships with the child's educational team. In most cases, school systems require that a child complete a formal psychoeducational assessment prior to implementation of an education plan. Some schools prefer to conduct the psychoeducational assessments themselves, with the assistance of a licensed or certified school psychologist. Families also have the option of having the assessment completed by a licensed psychologist or neuropsychologist in the community. For children with rare disorders and/or intensive care needs, having the assessment completed by a provider specializing in pediatric psychology can be beneficial, as this type of provider may have more specialized training in addressing the specific needs often found among children with unique genetic or medical disorders. These assessments are often completed in follow-up to earlier developmental assessments, and much like developmental evaluations, they often begin with interviews regarding the child's developmental history, current level of functioning, and specific concerns from family members and others. Most psychoeducational evaluations include formal assessments of cognitive functioning, adaptive functioning, academic achievement, and emotional and behavioral functioning. Depending on the primary presenting concerns, the assessment may also include evaluation of attention and impulsivity, memory, executive functioning, speech and language, and/or motor functioning. Once the assessment is complete, a report will be written and provided to the primary caregiver(s). As with developmental assessments, a typical report will consist of an overview of the child's medical, developmental, family, and social history, a detailed description of the assessment results, a summary of results with any associated diagnoses, and a list of recommendations and resources aimed at helping meet both the child and the family's needs.

Examples of Recommendations from Psychoeducational Assessments

A variety of recommendations can be found within the contents of a psychoeducational assessment report. These recommendations will be specific to each child's age, cognitive and developmental needs, cultural and language background, and available services and resources. As with developmental assessments, if significant deficits are present, the first recommendation made is likely to suggest that primary caregivers provide the assessment report to the school and request that a meeting be held to *discuss developing an IEP or 504 Plan*. If such a plan already exists, the report may advise that the school consider modifying or updating the current plan to best meet the child's current needs. Although not an exhaustive list, below are examples of recommendations that may be included in a psychoeducational assessment report.

Recommendation for Special Education Services or Resource Room Assistance

1) The results of this assessment indicate that the child displays significant cognitive and/or learning deficits. It is recommended that the child participate in special educational services and/or have access to resource room assistance to help support his/her significant educational needs.

Recommendations to Address Problems with Inattention and Hyperactivity

2) The following recommendations are provided to address the child's identified problems with inattention, distractibility, and hyperactivity.
   a. The child may benefit from taking tests in the resource room or library, where he/she can work without distractions.
   b. Avoid numerous directions or assignments. Allow the child to finish one assignment or direction at a time before going on to the next.
   c. Maintain a predictable classroom routine; keep the daily schedule as consistent as possible. Prepare the child ahead of time when you know that the routine must be changed or when transitions are going to take place.
   d. Allow the child to sit near the front of the classroom; stand in close proximity to the child while teaching. This will help keep him/her focused on the classroom activities.
   e. Before addressing the child, speak his/her name and make eye contact; keep oral directions short and uncomplicated. Ask him/her to repeat the directions until it is certain that he/she understands what is being asked.
   f. Be aware of the child's frustration level. Knowing when the child is about to lose focus or become frustrated may prevent inappropriate behavior and feelings of failure. Do not be afraid to discuss this with the child so that both of you can identify the factors that lead to frustration.

g. Allow the child to take breaks from schoolwork throughout the day. This will help decrease frustration and increase learning and productivity. Children with significant attention problems may need to take multiple breaks each hour.
h. As the child ages, encourage the utilization of assignment notebooks. This will promote organizational skills and increase the likelihood that assignments will be completed successfully. Children will fine motor problems may benefit from using an audio recording device to record assignments.

Recommendations to Address Problems with Mathematics Achievement
3) The following recommendations are provided to address the child's deficits in mathematics achievement:
   a. The child should receive remedial, one-on-one instruction in mathematics.
   b. It will be beneficial to ensure that the child has fully automatized his/her math facts before attempting to have him/her learn more abstract, problem-solving concepts. The better his/her understanding of basic math concepts (i.e., adding, subtracting, multiplying, dividing), the easier it will be for him/her to apply basic knowledge to higher level math problems and to complete math problems efficiently. Utilizing flashcards, charts, and computer programs may assist the child in learning his/her basic math facts and increasing the speed with which he/she is able to recall and apply these facts.
   c. Based on measured visual-spatial difficulties, the child may benefit from math worksheets that include structured workspace. Consistency in presentation is important so that examples should be written using either horizontal or vertical alignment, not both. Graph paper may also help with organizational efforts.
   d. Any difficulties with reading may also impact the child's ability to successfully complete mathematical word problems. Therefore, his/her parents and teachers are encouraged to read word problems to the child, to help him/her read through problems aloud, and/or to provide pictures that accompany word problems. The child should be taught specific strategies for identifying important pieces of information in the problem and determining the operation needed to solve the problem.
   e. Providing manipulative objects and utilizing them in instruction (e.g., rulers, beads, blocks) will likely improve the child's opportunities for success in math.
   f. At home, enjoy time as a family, engaging in tasks that encourage learning. Spend time playing structured age-appropriate games/activities that require visuo-spatial reasoning (e.g., Legos/blocks, puzzles, mazes, etc.).
   g. At the child ages, it will be especially important to focus on practical mathematical skill development such as telling time, reading thermometers and car gauges, using money, maintaining a checkbook, and understanding basic banking and credit principles.

Recommendations to Address Problems with Reading and Writing Achievement
4) The following recommendations are provided to address the child's deficiencies in reading and written expression:
   a. The child should receive remedial, one-on-one instruction in reading and written language.

b. Prepare a copy of the homework assignments and hand it to the child at the end of the day. The goal is to create a comfortable and successful environment. In this case, having the child accomplish the homework is more important than the difficulty encountered in copying his/her assignments.
c. Provide audiotaped copies of text books so that comprehension of class materials is not negatively influenced by reading deficits. This provision will also help the child's parent(s) assist him/her in completing course assignments.
d. The child may benefit from oral testing and from having test questions and items read to him/her so that his/her knowledge of course material is being assessed rather than her reading ability. Worksheet instructions should also be read aloud to the child.
e. For children with significant motor problems that deter hand written activities, consider allowing the use assistive devices such as computers and tablets to complete assignments.
f. Encourage the child's appreciation for reading by allowing him/her to choose age appropriate reading materials (books, comic books, magazines) and by reading with him/her, discussing the characters, exciting parts of the story, etc. The child may enjoy picking out books-on-tape from his/her local library and following along in the books as the stories are read to him/her. This strategy may be particularly helpful for improving reading fluency.
g. At home, enjoy time as a family, engaging in activities that encourage reading and writing skills (e.g., Boggle, Scrabble, Pictionary, word finds, etc.). Allow the child to choose family activities among a pre-determined list of options. Allowing him/her to determine the activity will give him/her a sense of control and encourage him/her to take an active role in his/her own learning.

Improving Confidence and Effort

5) The following recommendations are provided as methods for encouraging the child's continued engagement and effort in the classroom and when completing homework:
   a. Focus on building academic self-confidence. The child may show a strong desire to learn but need more time and more intensive instruction than other students to accomplish and master tasks. It will be important to promote confidence in his/her ability to learn as he/she ages so that he/she does not become discouraged by his/her cognitive and academic weaknesses.
   b. Try to identify the child's strengths that can be publicly announced or praised. In this way, the child's peers will perceive him/her positively, and he/she will continue to seek out positive attention.
   c. Address the child in a calm, clear tone when encouraging academic behaviors. If he/she feels overly pressured to accomplish academic tasks, he/she is more likely to feel anxious and lose confidence. At the same time, do not allow the child to avoid participation in academic work, as this may inadvertently increase anxiety related to school performance.

Addressing Behavioral Concerns within the Home

6) Specific behavioral interventions can be applied in the home to promote the child's social and emotional well-being. The following strategies and techniques are recommended:

   a. Develop a consistent schedule within the home. A schedule builds a sense of safety, reduces anxiety, sets reasonable expectations, and breaks things down into manageable components. Keeping the child on a routine will help him/her manage his/her behaviors and give him/her the best chance to succeed. He/she will be more invested in the schedule if he/she is able to help create it. The schedule needs to be posted prominently in the home. Although weekends tend to be more variable than weekdays, a schedule needs to be developed for the weekends with consistent bedtimes and hygiene routines. While being consistent, it is also important to foster flexibility and to ensure that the child does not become overly reliant on routine and resistant to change.

   b. Develop a list of household rules. Try to keep this list to no more than 5 of the most important rules, and allow the child (and his/her siblings) to help create the list. Specific age-appropriate consequences for breaking each rule should be written down and discussed so that the child will be aware of what the consequence will be if he/she disobeys.

   c. Always address the child in a calm, clear tone when redirecting him/her or encouraging academic behaviors. Avoid yelling and using loud tones of voice or physical discipline. While it is important to use firm tones so that the child knows what is expected of him/her, yelling and/or harsh tones will likely result in defiant behaviors. If he/she feels overly pressured to accomplish tasks, he/she is more likely to feel anxious and lose confidence.

   d. Create a Focus Zone within the home and school. This is a place where the child can go to calm down or to have quiet time. A Focus Zone could be a small area with a desk or table that is within sight and sound supervision. He/she should be encouraged to use the space, and it should not be considered a punishment. Things to have within the Focus Zone include: 1) Art Materials: Paper, crayons, and beads; 2) Puzzles and age-appropriate games; 3) Toys that require the child to put things together such as Legos; 4) Relaxing music; and 5) Comfortable seat, pillows, etc. TV and video games are not recommended. The Focus Zone should not be used as playroom. Encourage the child to use this area to calm down, and then return to his/her normal activities.

   e. Daily exercise and outdoor activities will allow the child to expel excess energy and calm down.

   f. If he/she wets the bed, have him/her complete the appropriate hygiene and assist him/her in changing his/her bedding. Avoid punishing him/her for this behavior. Simply have him/her help clean up any mess that has been made and then move on.

   g. Consequences for refusing to listen can include such things as loss of free time, early bed time, loss of fun outings, and loss of access to toys or video games. He/she should have the opportunity to earn these privileges back. The child should always be held accountable when he/she breaks rules. Avoid using corporal punishment, as this may result in increased acting out behaviors.

h. Children respond well to praise and compliments. When the child does something positive, be sure to acknowledge him/her and possibly allow him/her to earn rewards. This is especially important with school work and following household rules and expectations.
i. When the child refuses to do what is asked of him/her, inform him/her of the potential consequences of his/her actions and give him/her two to three choices for appropriate ways to behave if possible. This will assist the child in feeling as though he/she is maintaining some sense of power and control. Enforce the consequences immediately if he/she does not do what is asked.
j. Behavior management books such as *1-2-3 Magic* by Thomas Phelan and *S.O.S.: Help for Parents* by Lynn Clark are recommended to assist in reducing oppositional, defiant, and aggressive behaviors.

Promoting Healthy Weight and Physical Activity

7) Children with NDs are at high risk for problems related to obesity, beginning in the middle childhood years. While this may be related to metabolic problems, it will be important to promote healthy diet and exercise behaviors in the child. The family may benefit from working with a dietician in learning about portion control and how to develop healthy meal plans. The child's weight should be closely monitored and his/her eating habits should be closely supervised as much as possible. He/she should be praised for making healthy food choices.

8) The child should be encouraged to participate in physical activity on a regular basis. It will be important to identify exercises and activities that are enjoyable for the child so that he/she is more motivated and interested in maintaining them over time. He/she may enjoy karate, yoga, swimming, playing tag, taking walks with a friend or family member, gardening, participating in community service activities that require some physical exertion, dancing, or bowling, for example, He/she should be praised for his/her efforts, and physical activity logs and pedometers may be particularly helpful for monitoring. If significant physical limitations are present, the child and family may benefit from consulting with a physical therapist.

Promoting Social Skill Development

9) The following recommendations are being made to promote the child's social skill attainment.
   a. Use role-playing or social stories to teach new skills or desired interactions with others.
   b. Practice initiating and maintaining conversations by teaching the child how to shake hands, introduce himself/herself, ask reciprocal questions, and maintain eye contact.
   c. Look for times throughout the day to help the child better understand perspective taking. For example, ask the child to identify emotions of people in television shows or storybooks.
   d. Have the child participate in clubs, volunteer activities, library reading groups, school groups, or other activities that the child enjoys that will encourage him/her to practice socializing with other children his/her age.

    e. The child would benefit from participating in a social skills group. Such groups may be offered through the child's school or through a local mental health clinic.

Similar to developmental assessments, the final recommendation in a psychoeducational or neuropsychological assessment report is likely a statement regarding when the child and family should return for a follow-up assessment. It may also include recommendations regarding referrals to other disciplines, including speech/language, occupational, and physical therapists, psychologists or behavioral specialists, nutritionists, or sleep medicine clinics, for example.

CHALLENGES, ASSESSMENTS, AND INTERVENTIONS: THE TEENAGE YEARS AND BEYOND

"In my opinion the parents with young Williams children all think they are going to be better as adults than for the most part they really are going to be. I think [families are given] too optimistic of a rosy future for those with children. It's good to be encouraging and positive, but you need to sprinkle it with a dose or realism."

Parent of an individual diagnosed with WS

Developmental Challenges

As those with NDs become teenagers, additional challenges emerge for individuals and caregivers. As is common among those with NDs, challenges encountered during infancy, early childhood, and middle childhood may continue to exist, improve, or worsen over time. With this in mind, therapies and resources already in place prior to entering adolescence may continue to be required (e.g., school-based academic accommodations), while others may no longer be necessary (e.g., feeding clinics, speech and language therapy). During adolescence (i.e., approximately ages 11 to 18) and beyond, common concerns include issues related to sexual development, romantic relationships, and vocational planning. Many caregivers must also make considerations for semi-independent or community-based living and determine how to best address legal concerns such as guardianships and advanced care directives.

Sexual Development and Romantic Relationships

Addressing sexual development and romantic relationships can be a difficult topic for caregivers, regardless of whether or not their adolescent is diagnosed with a ND (Lesseliers and Van Hove, 2002). When the adolescent has a ND, additional challenges and safety concerns exist. The literature has discussed two common and contradictory perceptions when it comes to addressing sexuality among those with NDs (McCarthy, 1999). The first suggests that those with NDs need to be protected from society due to the inherent vulnerabilities that exist in a sexually provocative world. This could be interpreted to mean that the topic of sexuality and romantic relationships should be avoided, with the somewhat misguided presumption that this will protect individuals with NDs from desiring sexual interactions and/or being victimized. The second view acknowledges that most individuals with NDs will want to engage in sexual relationships, just like most individuals without NDs (McCarthy, 1999; Melberg-Schwier and Hingsburger, 2000). Unfortunately, normative sexual desire, combined with poor social boundaries and reduced intellectual ability, may lead those with NDs to pursue inappropriate and perhaps dangerous sexual encounters, making ongoing sexual education and discussion imperative.

In further considering the second (and more commonly accepted) viewpoint, primary caregivers are then charged with determining how and when to begin discussing sexual development and romantic desires with their child with a ND (Lesseliers and Van Hove, 2002; Thorin and Irving, 1992). This has been identified as a significant source of stress for primary caregivers, who are often unsure of what information to provide, how to present the information in a way that will be understandable, and when to begin discussions. Depending upon the level of intellectual, behavioral, and/or emotional impairment, there are also numerous questions regarding whether to "allow" romantic and potentially sexual relationships. Appropriate methods of pregnancy prevention must also be explored. In some cases, adolescents and adults with NDs will be reasonably well-supervised within their school and living environments. However, completely negating opportunities for sexual contact is nearly (if not completely) impossible, making it even more important that sexual education and social skills training are provided in a timely and developmentally sensitive manner.

Many primary caregivers struggle to acknowledge that their child with a ND may want to engage in sexual interactions (Melberg-Schwier and Hingsburger, 2000; Lesseliers and Van Hove, 2002). Picking up on any cues related to potential sexual interest (e.g., flirting behaviors, masturbation, wanting to watch television or movies with sexual content) displayed by the adolescent may be in important first step in promoting awareness for parents. These cues can also act as conversation starting points. As compared to parents, professionals working with individuals with NDs have been found to be more likely to notice sexual interest and behaviors. Additionally, while parents may be less inclined to acknowledge sexual interests, many professionals believe that those with NDs, like all other individuals, have a fundamental right to sexual expression. With this in mind, professionals are likely to work with individuals with NDs to normalize their sexual desires, discuss independent decision-making, and learn self-advocacy and appropriate social boundaries. A primary goal is to help primary caregivers feel capable of openly discussing issues surrounding intimacy and sexuality. In this way, medical and/or psychological professionals may act as a valuable resource in helping primary caregivers address sexual development and romantic relationships in their adolescent and adult children with NDs.

Life Skills and Vocations

Many individuals with significant NDs, such as SMS, WS, or DS, want to participate in work-related activities. Engaging in work activities allows individuals with NDs to find purpose and self-fulfillment, interact with and contribute to the community, and build self-esteem and life skills. What constitutes successful vocational attainment depends on the goals of the individual and what opportunities are available (Smith, Wilson, Webber, and Graffam, 2004). Vocational success may be dictated by the number of hours and environments in which it is feasible for the individual to work; employer expectations; and the cognitive, developmental, behavioral/emotional, physical, and medical problems of the individual. The American Association of Intellectual and Developmental Disabilities (AAIDD) stipulates that those with such challenges must be afforded opportunities that promote well-being in a variety of environments, including employment settings (AAIDD, 2010, 2012).

Historically, those with significant NDs have been perceived as unable to work (Marks, 1999; Oliver, 1990; Smith et al., 2004), and until recently, have often been excluded from work environments and society at large unless needed to fill a void in the workforce. For example, throughout much of the 20th century, those with NDs were called upon to work during times of war, when labor shortages existed, and were returned to institutions when the wars ended. Although much has changed with respect to how those with NDs are supported, stigmas still exist that can make employment an ongoing challenge. Statistics suggest that individuals with NDs are much less likely to be employed than those without such a disability (Smith et al., 2004). This is an important statistic to consider, especially given that community-based employment is associated with increased quality of life (Eggleton et al., 1999). In the U.S., all individuals with disabilities are protected by anti-discrimination legislation that requires that employers provide reasonable accommodations that allow the individual to complete his/her work-related tasks (Smith et al., 2004). These laws indicate that those with NDs should be able to work in an environment that supports satisfactory work experience such that no discrimination should exist in hiring practices; however, employment rates continue to be low. Employers who are more likely to employ those with NDs have been found to demonstrate greater awareness of anti-discriminatory processes and are more likely to favor social justice. Person-environment fit has also been found to be particularly important in that it is not only salient that the person be able to perform his/her job but that he/she feels accepted and valued as a member of the work team (Hagner, 1992). Social skills have been described as a predictor of whether or not an individual will be accepted in the work place, and intervention studied have shown that many individuals with NDs can be taught specific task-related social skills, such as asking for assistance and using verbal problem-solving strategies (Holmes and Fillary, 2000; Martella et al., 1993).

"Natural supports" are defined as "assistance provided by people, procedures, or equipment in a given workplace that (a) leads to desired personal and work outcomes, (b) is typically available or culturally appropriate in the work place, (c) is supported by resources from within the work place, facilitated to the degree necessary by human service consultation" (Butterworth et al., 1996, p. 106). These "natural supports" are imperative in helping those with NDs succeed in the workplace and may require co-worker training, on-site job coaches, and community-based partnerships. Job coaches or job instructors can help individuals break down work tasks, establish methods of performing tasks successfully, provide prompts, and build independence and self-confidence (Callahan and Garner, 1997). While the supports can require extensive time and training to implement, they should not deter employers from hiring individuals with specialized needs. Through partnerships with community-based agencies, such as rehabilitation services, employers may be able to offer specially created or "carved jobs," that enable the individual to be successful in the workplace (Gilbride and Hagner, 2005, p. 295).

Vocational Assessments and Planning

As discussed in the previous section, as individuals with NDs age, it is important to consider how to best plan for vocational goals. A formal vocational assessment can provide a helpful starting point for taking steps towards vocational planning. Such an assessment can be completed through a state-run vocational rehabilitation services program or through most mental health clinics that specialize in meeting the needs of adolescents and young adults. School systems will often be equipped to help families facilitate this process as well. Most vocational assessments will be conducted by a licensed psychologist, school psychologist, or psychological examiner. Again, as with developmental and psychoeducational assessments, family and other support persons are typically asked to participate in an interview regarding the child's current level of functioning and related concerns. This interview will be followed by a formal assessment of cognitive functioning, vocational interests, personality, adaptive functioning, and behavioral and emotional functioning. Depending on specific presenting concerns and the overall purpose of the evaluation, the assessment may also include an evaluation of academic achievement, memory, attention, and/or executive functioning, much like a psychoeducational evaluation. In medical settings, the assessment may also include additional measures of functional competence that address medication adherence and schedules, as well as awareness of medical factors associated with the ND. Once the assessment is complete, a report will be written and provided to the individual and/or primary caregivers. As with other assessment reports, a typical vocational assessment report will consist of an overview of the individual's medical, developmental, family, and social history, a detailed description of the assessment results, a summary of results with any associated diagnoses, and a list of recommendations and resources aimed at helping address the individual's vocational and life skill needs.

Examples of Recommendations Provided in Vocational Assessments

The following are examples of recommendations that may be made as part of a vocational assessment for an individual with a ND. The specific recommendations made will vary substantially depending upon the severity of intellectual disability, learning disorders, and problems with adaptive functioning, medical limitations, and/or mood and behavioral problems that exist. However, in general, there will be a recommendation to provide the assessment report to a either the individual's school or local vocational rehabilitation services, who can then provide additional help in facilitating vocational placements and supervision (if needed). Additionally, the recommendations may include further suggestions for online vocational exploration, vocational counseling, and/or job shadowing.

Referral to Vocational Rehabilitation Services
1) The individual is encouraged to share the results of this assessment with Vocational Rehabilitation Services and/or to provide a copy of the results to administrative officials at his/her current educational facility. Vocational Rehabilitation Services may be especially helpful in facilitating the individual's ongoing vocational development.

Options for Additional Vocational Exploration
2) The individual can take advantage of the following career resources to continue with his/her vocational exploration:

    a. O*NET Online (http://online.onetcenter.org/): O*NET Online provides comprehensive information on key attributes and characteristics of workers and occupations. On this site, the individual can take a free skills search assessment that will provide additional information on the types of careers for which he may be well-suited.

    b. Occupational Outlook Handbook (http://www.bls.gov/oco/): The Occupational Outlook Handbook provides the most up-to-date information available on hundreds of jobs and includes information on the amount of training and education needed, earnings, expected job prospects, and work conditions.

Vocational Counseling

3) Vocational counseling, which may be available through his/her school, is recommended to assist the individual as he or she continues to explore vocations of interest. In addition to facilitating the development of a specific vocational path and the steps that need to be taken to further his/her vocational development, engaging in such counseling will allow the adolescent to consider how his/her personal values, cognitive/academic strengths and limitations, and openness to new ideas influence his/her ability to obtain a satisfying vocation.

Vocational Shadowing

4) Once vocational interests have been solidified, it may be beneficial to shadow professionals in vocations that the individual wants to pursue. This will allow the individual to network with others in fields of interest and get an in-depth view of what the vocation entails on a day-to-day basis.

Vocational assessments may also result in other recommendations offered to promote the quality of life of the individual and/or his/her family. For example, recommendations may be given to promote adaptive functioning. Again, the examples below represent areas that may need to be addressed in adolescence or adulthood and do not represent an exhaustive list that will meet all individual needs.

Adaptive Functioning Skills

5) The following recommendations are provided to the individual and his/her primary caregivers to promote development of adaptive functioning skills:

    a. Focus on developing practical mathematics skills, such as counting money, making correct change, and understanding basic banking and credit principles.

    b. Practice setting longer-term goals (e.g., work-related goals, social goals) and how to break these larger goals into smaller goals that can be achieved in a reasonable amount of time.

    c. Continue to encourage writing skills by having the individual write short notes or letters to friends. This will help him/her maintain the writing skills and fine motor dexterity he/she has developed thus far.

d. Assist the individual in taking more control over his/her medication adherence. Although the individual may need to be supervised in doing this, using pills boxes or cell phone/watch alarms may help the adolescent monitor his/her own medications more independently.

Community Living

Individuals with SMS, WS, and DS typically experience pervasive problems with daily living skills, or adaptive functioning, to the extent that they will require some level of monitoring throughout their lives and are unable to live independently as adults (Schubert, 2009). Deinstitutionalization has created an impetus for policymakers and researchers to focus on more appropriate long-term living arrangements for individuals with significant disabilities as they reach adulthood (Emerson, 2004). With this in mind, community integration has now become the primary goal, with its emphasis on independent or semi-independent living (Racino, 1995). Successful community integration implies that individuals with NDs have the opportunity to not only reside in the community, but to work and recreate in ways that are similar to those without NDs. Many individuals with NDs who are unable to live independently will reside in publicly-funded, supportive housing programs that provide supervised living and supportive services (Wong and Stanhope, 2009). Community-based care following deinstitutionalization has been greatly influenced by Wolfensberger's normalization principle (Flynn and Aubry, 1999; Wolfensberger, 1983). This principle stems from Nirje's work on social role valorization and indicates that individuals with NDs need to be integrated into culturally-rich normative community settings (Flynn and Aubry, 1999). Within these settings, quality of life will be improved if individuals can actively participate in socially valued roles and interactions.

The principle argues that institutions are harmful, because they perpetuate atypical behavioral interactions and ways of functioning, which in turn increases public stigmas regarding those with disabilities. Competence and self-worth are believed to be enhanced via participation within the larger society. Residential settings can vary widely (Wong and Stanhope, 2009).

They may include intensive therapeutic care with extensive treatment and rehabilitation, small group living scenarios emphasizing peer relationships and community involvement, living with a surrogate family, or residing with family members with in-home supportive services. Some residential settings serve to transition those with mild to moderate NDs to independent living. Others are structured to offer long-term supervised care in a supportive atmosphere.

Programs such as the 1981 Home and Community Based Services Waiver have effectively reduced the number of people residing in larger institutional settings (i.e., settings with more than 15 individuals) by providing Medicaid funding for non-institutional services. As of 2004, 83.5% of individuals with NDs were residing in settings with 15 people or less; nearly half (46.2%) were residing in settings with 3 people or less (Prouty, Smith, and Lakin, 2005).

Home-based supports tend to be a newer avenue of support (Wong and Stanhope, 2009). These allow individuals to remain in their own home environments while offering daily or weekly therapies and respite care for family members.

Guardianships, Alternatives to Guardianships, and Advance Care Directives

As children with neurodevelopmental disorders (NDs) move through adolescence, society also begins to presume adulthood. The following information has been gathered from various U.S. state specific sources. Although specific details differ by state, a person with or without a ND is generally considered an adult if any one of the following criteria are met: 1.) the individual has been emancipated by a court of law, 2.) the individual is 18 years of age or older, or 3.) the individual has been married. In some states, an individual is also considered emancipated if she has been pregnant. It is important to remember that once people meet the definition of adulthood, whether or not they have a ND, it is assumed that they should be able to make informed decisions by the legal system, health care providers, governmental agencies and society in general. Parents who have had de facto natural guardianship of their child do not automatically retain guardianship or legal decision making authority for the adult. This has special implications for adults with NDs.

The only legal alternative available to caregivers to retain guardianship of an adult is to initiate a court proceeding, which can be costly and may be unnecessary depending upon the severity of the ND and the needs of the individual. Such a proceeding seeks to determine whether the adult's ND severely impacts his/her decision making ability to such an extent that he/she is in need of protection. This, however, does not need to be the first course of action for an adult with a ND (O'Sullivan, 1999), even for people with severe limitations in cognitive function and decision-making abilities. There may be multiple ways for family members to continue supporting the individual in decision-making endeavors without seeking formal adult guardianship. For example, unless the person with ND has elected otherwise, family members are still able to attend and participate in Individualized Education and Support Planning meetings and may be able to give needed medical consents as next of kin.

With changes in privacy laws such as the *Health Insurance Portability and Accountability Act of* 1996, it has become more difficult for parents to gain access to the health records of their adult children (HIPAA, 1996). However, there are ways for caregivers to initiate conversations with the adult child and the healthcare provider team to discuss how medical decisions will be made. A discussion including the individual with a ND, the caregiver, and the individual's provider often results in a plan that is agreed to by all parties. This may include the completion of releases of information that allow the caregiver to continue communicating directly with the healthcare provider or those that allow the caregiver to continue obtaining medical information. The primary stipulation in allowing the individual with the ND to complete release forms is ensuring that consent has been provided through an informed process. In non-emergent situations, providers have an obligation to obtain informed consent from service recipients and to make every effort to present the information in language and terms that is understandable (Beauchamp and Childress, 1994). Formal cognitive assessments may be needed to determine whether the individual with the ND has the cognitive capacity to provide informed consent for medical care and/or sign release forms allowing caregivers permission to continue actively participating in care.

Guardianship Alternatives

Individual state processes vary, but in general, procedures are available to ensure that caregivers and other family members can exercise certain authorities without undergoing a full guardianship procedure (Dinerstein, 2006). Some of these procedures are detailed below, but caregivers and family members should discuss the best course of action with the service providers who provide routine support to the individual with ND, such as physicians and social service agencies, before proceeding. Individual state offices typically publish regulations governing decision making that impact people with NDs (Pennsylvania Code Title 55, ch.6000 subchapter R, 2011). Similarly, state specific advocacy groups (Disability Rights Texas, 2011) also have publications and staff available that provide education regarding state-specific options. These referenced sources outline the following potential alternatives to guardianship.

Representative Payee. People with NDs who qualify for benefits under the Social Security Administration (SSA) but who are unable to manage their fiscal affairs can participate in the representative payee program. This program provides for the management of Social Security and Supplemental Security Income payments to people with NDs, who are not capable of independently managing their payments. In most cases, a family member or friend serves as the representative payee, but an agency, such as a supports provider, can also serve in this capacity. The representative payee helps a person with NDs manage his/her benefits and has certain responsibilities, such as ensuring that the benefits are used as intended, saving any remaining benefits amounts, and maintaining adequate financial records. More information is available from the SSA (www.ssa.gov).

Power of Attorney (POA). The execution of a POA enables an individual to act on behalf of another person in certain situations. Consent for the POA must be given by an individual who understands the process and the ramifications of giving another person the authority to make decisions on their behalf. An attorney should be consulted about the possible uses of a POA. There are jurisdictional differences, but a POA typically remains active if an individual is no longer able to understand the POA process, and it carries broad authority beginning the day the document is executed. This type of POA is called a durable POA. The POA process is much less costly and cumbersome than a full guardianship determination, and most families of people with ND who get a POA execute a durable POA and not a limited POA. The latter can be used for brief periods of time where an individual is not available to act on their own behalf. Many healthcare and service providers, as well as governmental agencies, will accept a POA in situations requiring decisions related to accessing records. If a POA is executed, caregivers should provide copies to service providers and governmental agencies such as the SSA.

Health Care Proxy (HCP). A HCP appoints another individual, or agent, to make healthcare decisions for a person in the event that the person becomes unable to make such decisions. Again, states differ widely in the extent of authority of the HCP and the process by which a HCP can be appointed. Generally, an HCP is executed by a person who is appointing a trusted friend or family member to make medical decisions in the event that the individual executing the document becomes incapacitated, or unable to do so. Most jurisdictions leave the decision of incapacitation to the primary physician.

Some jurisdictions also recognize health care representatives and health care agents, the former only requiring an agreement drafted between the two parties, while the latter requires the services of a notary. Some states have also enacted statutes that give default decision-making authority to certain individuals, such as family members, in a prescribed, hierarchical arrangement. Typically, people who work for agencies that support people with NDs are not able to serve in this capacity for a particular individual, except as a last resort, unless the agency employee also happens to be a family member. Likewise, certain rules may apply for individuals residing in state administered developmental centers. State or county offices that are responsible for administering programs for people with developmental disabilities are often the best resource for specific information.

Advanced Directives (AD). In instances where a HCP has been appointed, an individual also usually executes an AD. This is a separate legal document that contains instructions to healthcare providers and that specifies what procedures are desired or not desired in the event that the person becomes unable to make such decisions on their own behalf. The use of dialysis, respirators, cardio pulmonary resuscitation (CPR) techniques, tube feedings, and organ donation all can be expressly addressed in an AD. Discussing these issues with a family member with a ND can be difficult, but it can prevent scenarios during which caregivers are asked to make these decisions quickly during a time of crisis. In addition, certain decisions that an individual can make for himself/herself as part of an AD cannot be made once the person is unable to make the decision for himself/herself, even if a legal guardian has been appointed. The contents of an AD for people with ND can become controversial, and an attorney should be consulted when formulating such a document. For example, in most jurisdictions, a person acting on behalf of another cannot decline life sustaining treatment for another individual, unless the other individual meets specific criteria for a "terminal condition." This is true even for a person who is a court appointed legal guardian.

Adult Guardianship

In most cases and situations, use of the above procedures is sufficient to support people with NDs in managing their own lives. On occasion, legal guardianship is the only alternative. A guardian is a person or an agency that has been appointed by a court to act on behalf of another person. This ultimately removes that person's right of self-determination. A court appointed guardian can be a single person, or in some instances, more than one person can act as co-guardians. In guardianship proceedings that appoint co-guardians, special attention should be given to whether consent from both parties is needed, or if one or the other party can consent independently. It is also possible to include guardian succession in a decision. A guardianship decision, or decree, once rendered, can only be modified by the court.

For the guardianship determination to proceed, an attorney must be engaged by the person petitioning the court for guardianship. In addition, an attorney may be appointed by the court to represent the interests of the individual with a ND. Before the court proceedings, the individual with a ND will need to be evaluated by a licensed clinician to determine his/her current competence, or ability to make decisions. Part of this evaluation will include a determination of potential risk to the person should a guardian not be appointed. This evaluation, depending on the jurisdiction, can be completed by a licensed psychologist, a psychiatrist, or a primary care physician. A court date will be determined, and all parties involved may receive a summons to appear in court, including close family members. In certain circumstances, a physician or psychologist can attest that the presence of the person with the ND would not be in the person's best interest, and an exception to attendance can be made. During the hearing, the hearing master or judge will listen to the evidence, witnesses may be called to testify, and both attorneys will have the opportunity to ask the witnesses questions. A determination is then made, granting either general or limited guardianship. General Guardianship is sometimes referred to as 'plenary' guardianship and may be appropriate for individuals with NDs who have been found generally incapable of decision making in all aspects of their lives. Limited Guardianship can cover specific decision making circumstances. Specific circumstances include issues arising in residential, educational, financial, health care, legal, and/or job related settings.

A legal guardianship determination transfers the rights of the individual to the guardian, and, therefore, is the most restrictive alternative. The concept of "support," which enables an individual to participate in decision making, has supplanted "surrogacy," or making decisions on behalf of an individual, as the method of choice for meeting the needs of individuals with NDs (AAIDD, 2010, 2012). As such, professional and family organizations, such as the American Association on Intellectual and Developmental Disabilities (AAIDD) and The ARC, have issued a joint position statement on guardianship that recommends such an action as a last resort measure (AAIDD and The ARC, 2012).

PRIMARY CAREGIVERS AND SIBLINGS: CHALLENGES, BENEFITS, AND FAMILY WELL-BEING

Primary Caregivers

"I can only speak to what it has been like for our family. Our child with Down syndrome…has taught our family so many lessons; the most important for me has been acceptance and unconditional love. When I am at my worst, [he] opens his arms to me in an embrace. He loves me, holds me, and shows me the power of unconditional love. Because of his example, I have been able to offer that to my other children. [He] has shown us the importance of inclusion and the beauty of every single person, regardless of ability. He has shown us the joy woven throughout each day and the importance of learning things in small steps instead of giant gulps. He has shown me what it is like to be genuinely joy-filled for someone else's achievement or special moment. His level of compassion and empathy are incredible and often humbling. We also have witnessed the pain of being different and the difficulties that our society has with people who are different."

Parent of 11 year-old child with DS and 11 year-old child without DS

"We still do not have a good handle on how to care for him; we just want his quality of life to be as good as we can make it, but that remains a mystery."

Parent of a child diagnosed with WS

Parenting a typically developing child is a monumental task that requires tremendous time, emotional, and financial commitments. In addition to meeting these typical child care needs, caregivers of individuals who are diagnosed with one or more NDs also face a number of unique and often unexpected challenges, which may include added financial burdens due to medical care costs and specialized therapies, advocating for educational needs, and determining how to provide for their child as they age (Davies, Howlin, and Udwin, 1997). Caregivers of children diagnosed with SMS, WS, or DS must learn to cope with and readily adapt to the physical and behavioral features of the syndrome as they emerge across the lifespan. Many of these challenges have been discussed throughout the course of this chapter and may include any number of problems, such as feeding, sleep, and other developmental concerns; motor and/or language deficits; intellectual disability; significant maladaptive behaviors; social deficits; learning and attention problems; and learning to cope with complex medical problems (Pober, 2010).

Primary caregivers must not only manage individual child needs, but simultaneously address these challenges while working to provide the best quality of life possible for the entire family system (Silver, Westbrook, and Stein, 1998). The significant demands of the direct support role leads to a high degree of stress and burden (Fidler, Bailey, and Smalley, 2000). For example, questionnaires completed by parents of 36 children with SMS showed that the degree of maladaptive behavior displayed by the child with SMS was the best predictor of parental stress and pessimism (Hodapp et al., 1998). The burden is then compounded by the knowledge that the direct support role will continue throughout the course of the child's life, as most individuals with SMS, WS, or DS will be unable to live independently as adults (Davies, Howlin, and Udwin, 1998; Udwin, Webber, and Horn, 2001). Over time, the associated burdens can lead to problems with primary caregiver well-being (Graham, Ballard, and Sham, 1997; Hasselkus, 1988), especially given that the direct support role is unrelenting and oftentimes unexpected (Eicher and Batshaw, 1993).

Research exploring primary caregiver well-being and NDs continues to emerge. Established literature cites the importance of social support in promoting the psychological and physical health of these primary caregivers (Barakat and Linney, 1992; Erickson and Upshur, 1989). With the intensity of caregiver demands associated with supporting a child with SMS, WS, or DS, it may be expected that primary caregivers would display poor self-care behaviors or demonstrate coping difficulties. In fact, one study of SMS caregiver well-being supported this statement with findings suggesting that maternal caregiver well-being was directly impacted by perceived child health vulnerability, caregiver satisfaction, and benefit finding (Foster et al., 2010). Paternal caregiver well-being was most influenced by depressive symptoms and benefit finding. Overall, this study found significantly increased rates of depressive and anxiety symptoms, disrupted sleep, and difficulties maintaining annual physical exams among both mothers and fathers providing direct support to individuals with SMS. These findings and other similar studies have identified an increased need for counseling services for these caregivers (Foster et al., 2010; Scallan et al., 2010).

Resources for Primary Caregivers

The following resources are provided to help primary caregivers address the personal needs and challenges of providing direct support to individuals with NDs.

Books and other written resources: There are a number of books and other written resources available to caregivers raising children with NDs. Although certainly not exhaustive, this list provides a sampling of available written works that have been recommended by others raising children with specialized needs.

1) *Swan Mothers: Discovering our True Selves by Parenting Uniquely Magnificent Children* by Natalia Erehnah (2012)
2) *You Will Dream New Dreams: Inspiring Personal Stories by Parents of Children with Disabilities* by Kim Schive and Stanley D. Klein (Editors) (2001)
3) *A Different Kind of Perfect: Writings by Parents Raising a Child with Special Needs* by Cindy Dowling and Neil Nicoll (Editors) (2006)

4) *The Elephant in the Playroom: Ordinary Parents Write Intimately and Honestly about the Extraordinary Highs and Heartbreaking Lows of Raising Kids with Special Needs* by Denise Brodey (2007)
5) *Where We Going Daddy?* by Jean-Louis Fournier (2010)
6) *When your Child has a Disability* by Mark L. Batshaw MD (2000)
7) *Special Children, Challenging Parents: The Struggles and Rewards of Raising a Child with a Disability* by Robert A. Naseef (2001)

Online resources and networks: There are also a number of online resources available to caregivers. The following includes a list of general resources as well as more specialized online supports for those caring for individuals with SMS, WS, and DS.

1) General Online Supports and Networks
   a. Parents Helping Parents (www.php.com)
   b. Parent to Parent USA (www.p2pusa.org/p2pusa/SitePages/p2p-links.aspx)
   c. Alliance of Genetic Support Groups (www.geneticalliance.org/)
   d. Exceptional Parent Magazine (www.eparent.com/)
   e. Siblings of Kids with Special Needs, University of Michigan Health System (www.med.umich.edu/yourchild/topics/ specneed.htm)

2) Smith-Magenis syndrome
   a. Parents and Researchers Interested in Smith-Magenis syndrome (PRISMS; www.prisms.org)
   b. Smith-Magenis syndrome: National Institutes of Health, Genetics Home Reference (ghr.nlm.nih.gov/condition/smith-magenis-syndrome)

3) Williams syndrome
   a. Williams syndrome Association (www.williams-syndrome.org)
   b. Williams syndrome: PubMed Health (www.ncbi.nlm.nih.gov/pubmedhealth/ PMH0002105/)
   c. Williams syndrome: National Institutes of Health, Genetics Home Reference (ghr.nlm.nih.gov/condition/williams-syndrome)

4) Down syndrome
   a. National Down syndrome Society (www.ndss.org)
   b. National Association for Down syndrome (www.nads.org)
   c. Down syndrome: PubMed Health (www.ncbi.nlm.nih.gov/pubmedhealth/ PMH0001992/)

Finding individual and family therapists. There are many approaches to seeking out individual and/or family counseling services. Depending on the primary caregiver's comfort level, it may be beneficial to ask his/her primary care physician or the family's pediatrician about referral sources for therapy. Physicians are often well-networked within their respective communities and may be able to identify appropriate mental health professionals. As discussed in previous sections of this chapter, many children and adolescents with NDs participate in a variety of specialized therapy services. The professionals conducting these therapies may also be able to provide referrals for primary caregivers interested in engaging in psychotherapy. Alternately, individuals with medical insurance can go to the insurance company's website to find out more about the mental health benefits that are available to them and providers in their area. Depending upon the specific goals of therapy, it may be beneficial for the caregiver to seek out a therapist with a background in health psychology, as these care providers are more likely to have training in addressing caregiver needs. It is recommended that primary caregivers *consider asking potential therapists about their area of expertise* to help determine whether the therapist will be a good fit in meeting the person's needs (Martin, 2006; Stoppler, 2005). The following additional questions may also be helpful to ask potential therapists when determining who to see:

1) What is your approach to therapy? How are therapy sessions conducted (individually, group, family, etc.)?
2) What are my treatment options? How long can I expect treatment to take?
3) What are your views on the utilization of medication to treat mental health concerns?
4) Are there any alternative therapies or options to consider (e.g., changes in diet or exercise, biofeedback, acupuncture) that may be beneficial?
5) What is your level of education? What type of licensure do you have?
6) What are the costs for your services? What insurance do you accept? Are there alternate payment options?
7) What policies are in place for cancellations and/or emergencies?
8) What are the hours you are available? How often do I need to be seen for therapy?

Siblings

"My sister is very strong willed and knows what she wants to do. She doesn't let others influence what she does. She has a set plan in her mind and that's what she sticks to, and I love and hate that about her. Growing up with [my sister] was hard because I never understood why [she] was getting so much more attention from my parents. As well as why she got away with so much stuff. She did something and would get sent to her room for an hour, and I did the same thing and got grounded for two weeks, which seemed very unfair at the time. Now I understand it more...I still don't like it, but I understand why."

16 year-old sibling of 22 year-old diagnosed with DS

"I was 13 years old when [my sister] was born. She did change our lives considerably. It was stressful going thru junior high school and high school with her, as I was her main caregiver, because both my parents worked. When I came home from school, my responsibility was to care for both of my sisters. My younger sister was 8 years old when [our sister] was born, and she admits to being ashamed of her. She would not bring her girlfriends to the house because of [our sister]. I, on the other hand, being the oldest sibling, was involved in her life, to the extent that I used to babysit other developmentally disabled children who went to the same training center as [our sister]. She was certainly a challenge. Our parents are deceased now, and my younger sister and I are [our sister]'s conservators. It has been very hard in the later years, as we are both involved in her life and her care. She has now been diagnosed with Alzheimer's making this much more challenging to deal with. I would say that [our sister] has definitely changed our lives. Everyone in our direct family knows, loves, and understands [our sister], even the youngest of my grandchildren. [Our sister] has the mental age of 4 years old is 51 years old chronologically and has Alzheimer's...we are learning more every day, and each day has its own challenges."

64 year-old sibling of 51 year-old with DS

"My responsibility for him is scary. I get stressed trying to keep him out of trouble and safe. I enjoy his hugs and his nickname for me because I know he loves me. He misses me when I am gone and expresses his joy to see me; that always makes me feel good. He teaches me patience, and he is very loving so he is easy to care about. He shows love and acceptance toward me and so I feel the same toward him. He has directed me to a goal for myself to be an advocate for the disabled. I also have gained a desire to learn sign language and other skills to work with the disabled."

17 year-old sibling of 15 year-old with SMS

"It is TOUGH growing up with a SMS sibling. 'Fair' is not part of the equation. Do not get to do many things because of sibling. Do not get to do things with both parents...one is always with the SMS individual. Embarrassing situations. Hard to have friends over. Don't get to do casual trips. Everything must be planned out."

Parent of a 17 year-old without SMS and a 15 year-old with SMS

It is important to consider the dynamic of the family and how family members both positively and negatively influence one another when determining how to best promote quality of life among the entire family, while effectively caring for a child with a ND. Research in this area has focused primarily on children with disabilities and their parents, while the way other children in the family are influenced has been often overlooked. Siblings of individuals with disabilities have unique experiences, concerns, benefits, and intra-familial relationship factors that directly result from living with a sibling with a disability. Conway and Meyer (2008) found that siblings experience many of the same emotional concerns as parents and other caregivers who provide direct support, including feelings of isolation and guilt, support demands, a need for information, and concerns about the future of the individual with a disability. In addition to these concerns, siblings may face unique issues not faced by their parents, such as resentment and embarrassment, social problems, and a pressure to achieve. While potential negative emotions and experiences have been reported, a number of positive experiences have also been acknowledged. One study on families with children with Down syndrome and Rett syndrome found that siblings demonstrated increased tolerance, better awareness of differences, and greater maturity when compared to peers (Dyke, Mulroy, and Leonard, 2009). Siblings of children with NDs have also been described as having an especially caring and compassionate nature (Dyke et al., 2009). It should be noted that siblings' experiences vary depending on the type of illness or condition their sibling has. For example, siblings of individuals with SMS need to learn to adjust to and to cope with their sibling's severe maladaptive behaviors (Moshier et al., 2012). By comparison, siblings of individuals with WS or DS will likely experience the unique challenges and benefits associated with living with an individual who has significant medical and/or psychiatric problems. The typically developing sibling may feel that he or she has less in common with the sibling with SMS, WS, or DS, resulting in greater emotional separation between the siblings.

In addition to influencing the sibling relationship, the presence of a child with a disability in the family affects the relationship between the well-sibling and his/her parents (Moshier et al., 2012; Neece, Blacher, and Baker, 2010; Schuntermann, 2009). The greater the number and severity of stereotypic and self-injurious behaviors displayed by a child with SMS, the more time parents must spend addressing them and providing direct attention to the child with the disability (Moshier et al., 2012). In families of children with WS, parents may need to spend large quantities of time attending to the psychiatric concerns of the child with WS (Leyfer, Woodruff-Borden, and Mervis, 2009). Similarly, the presence of a child with DS in a family means that parents will likely spend more time addressing medical concerns for that child (Graff et al., 2012). This results in less time available for the parent to spend with the sibling (Schuntermann, 2009). Furthermore, the more difficult a child's temperament, the more pronounced the degree of differential parenting, defined as the extent to which a parent's expectations, treatment of, and quality of time spent with a child with a disability differs with regards to other children in the family (Rivers and Stoneman, 2008). Research has found that families of children with disabilities tend to show greater rates of differential parenting than families of children without disabilities. Siblings' responses to differential parenting range from resentment and anger to acceptance. Studies have found differential parenting to be associated with negative sibling outcomes, such as greater competition and increased conflict (Rivers and Stoneman, 2008; Taylor, Fuggle, and Charman, 2001). However, children who are able to understand why they are being treated differently from their sibling, and perceive this as being fair, tend to be more accepting of the parenting differences.

Resources for Siblings

The following resources are provided to help support siblings in addressing personal needs and challenges.

Books and other written resources: There are a number of books and other written resources available to siblings of individuals with NDs. This list provides a sampling of available written works that have been recommended by others living with and/or caring for those with NDs.

1) *A Boy Alone* by Karl Taro Greenfeld (2009)
2) *At Home in the Land of Oz: Autism, My Sister, and Me* by Anne Clinard Barnhill (2007)
3) *Brothers and Sisters* by Laura Dwight (2007)
4) *Brothers and Sisters of Disabled Children* By Peter Burke (2003)
5) *Thicker than Water: Essays by Adult Siblings of People with Disabilities* from Woodbine House (Editors) (2009)
6) *The Sibling Slam Book*: *What It's Really Like to have a Brother or Sister with Special Needs* by Don Meyer and David Gallagher (2005)

Online resources and networks: There are also a limited number of online resources available to siblings of individuals with NDs.

1) Sibling Support Project (www.siblingsupport.org)
2) Kids Health (www.kidshealth.org)

Finding individual and family therapists. Siblings of individuals with NDs may benefit from seeking professional assistance to help support appropriate coping and adjustment. It can be helpful for siblings to have a safe and confidential environment in which they can voice frustrations, ask questions regarding their sibling's diagnosis and prognosis, learn to strengthen relationships with siblings and parents, assess benefits, and improve their quality of life. It can be especially beneficial for siblings to have such supports during naturally developmentally stressful times such as the teenage years or when transitioning into adult caregiver roles. It is recommended that children and adolescent siblings seek out therapy with professionals specializing in NDs, such as pediatric psychologists. Many hospitals and communities also offer Sibshops, or group-based support systems, for siblings. A list of Sibshops can be found at www.siblingsupport.org/sibshops/index_html.

CONCLUSION

The ever-changing needs of individuals with NDs necessitate substantial specialized support, intervention, and resources across the lifespan. As these individuals age, each developmental period presents unique challenges for primary caregivers, who must learn to cope in such as way that promotes individual well-being and the family's overall quality of life. Understanding the potential concerns that may arise can help caregivers prepare to meet developmental needs in an active and adaptive manner. For infants and young children, developmental assessments can be utilized to indentify strengths and weaknesses in such a way that leads to individualized therapies (e.g., speech and language, occupational, physical, and behavioral therapies) and initial academic planning. In middle childhood, psycho-educational evaluations and the resulting recommendations provided can further assist families in developing academic plans (e.g., IEPs) and continuing necessary therapies. Additionally, challenges with social skills and peer relationships may need to be continuously addressed. Throughout adolescence and beyond, challenges with puberty and romantic relationships, vocations, and adult living arrangements all need to be addressed. Vocational assessments can offer assistance in determining appropriate job-related skills and settings. Considerations also need to be made with respect to individual decision-making capacities and whether guardianships or alternative to guardianships need to be pursued. This can often be a cumbersome and involved process for caregivers, including adult siblings, who often are charged with transitioning into caregiver responsibilities as parents age. Due to the intense demands associated with caring for an individual with a ND, caregiver and sibling needs must be considered and supportive resources implemented.

REFERENCES

American Association of Intellectual and Developmental Disabilities. (2010). *Intellectual disability; Definition, classification, and systems of supports.* Washington, D.C.: Author.

American Association of Intellectual and Developmental Disabilities. (2012). FAQ on Intellectual Disability. Retrieved from http://www.aamr.org/ content_104.cfm?navID=22.

American Association of Intellectual and Developmental Disabilities and The ARC. (2012). *Joint Position Statement of AAIDD and The Arc*: Author. Retrieved from http://aaidd.org/content_159.cfm?navID=31.

American Psychiatric Association. (2000). *Diagnostic and statistical manual of mental disorders* (4th ed., text rev.). Washington, DC: Author.

Annaz, D., Remington, A., Milne, E., Coleman, M., Campbell, R., Thomas, M., and Swettenham, J. (2010). *Atypical development of motion processing trajectories in children with autism*. Retrieved from psyc.bbk.ac.uk.

Bagwell, C. L., Schmidt, M. E., Newcomb, A. F., and Bukowski, W. M. (2001). Friendship and peer rejection as predictors of adult adjustment. *New Directions for Child and Adolescent Development, 91*, 25-49. doi:10.1002/cd.4.

Barakat, L. P., and Linney, J. A. (1992). Children with physical handicaps and their mothers: The interrelation of social support, maternal adjustment, and child adjustment. *Journal of Pediatric Psychology, 17*, 725-739. doi:10.1093/jpepsy/17.6.725.

Beauchamp, T. L., and Childress, J. F. (1994). *Principles of biomedical ethics.* New York: Oxford University Press.

Bierman, K. L. (2004). *Peer rejection: Developmental processes and intervention strategies.* New York, NY: The Guilford Press.

Borg, I., Delhanty, J. D., and Baraitser, M. (1995). Detection of hemizygosity at the elastin locus by FISH analysis as a diagnostic test in both classical and atypical cases of Williams syndrome. *Journal of Medical Genetics, 32*, 692-696. doi:10.1136/jmg.32.9.692.

Burn, J. (1986). Williams syndrome. *Journal of Medical Genetics, 23*, 398-395. doi: 10.1136/jmg.23.5.389.

Butterworth, J., Hagner, D., Kiernan, W. E., and Schalock, R. L. (1996). Natural supports in the workplace: Defining an agenda for research and practice. *Journal of the Association for Personas with Severe Handicaps, 21*(3), 103-113.

Callahan, M., and Garner, J. (1997). Keys to the workplace: Skills and supports for people with disabilities. Baltimore, MD: Brookes.

Cambiaso, P., Orazi, C., Digilio, M.C., Loche, S., Capolino, R., Tozzi, A.,…, and Cappa M. (2007). Thyroid morphology and subclinical hypothyroidism in children and adolescents with Williams syndrome. *Journal of Pediatrics, 150*, 62–65. doi:10.1016/j.jpeds.2006.10.060.

Canfield, M. A., Ramadhani, T. A., Yuskiv, M. P., Davidoff, M. J., Petrini, J. R., Hobbs, C. A., …, and Correa, A. (2006). Improved national prevalence estimates for 18 selected major birth defects—United States, 1999-2001. *Mortality and Morbidity Weekly Review,* 1301-1305.

Children's Health Care of Atlanta (2012). Your child's occupational therapy evaluation. Retrieved from http://www.choa.org/childrens-hospital-services/rehabilitation/locations/~/media/CHOA/Documents/Services/Rehabilitation/What-to-Expect-OT.pdf.

Clibbens, J. (2001). Signing and lexical development in children with Down syndrome. *Down syndrome Research and Practice, 7,* 101-105. doi:10.3104/reviews.119.

Colley, A., Leversha, M., Voullaire, L., and Rogers, J. (1990). Five cases demonstrating the distinctive behavioral features of chromosome deletion 17(p11.2) (Smith-Magenis

Syndrome). *Journal of Pediatrics and Child Health, 26,* 17-21. doi:10.1111/j.1440-1754.1990.tb02372.x

Comer, R. (2013). *Abnormal Psychology* (8th ed). New York, NY: Worth Publishers.

Conway, S., and Meyer, D. (2008). Developing support for siblings of young people with disabilities. *Support for Learning, 23*(3), 113-117. doi:10.1111/j.1467-9604. 2008 .00381.x.

Cooper-Brown, L., Copeland, S., Dailey, S., Downey, D., Peterson, M. C., Stimson, C., and Van Dyke, D. C. (2008). Feeding and swallowing dysfunction in genetic syndromes. *Developmental Disabilities Research Reviews, 14,* 147-157. doi: 10.1002/ddrr.19.

Davies, M., Howlin, P., and Udwin, O. (1997). Independence and adaptive behavior in adults with Williams syndrome. *American Journal of Medical Genetics, 70,* 188-195. doi:10.1002/(SICI)1096-8628(19970516)70:2<188::AID-AJMG16>3.0.CO;2-F.

Davies, M., Udwin, O., and Howlin, P. (1998). Adults with Williams syndrome. Preliminary study of social, emotional and behavioural difficulties. *British Journal of Psychiatry, 172,* 273-276. doi:10.1192/bjp.172.3.273

Dinerstein, R. D. (2006). Guardianship and its Alternatives for Adults with Down Syndrome. In S. M. Pueschel, (Ed.), *Adults with Down Syndrome.* Baltimore, MD: Paul H. Brookes.

Disability Rights Texas (2011). *Guardianship for Texans with disabilities* (13th ed.). Austin, TX: Disability Rights Texas.

Dyke, P., Mulroy, S., and Leonard, H. (2009). Siblings of children with disabilities: Challenges and opportunities. *Acta Paediatrica, 98*(1), 23-24. doi: 10.1111/j.1651-2227.2008.01168.x.

Dykens, E. M. (2003). Anxiety, fears, and phobias in persons with Williams syndrome. *Developmental Neuropsychology, 23,* 291–316. doi:10.1207/S15326942DN231and2_13.

Dykens, E. M., and Smith, A. (1998). Distinctiveness and correlates of maladaptive behavior in children and adolescents with Smith-Magenis syndrome. *Journal of Intellectual Disability Research, 42,* 481-489. doi:10.1046/j.1365-2788.1998.4260481.x.

Dykens, E. M., Finucane, B., and Gayley, C. (1997). Brief report: Cognitive and behavioral profiles in persons with Smith-Magenis syndrome. *Journal of Autism and Developmental Disorders, 27,* 203-211. doi:10.1023/A:1025800126086.

Dykens, E. M., Hodapp, R., and Finucane, B. (2000). *Genetics and Mental Retardation Syndromes. A New Look at Behavior and Interventions.* Baltimore, MD: Paul H. Brooks Publishing Company.

Edelman, E. A., Girirajan, S., Finucane, B., Patel, P. I., Lupski, J. R., Smith, A. C., and Elsea, S. H. (2007). Gender, genotype, and phenotype differences in Smith-Magenis syndrome: a meta-analysis of 105 cases. *Clinical Genetics, 71*(6), 540-550. doi:10.1111/j.1399-0004.2007.00815.x.

Eggleton, I., Roberston, S., Ryan, J., and Kober, R. (1999). The impact of employment on the quality of life of people with an intellectual disability. *Journal of Vocational Rehabilitation, 13,* 95-107.

Eicher, P. S., and Batshaw, M. L. (1993). Cerebral palsy. *Pediatric Clinics of North America, 40,* 537-551. Retrieved from www.pediatric.theclinics.com/

Ekstein, S., Glick B., Weill M., Kay B., Berger I. (2011). Down syndrome and Attention-Deficit/Hyperactivity Disorder (ADHD). *Journal of Child Neurology, 26,* 1290–1295. doi:10.1177/0883073811405201.

Elcioglu, N., Mackie-Ogilvie, C., Daker, M., and Berry, A. C. (1998). FISH analysis in patients with clinical diagnosis of Williams syndrome. *Acta Paediatrica. 87*, 48– 53. Retrieved from www.wiley.com/bw/ journal.asp?ref=0803-5253.

Elsea, S.H., and Girirajan, S. (2008). Smith-Magenis Syndrome. *European Journal of Human Genetics, 16*, 412-21. doi:10.1038/sj.ejhg.5202009.

Emerson, E. (2004). Cluster housing for people with intellectual disabilities. *Journal of Intellectual Disability and Developmental Disability, 29*(3), 187–197. doi:10.1080/13668250412331285208.

Emery, A. H., and Rimoin, D.L, (1996). *Principles and Practice of Medical Genetics* (3rd ed.). New York, NY: Churchill Livingstone.

Erickson, M., and Upshur, C. (1989). Caretaking burden and social support: A comparison of mothers of children with and without disabilities. *American Journal on Mental Retardation, 94*, 250-258. Retrieved from www.aaiddjournals.org/.

Fidler, D. J., Bailey, J. N., and Smalley, S. L. (2000). Macrocephaly in autism and other pervasive developmental disorders. *Developmental Medicine and Child Neurology, 42*, 737–740. doi:10.1017/S0012162200001365.

Flynn, R. J., and Aubry, T. D. (1999). Integration of persons with development or psychiatric disabilities: conceptualization and measurement. In R. J. Flynn, and R. Lemay (Eds.), *A quarter century of normalization and social role valorization: Evolution and impact* (pp. 3–16). Ottawa, CAN: University of Ottawa Press.

Foster, R. H., Kozachek, S., Stern, M., and Elsea, S. H. (2010). Caring for the caregivers: An investigation of factors related to well-being among parents caring for a child with Smith-Magenis syndrome. *Journal of Genetic Counseling, 19*, 187-198. doi:10.1007/s10897-009-9273-5.

Fowler, A. E. (1990). Language abilities in children with Down syndrome: Evidence for a specific syntactic delay. In D. Cicchetti and M. Beeghly (Eds.), *Children with Down Syndrome: A Developmental Perspective*. Cambridge: Cambridge University Press.

Froehlich, T. E., Lanphear, B. P., Epstein, J. N., Barbaresi, W. J., Katusic, S. K., and Kahn, R. S. (2007). Prevalence, recognition, and treatment of attention-deficit/hyperactivity disorder in a national sample of US children. *Archives of Pediatrics and Adolescent Medicine, 161*(9), 857-864. doi:10.1001/archpedi.161.9.857.

Geisthardt, C. L., Brotherson, M., and Cook, C. C. (2002). Friendships of children with disabilities in the home environment. *Education and Training in Mental Retardation and Developmental Disabilities, 37*(3), 235-252.

Gilbride, D., and Hagner, D. (2005). People with disabilities in the workplace. R. Parker, E. Symanski, and J. Patterson (Eds.) *Rehabilitation Counseling: Basics and Beyond* (4th Ed.), pp. 281-306). Austin, TX: Pro-Ed.

Graff, C., Mandleco, B., Dyches, T., Coverston, C. R., Roper, S., and Freeborn, D. (2012). Perspectives of adolescent siblings of children with Down syndrome who have multiple health problems. *Journal of Family Nursing, 18*(2), 175-199. doi:10.1177/1074840712439797.

Graham, C., Ballard, C., and Sham, P. (1997). Carers' knowledge of dementia, their coping strategies and morbidity. *International Journal of Geriatric Psychiatry, 12*, 931-936. doi:10.1002/(SICI)1099-1166(199709)12:9<931::AID-GPS666>3.0.CO;2-8.

Grandjean, P., and Landrigan, P. J. (2006). Developmental neurotoxicity of industrial chemicals. *Lancet, 368*, 2167-2178. doi:10.1016/S0140-6736(06)69665-7.

Greenberg, F., Lewis, R., Potocki, L., Glaze, D., Parke, J., Killian, J., ..., Lupiski, J. (1996). Multi-disciplinary clinical study of Smith-Magenis syndrome: (deletion 17p11.2). *American Journal of Medical Genetics, 62*, 247-254. doi:10.1002/(SICI)1096-8628(19960329)62:3<247::AID-AJMG9>3.3.CO;2-9.

Grupp-Phelan, J., Harman, J. S., and Kelleher, K. J. (2007). Trends in mental health and chronic condition visits by children presenting for care at U.S. emergency departments. *Public Health Reports, 122*(1), 55-61. doi:10.1016/j.jaac.2011.08.011.

Hagner, D. C. (1992). The social interactions and job supports of supported employment. In J. Nisbet (Ed.), *Natural supports in school, at work, and in the community for people with disabilities* (pp. 217-239). Baltimore: Paul H. Brookes Publishing Co.

Hasselkus, B. R. (1988). Meaning in family caregiving: Perspectives on caregiver /professional relationships. *Gerontologist, 28*, 686–691. doi:10.1093/ geront/28.5.686.

Health Insurance Portability and Accountability Act of 1996, Pub. L. No. 104-191, 110 Stat. 204 (1996).

Heiman, T. (2000). Friendship quality among children in three educational settings. *Journal of Intellectual and Developmental Disability, 25*, 1-12. doi:10.1080/132697800112749.

Hemmeter, M. (2000). Classroom-based interventions: Evaluating the past and looking toward the future. *Topics in Early Childhood Special Education, 20*(1), 56-61. doi:10.1177/027112140002000110.

Hodapp, R. M., Fidler, D. J., and Smith, A.C. (1998). Stress and coping in families of children with Smith-Magenis syndrome. *Journal of Intellectual Disability Research, 42*, 331-340. doi:10.1046/j.1365-2788.1998.00148.x.

Holmes, J. and Fillary, R. (2000). Handling small talk at work: Challenges for workers with intellectual disabilities. *International Journal of Disability, Development and Education, 47*, 273-291. doi:10.1080/713671114.

Jones, K. L. (2006). *Smith's recognizable patterns of human malformation* (6th ed.). Philadelphia: Elsevier Inc.

Kelleher, K. J., McInerny, T. K., Gardner, W. P., Childs, G. E., and Wasserman, R. C. (2000). Increasing identification of psychosocial problems: 1979-1996. *Pediatrics, 105*(6), 1313-1221. doi:10.1542/peds.105.6.1313.

Laje, G., Bernert, R., Morse, R., Pao, M., and Smith, A. C. (2010). Pharmacological treatment of disruptive behavior in Smith-Magenis syndrome. *American Journal of Medical Genetics Part C: Seminars in Medical Genetics, 154C*(4), 463–468. doi:10.1002/ ajmg.c.30282.

Lesseliers, J., and Van Hove, G. (2002). Barriers to the development of intimate relationships and the expression of sexuality among people with developmental disabilities: Their perceptions. *Research and Practice for Persons with Severe Disabilities, 27*(1), 69-81. doi:10.2511/rpsd.27.1.69.

Levitin, D. J., Cole, K., Lincoln, A., and Bellugi, U. (2005). Aversion, awareness, and attraction: investigating claims of hyperacusis in the Williams syndrome phenotype. Journal Child Psychology and Psychiatry, 46 (5), 514-523. doi: 10.1111/j.1469-7610.2004.00376.x.

Leyfer, O. T., Woodruff-Borden, J., Klein-Tasman, B., Fricke, J., and Mervis, C. (2006). Prevalence of psychiatric disorders in 4-16 year olds with Williams syndrome. *American Journal of Medical Genetics, 141B*, 615-622. doi:10.1002/ajmg.b.30344.

Leyfer, O., Woodruff-Borden, J., and Mervis, C. B. (2009). Anxiety disorders in children with Williams syndrome, their mothers, and their siblings: Implications for the etiology of anxiety disorders. *Journal of Neurodevelopmental Disorders, 1*(1), 4-14. doi:10.1007/s11689-009-9003-1.

Marks, D. (1999). *Disability: Controversial debates and psychosocial perspectives.* London: Routledge.

Martella, R., Marchand-Martella, N., and Agran, M. (1993). Using a problem-solving strategy to teach adaptability skills to individuals with mental retardation. *Journal of Rehabilitation, 59*(3), 55-60.

Martens, M. A., Wilson, D. C., and Reutens, J. (2008). Research Review: Williams syndrome: a critical review of the cognitive, behavioral, and neuroanatomical phenotype. *Journal of Child Psychology and Psychiatry and Allied Disciplines, 49,* 576-608. doi:10.1111/j.1469-7610.2008.01887.x.

Martin, B. (2006). Questions to Ask Your Therapist. *Psych Central.* Retrieved from http://psychcentral.com/lib/2006/questions-to-ask-your-therapist/.

Martin, S. C., Wolters, P. L., and Smith, A. C. (2006). Adaptive and maladaptive behavior in children with Smith-Magenis syndrome. *Journal of Autism and Developmental Disorders, 36,* 541-552. doi:10.1007/s10803-006-0093-2.

McCarthy, M. (1999). *Sexuality and women with learning disabilities.* London: Jessica Kingsley Publishers.

Melberg-Schwier, K., and Hingsburger, D. (2000). *Sexuality: Your sons and daughers with intellectual disabilities.* London: Jessica Kingsley Publishers.

Mervis, C. B., Robinson, B. F., Bertrand, J., Morris, C. A., Klein-Tasman, B. P.. and Armstrong S. C. (2000). The Williams syndrome cognitive profile. *Brain and Cognition,* 44, 604–628. doi:10.1006/brcg.2000.1232.

Meyer-Lindenberg, A., Mervis, C. B., and Berman, K.F. (2006). Neural mechanisms in Williams syndrome: A unique window to genetic influences on cognition and behaviour. *Nature Reviews Neuroscience,* 7, 380–393. doi:10.1038/nrn1906.

Miller, J. F. (1992). Development of speech and language in children with Down syndrome. In I. T. Lott and E. E. McCoy (Eds.), *Down Syndrome: Advances in Medical Care.* New York: Wiley-Liss.

Miller, J. F. (1999). Profiles of language development in children with Down syndrome. In J. F. Miller, M. Leddy and L. A. Leavitt (Eds.), *Improving the Communication of People with Down Syndrome* (pp. 11-39). Baltimore: Paul H. Brookes.

Moshier M. S., York T. P., Silberg J. L., and Elsea S. H. (2012). Siblings of individuals with Smith-Magenis syndrome: An investigation of the correlates of positive and negative behavioral traits. *Journal of Intellectual Disabilities Research, 56,* 996-1007. doi: 10.1111/j.1365-2788.2012.01581.x.

Nakamura, M., Mizuno, S., Douyuu, S., Matsumoto, A., Kumagai, T., Watanabe, S., and Kakigi, R. (2009). Development of visuospatial ability and kanji copying in Williams syndrome. *Journal of Pediatric Neurology, 41,* 95-100. doi:10.1016/ j.pediatrneuro l.2009.02.005.

National Center for Learning Disabilities. (2012). *Section 504 and the IDEA comparison chart.* Retrieved from http://www.ncld.org/disability-advocacy/learn-ld-laws/adaaa-section-504/section-504-idea-comparison-chart.

Neece, C. L., Blacher, J., and Baker, B. L. (2010). Impact on siblings of children with intellectual disability: The role of child behavior problems. *American Journal on Intellectual and Developmental Disabilities, 115*(4), 291-306. doi:10.1352/1944-7558-115.4.291.

Newschaffer, C. J., Falb, M. D., and Gurney, J. G. (2005). National autism prevalence trends from United States special education data. *Pediatrics, 115*(3), 277-282. doi:10.1542/peds.2004-1958.

Odom, S. L., Zercher, C., Li, S., Marquart, J. M., Sandall, S., and Brown, W. H. (2006). Social acceptance and rejection of preschool children with disabilities: A mixed-method analysis. *Journal of Educational Psychology, 98*, 807-823. doi:10.1037/0022-0663.98.4.807.

Oliver, M. (1990). *The politics of disablement: A sociological approach.* New York, NY: St. Martin's Press.

O'Sullivan, J. L. (1999). Adult guardianship and alternatives. In R. D. Dinnerstein, S. H. Herr and J. L. O'Sullivan (Eds.), *A Guide to Consent.* Washington, DC: AAMR.

Pastor, P., and Reuben, C. (2009). Mental retardation, other developmental delay, down syndrome, autism, learning disability, and attention-deficit/hyperactivity. *National Health Interview Survey, 2001-2006.*

Pennsylvania Code. (2011). *Procedures for Surrogate Health Care Decision Making.* Title 55, Pa.B. 6000, Subchapter R. Retrieved from http://www.pacode.com/secure/data/055/chapter6000/subchapRtoc.html.

Peoples, R., Frankie, Y., Wang, Y.K., Perez-Jurado, L., Paperna, T., Cisco, M., and Francke, U. (2000). A physical map, including a bac/pac clone contig, of the Williams-Beuren syndrome–deletion region at 7q11. 23. *American Journal of Human Genetics, 66*, 47-68. doi:10.1086/302722.

Physical Therapyworks (2012). *Evaluation.* Retrieved from http:// www.physical therapy works.com/evaluation.htm.

Pober, B. R. (2010). Williams-Beuren Syndrome. *New England Journal of Medicine, 362*, 239- 252. doi:10.1056/NEJMra0903074.

Prior, M. (2003). Is there an increase in the prevalence of autism spectrum disorders? *Journal of Pediatrics and Child Health, 39*(2), 81-82. doi:10.1046/j.1440-1754.2003.00097.x.

Prouty, R. W., Smith, G., and Lakin, K. C. (2005). Executive summary. In R. W. Prouty, G. Smith, and K. C. Lakin (Eds.), *Residential services for persons with developmental disabilities: Status and trends through 2004.* Minneapolis: University of Minnesota, Research and Training Center on Community Living, Institute on Community Integration.

Racino, J. A. (1995). Community living for adults with developmental disabilities: A housing and support approach. *Journal of the Association for Persons with Severe Handicaps, 20*(4), 300–310.

Reynolds, C., and Goldstein, S. (1999). *Handbook of neurodevelopmental and genetic disorders in children.* New York: The Guilford Press, pp. 3-8.

Rillotta, F., and Nettelbeck, T. (2007). Effects of an awareness program on attitudes of students without an intellectual disability towards persons with an intellectual disability. *Journal of Intellectual and Developmental Disability, 32*(1), 19-27. doi:10.1080/13668250701194042.

Rivers, J. W., and Stoneman, Z. (2008). Child temperaments, differential parenting, and the sibling relationships of children with autism spectrum disorder. *Journal of Autism and Developmental Disorders, 38;* 1740-1750. doi: 10.1007/s10803-008-0560-z.

Rondal, J. A., and Comblain, A. (1996). Language in adults with Down syndrome. *Down Syndrome: Research and Practice, 4,* 3-14. doi:10.3104/reviews.58.

Rutter, M. (2005). Incidence of autism spectrum disorders: changes over time and their meaning. *Acta Paediatrica, 94*(1), 2-15. doi:10.1080/08035250410023124.

Scallan, S., Senior, J., and Reilly, C. (2010). Williams syndrome: Daily challenges and positive impact on the family. *Journal of Applied Research in Intellectual Disabilities, 24,* 181-188. doi: 10.1111/j.1468-3148.2010.00575.x.

Schroeder, S. R. (2000). Mental retardation and developmental disabilities influenced by environmental neurotoxic insults. *Environmental Health Perspectives, 108*(Suppl. 3), 395-399. doi:10.2307/3454526.

Schubert, C. (2009) The genomic basis of the Williams-Beuren syndrome. *Cellular and Molecular Life Sciences, 66,* 1178-1197.

Schumann, C. M., Bauman, M. D., and Amaral, D. G. (2010). Abnormal structure or function of the amygdale is a common component of Neurodevelopmental Disorders. *Neuropsychologia, 49,* 745-759. Retrieved from www.sciencedirect.com/science/journal/00283932.

Schuntermann, P. (2009). Growing up with a developmentally challenged brother or sister: A model for engaging siblings based on mentalizing. *Harvard Review of Psychiatry, 17*(5), 297-314. doi:10.3109/ 10673220903299161.

Silver, E., Westbrook, L., and Stein, R. (1998). Relationship of Parental Psychological Distress to consequences of chronic health conditions. *Journal of Pediatric Psychology, 23,* 5-15. doi:10.1093/jpepsy/23.1.5.

Shokoohi-Yekta, M., and Hendrickson, J. M. (2010). Friendships with peers with severe disabilities: American and Iranian secondary students' ideas about being a friend. *Education and Training in Autism and Developmental Disabilities, 45*(1), 23-37.

Slosky, L., Foster, R.H., and Elsea, S. (2012). Caring for children with intellectual disabilities: A focus on Williams and Smith-Magenis syndromes. In D. F. Mancini and C. M. Greco (Eds.), Intellectual Disability: Management, Causes, and Social Perceptions. Hauppauge, NY: Nova Science Publishers, Inc.

Smith, A., Allenson, J., Elsea, S., Finucane, B., Haas-Givler, B., and Gropman, A. (2006). Smith-Magenis Syndrome. Gene reviews. University of Washington.

Smith, A. C., Boyd, K. E., Elsea, S. H., et al. (2012). Gene Reviews. In: Pagon, R. A. Pagon, T. D. Bird, C. R. T. D., Dolan, , C. R., et al., (Eds.), Smith-Magenis Syndrome. Retrieved from http://www.ncbi.nlm.nih.gov/ books/NBK1310/.

Smith, A., Dykens, E., and Greenberg, F. (1998). Sleep disturbance in Smith-Magenis syndrome. *American Journal of Medical Genetics, 81,* 186-191. doi:10.1002/(SICI)1096-8628(19980328)81:2<186::AID-JMG11>3.3.CO;2-A.

Smith, A., McGavran, L., Waldstein, G., and Robinson, J. (1982). Deletion of the 17 short arm in two patients with facial clefts and congenital heart disease. *American Journal of Human Genetics, 34,* A410. Retrieved from www.cell.com/AJHG/.

Smith, K., Wilson, C., Webber, L., and Graffam, J. (2004). Employment and intellectual disability: Achieving successful employment outcomes. *International Review of Research in Mental Retardation, 29,* 261-289. doi:10.1016/S0074-7750(04)29008-5.

Solish, A., Perry, A., and Minnes, P. (2010). Participation of children with and without disabilities in social, recreational and leisure activities. *Journal of Applied Research in Intellectual Disabilities, 23*(3), 226-236. doi:10.1111/j.1468-3148.2009.00525.x

Stagi, S., Bindi, G., Neri, A. S., Lapi, E., Losi, S., Jenuso, R. S., and Chiarelli, F. (2005). Thyroid function and morphology in patients affected by Williams syndrome. *Clinical Endocrinology, 63*, 456–460. doi:10.1111/j.1365-2265.2005.02365.x.

Staub, D. (1998). *Delicate threads: Friendships between children with and without special needs in inclusive settings.* Bethesda, MD US: Woodbine House.

Stoppler, M. (2005). Questions to Ask When Choosing a Mental Health Care Provider and Doctor. In: Shiel, W. C. (Ed.), *MedicineNet.* Retrieved from http://www.medicinenet.com/script/main/art.asp?articlekey=47440.

Stratton, R., Dobyns, W., Greenberg, F., DeSana, J., Moore, C., Fidone, G., ..., Ledbetter, D.(1986). Interstitial deletion of (17)(p11.2): Report of six additional patients with a new chromosome deletion syndrome. *American Journal of Medical Genetics, 24*, 421-432. doi:10.1002/ajmg.1320240305.

Stromme, P., Bjomstad, P. G., and Ramstad, K. (2002). Prevalence estimation of Williams syndrome. *Journal of Child Neurology, 17*, 269-271. doi:10.1177/088307380201700406.

Tager-Flusberg, H. (1999). Language development in atypical children. In M. Barrett (Ed.), *The Development of Language.* Hove: Psychology Press.

Taylor, V., Fuggle, P., and Charman, T. (2001). Well sibling psychological adjustment to chronic physical disorder in a sibling: How important is maternal awareness of their illness attitudes and perceptions? *Journal of Child Psychology and Psychiatry and Allied Disciplines, 42*, 953-963. doi:10.1111/1469-7610.00791.

Thorin, E. J., and Irvin, L. K. (1992). Family stress associated with transition to adulthood of young people with severe disabilities. *The Journal of the Association for Persons with Severe Handicaps, 17*(1), 31-39.

Tsai, S. W., Wu, S. K., Liou, Y. M., and Shu, S. G. (2008). Early development in Williams syndrome. *Pediatrics International, 50*, 221-224. doi:10.1111/j.1442-200X.2008.02563.x

Turnbull, A. P., Blue-Banning, M., and Pereira, L. (2000). Successful friendships of Hispanic children and youth with disabilities: An exploratory study. *Mental Retardation, 38*, 13-153.

Udwin, O., Webber, C., and Horn, I. (2001). Abilities and attainment in Smith-Magenis syndrome. *Developmental Medicine and Child Neurology, 43*, 823–828. doi:10.1017/S0012162201001499.

Udwin, O., and Yule, W. (1991). A cognitive and behavioural phenotype in Williams syndrome. *Journal of Clinical and Experimental Neuropsychology, 13*, 232–244. doi:10.1080/01688639108401040.

U.S. Department of Education (2007). *27th Annual (2005) Report to Congress on the Implementation of the Individuals with Disabilities Education Act, Vol. 1.* Washington, DC: Author.

Vignes, C., Godeau, E., Sentenac, M., Coley, N., Navarro, F., Grandjean, H., and Arnaud, C. (2009). Determinants of students' attitudes towards peers with disabilities. *Developmental Medicine and Child Neurology, 51*(6), 473-479. doi:10.1111/j.1469-8749.2009.03283.x

Visser, S. N., Bitsko, R. H., Danielson, M. L., Perou, R., and Blumberg, S. J. (2010). Increasing prevalence of parent-reported attention-deficit/hyperactivity disorder among children - United States, 2003 and 2007. *Morbidity and Mortality Weekly Report, 59*(44),1439-1443. Retrieved from http://www.cdc.gov/mmwr/

Wessel, A., Gravenhorst, V., Buchhorn, R., Gosch, A., Partsch, C. J., and Pankau, R. (2004). Risk of sudden death in the Williams-Beuren syndrome. *American Journal of Medical Genetics, 127*(3), 234–237.

Wiseman, F. K., Alford, K. A., Tybulewicz, V. L., and Fisher, E. M. (2009). Down Syndrome: Recent progress and future prospects. *Human Molecular Genetics, 18*(1), 75-83. doi:10.1093/hmg/ddp010.

Wolfensberger, W. (1983). Social role valorization: a proposed new term for the principle of normalization. *Mental Retardation, 21,* 234–239. doi:10.1352/1934-9556-49.6.435.

Wolters, P. L., Gropman, A. L., Martin, S. C., Smith, M. R., Hildenbrand, H. L., Brewer, C. C., and Smith, A. C. (2009). Neurodevelopment of children under 3 years of age with Smith-Magenis syndrome. *Pediatric Neurology, 41,* 250-258. doi:10.1016/j.pediatrneurol.2009.04.015.

Wong, Y. I., and Stanhope, V. (2009). Conceptualizing community: A comparison of neighbourhood characteristics of supportive housing for persons with psychiatric and developmental disabilities. *Social Science and Medicine, 68,* 1376-1387. doi:10.1016/j.socscimed.2009.01.046.

World Health Organization. (2005). WHO Executive Board Report – Control of Genetic Diseases. Retrieved from apps.who.int/gb/ebwha/ pdf_files/EB116/B116_3-en.pdf

In: Caregivers: Challenges, Practices and Cultural Influences
Editors: Adrianna Thurgood and Kasha Schuldt
ISBN: 978-1-62618-030-7
© 2013 Nova Science Publishers, Inc.

Chapter 2

THE FAMILY CAREGIVERS OF PATIENTS WITH CANCER: ROLES AND CHALLENGES

Sabrina Cipolletta
Department of General Psychology, University of Padua, Italy

ABSTRACT

Assisting a loved one with cancer implies assuming a role that may fit or contrast with the person's previous role, thereby allowing the person to adjust to the new role or provoking suffering. In order to explore the constraints and challenges this situation may pose, a research project was developed at the University of Padua (Italy). A first study explored if it was possible to identify different profiles of caregivers on the basis of their different ways of giving and receiving help. Fifty Italian family caregivers of patients with cancer completed the Beck Anxiety Inventory, the Beck Depression Inventory-II and Kelly's Dependency Grids. Cluster analysis was conducted on the indices derived from the three instruments. Three profiles emerged and were described on the basis of the balance/imbalance between the usual and present role of the caregiver. If there was congruence between the situation of giving help that the caregivers experienced and their personal role, then anxiety and depression decreased, otherwise they increased. The implications of the balance/imbalance between the usual and present role depended also on the typicality of the caregivers' experience, as related to their caring role. With a subsequent study, we aimed at investigating in depth the meaning and impact of cancer in patients and caregivers' lives and relationships. Thus, we carried out semi-structured interviews with eight patients admitted to a hospice in northern Italy and their family caregivers. We used interpretative phenomenological analysis to analyze the interview transcripts. We discovered a complex relationship between patients and caregivers' narrations, also influenced by their relationship with health professionals. These results suggest that personalized support to family caregivers may empower them, allowing them to find new ways to play their helping role.

Keywords: Cancer, caregiver, constructivism, dependency, narrations

A cancer diagnosis has a significant impact not only on patients, but also on family members. With cancer rapidly developing into a continuous care problem because of increasing incidence rates, longer survival times, and a trend toward outpatient treatment, providing support and managing care has placed added responsibilities on caregivers. Family caregivers are often the primary source of social and emotional support for patients and play a major role in how patients manage their illness. A family caregiver is a spouse, child, other relative, partner or friend who has a personal relationship with, and provides a broad range of assistance for an older adult with a chronic or disabling condition (Hudson and Payne, 2008).

Several studies have focused on the effects of oncological illness on the caregiver and highlighted that the diagnosis of cancer may cause emotional responses of shock, doubt, anxiety and depression (Bambauer et al., 2006; Stenberg, Ruland, and Miaskowski, 2010). The results of these studies confirm that conditions surrounding the illness can compromise the quality of family life, by modifying habits and social relationships and determining psychological tension, which becomes more intense when support is lacking. During the palliative phases of the patient's illness greater physical tension can lead to an increased burden imposed on the carer, to tiredness and to the limited time available to rest and to take care of oneself (Shyu, 2000). The diagnosis of cancer may also contribute to modify the family structure. The family's reaction will depend on various factors such as age, gender, the type of cancer, the patient's role in the family, the family's life cycle, the presence of conflicts among family members and the manner of expressing emotions (Società Italiana di Psico-Oncologia, 1998). Even when the caring experience is described as positive, it is a physically and emotionally stressful experience and can end up in psychological and physical suffering.

Most of the studies have analyzed the present caregiver's experience, the impact of this experience on health, on life and coping style (Gaugler, Kane, Kane, Clay, and Newcomer, 2005; Sales, 1991). They have especially underlined the negative consequences of caregiving, but some studies have also investigated the positive impact of tending to the ill person's needs, including improvement on measures of the caregiver's level of mastery, satisfaction, self-esteem (Nijboer, Triemstra, Tempelaar, Sanderman, and Van Den Bos, 1999), and intimacy with the person cared for (Gritz, Wellish, Siau, Wang, 1990). Some of the gains that are reported by caregivers include giving back to someone who has cared for them, the satisfaction of knowing that their relative is getting excellent care, a sense of personal growth, and gaining meaning and purpose in one's life (Haley et al., 2001). In a study with 1158 Italian caregivers (Morasso et al., 2008) negative, positive, and neutral experiences were highlighted. The negative experiences dealt with emotional suffering, care burden, powerlessness, anger, sense of void, characteristics of the patient or the caregiver, remorse and guilt, fear and breaking of family relationship. Six positive topics have been identified: sense of self-efficacy, personal growth, family cohesiveness, characteristics of the patient or of the illness, improved relationship with the ill family member and satisfaction with health-care service.

The different effect of caregiving depends on the kind of relationship with the patient, e.g. spousal caregivers may be especially vulnerable because of their own age, health, and willingness to sacrifice themselves for the care of their partner. Cultural values, personal attitudes and motivations may also impact caregiving experiences. Informal careving is primarily voluntary and related to bonds of attachment between family members, but can also be affected by cultural norms about family obligations, or feelings of guilt and obligation (Haley, 2003).

Exploring how caregivers ended up accepting this role and what implications this had would enable us to evaluate the burden placed on the caregiver on the basis of his/her subjective experience, rather than on the basis of the actual amount of assistance provided (Stenberg, Ruland, and Miaskowski, 2010). To this end a research project was developed at the Department of General Psychology of the University of Padua. In this chapter I shall discuss the results of a first quantitative study exploring if different levels of anxiety and depression in caregivers might be associated with different ways of giving and receiving help. Later I shall present a subsequent qualitative study we conducted to investigate in depth the meaning and impact of cancer in patients and caregivers' lives and relationships. Before that, I shall briefly introduce the theoretical framework that informed these studies.

UNDERSTANDING CAREGIVING FROM A CONSTRUCTIVIST PERSPECTIVE

Kelly's personal construct psychology may be useful to understand caregiver's experience because it focuses precisely on the personal ways of giving meaning to the world, which are the personal constructs. When they are implied in the maintenance of one's own survival they are called core constructs. Some of these, the dependency constructs, ensure our survival by allowing the satisfaction of our needs within our close relationships, as the satisfaction of the need for food, protection and care during our childhood testifies (Kelly, 1955; Walker, 1997). Contrary to the traditional perspective, which considers dependency as the opposite of independence, and which considers the latter a priori the mature route an individual should take, from the personal construct perspective everybody depends on somebody for something. The question then is how the person distributes his or her dependencies among relevant people. This enables us to move from an approach that risks confining people to pre-defined categories (dependent or independent) to an approach that focuses on the implications that certain choices may have.

Cases where dependency is concentrated on one particular person or thing makes us consider the more evident implications of poor dependency distribution; if the resource the person relies on to satisfy most of his or her needs runs out, the consequences can be very difficult since the person no longer knows where to look for satisfaction and may find him or herself with a gaping hole that cannot be filled. This is just as difficult for the person who refers indiscriminately to a resource or to another one in a given situation because resources end up all being substantially the same. Chiari et al. (1994) identified four paths of dependency on the basis of the person's distribution of dependency. The first is characterized by a high degree of dispersion of dependency and a tendency to relate to others on the basis of role rather than on dependency constructs. People belonging to this group try to understand others rather than expect them to behave in a certain manner. The second path is characterized by a low dispersion of dependency and by a high degree of dependency on a few people, in particular parents. In the dependency relationship people felt accepted and loved, thus self confident. People belonging to the third group are characterized by a high dependency on themselves, showing low self-confidence and low self-esteem. They felt rejected and unloved and construed themselves as being substantially different from others. The fourth path is characterized by the lowest dispersion of dependency and by a high dependency on the mother and on the self. People in this group felt comfortable in relationships, where they usually played a helping role, and described themselves as being reliable and accepted by others.

THE FIRST STUDY

As this short review has highlighted, the distribution of dependency is implied in the giving and receiving of help. For this reason we hypothesized it could be implied in the care giving experience.

The purpose of our first study was to verify if different levels of anxiety and depression corresponded to different ways of distributing dependency in caregivers. Moreover, we assumed that it was possible to distinguish between different profiles on the basis of the extent to which the caregivers felt they could rely on others, or on themselves for receiving help. Following the direction indicated by Chiari et al. (1994), we wanted to verify if these profiles would have changed depending on who the caregiver relied on, and who relied on the caregiver, also taking into account caregivers' dependency on their parents because their core role was developed within this relationship. In particular, we hypothesized that those situations in which there was an "imbalance" between the usual role of the caregivers and the situation they were living might have been characterized by higher levels of depression and anxiety. Conversely, if there was no imbalance, depression and anxiety levels would be lower. For example, a person who had always relied on him or herself probably would have found confirmation of his or her core role in the role of carer, and would have suffered less anxiety and depression.

These symptoms may be considered to be the expression (or the result) of Kellian transitions of threat, anxiety and guilt (Tobacyk and Downs, 1986; Winter, Bell, and Watson, 2010).

The unbalanced situation described above might lead caregivers towards experiencing a real or impending change in their construct systems, referred to as dimensions of transition by Kelly. Kelly (1955) defined guilt as the awareness of the dislodgment of self from one's core role. It is often associated with a range of clinical manifestations that are usually described as depression. Threat was defined by Kelly (1955) as the awareness of an imminent comprehensive change in one's core structures (in the present context the awareness of such change in one's core role or dependency relationships); and, anxiety as the awareness that the events with which one is confronted lie mostly outside the range of convenience of one's construct system. The latter two transitions may be expressed in what is commonly described as anxiety.

Method

Fifty family caregivers of oncology patients receiving day hospital treatment at a Research and Care Oncological Institute in Northern Italy participated in the research. They were 34 women and 16 men, aged between 27 and 83, who were mostly partners of patients' (64%) or children (20%).

We used Dependency Grids (Kelly, 1955; Walker, 2005; Beail and Beail, 1985) to investigate to whom the person would have turned for receiving help (Being Helped Grid) and whom they thought would have turned to them for help (Helping Grid), the Beck Anxiety Inventory (BAI; Beck and Steer, 1990) to assess caregiver's anxiety, and the Beck Depression Inventory-II (BDI II; Beck, Steer, and Brown, 1996) to assess depression in caregivers.

A hierarchical cluster analysis was carried out on the concatenated data as a whole using SPSS, via the Ward method. This method allowed us to group those data that imply the lower deviance increase within the cluster, ensuring the greatest inner cohesion. This analysis was conducted on two groups of data, the first derived from the BAI, BDI-II and the Being Helped Grid, the second derived from the BAI, BDI-II and the Helping Grid.

We used univariate ANOVA to test the effect of each variable, represented by each index, on the cluster formation and Bonferroni post-hoc analysis to identify the variables that significantly differentiated among clusters. We then applied a Chi Square test on case distribution among clusters of each of the two data sets to verify if there were significant differences due to gender and type of relationship between the patient and caregiver, and univariate ANOVA to test for any age effects.

Results

Results of this study shall not be presented in detail because they have been reported previously (Cipolletta, Shams, Tonello, and Pruneddu, 2011), but will be summarized for the distinctive characteristics of the three profiles highlighted by each of the two cluster analyses. The first profile derived from the first cluster analysis, which referred to the Being Helped Grid, was mainly composed of women. These women might have been wives or daughters, or they may have had another relationship with the patient. This group of people were characterized by high levels of depression and anxiety, and a relatively poor social network, since in their dependency grids there were not many people indicated as being important. Nevertheless dependency was differentiated enough because participants turned to some of them in some situations and to others in other situations. This group of people did not rely on themselves, nor on the mother or the patient, but could count on the father. They may be called "unbalanced atypical" caregivers because it is "atypical" that a person who cares for somebody cannot rely on him or herself. This creates an "unbalanced" situation, which is expressed in terms of high levels of anxiety and depression, between their usual role (to look for care) and their current role (to care).

The second profile, defined by the lowest anxiety and depression levels, also presented the highest number of resources the caregiver could rely on and a dependency which was more concentrated on the mother and on the patient than on the self or on the father. It is an unexpected profile, since we might expect that, due to their role, caregivers would rely less on the patient and more on themselves.

However, relying on others, most of all on the mother, probably allowed them to feel less depressed and anxious. Consequently, we may call these caregivers "balanced atypical".

The third profile was characterized by the lowest total dependency and the highest dependency on oneself. It can be defined as "typical" because caring is the usual role of the people belonging to this profile. The concentration of dependency on themselves allow caregivers of this group to trust in their helping role, preventing them from heading towards too much anxiety and depression. They are "balanced typical" caregivers and they constitute the profile that corresponds more to the third path of dependency identified by Chiari et al. (1994).

In regards to the person's helping role, as identified by the Helping Grid, we again found three profiles. The first was composed of people who believed that others rely on them for help, apart from the person they assisted. When compared to the other groups, these caregivers registered intermediate levels of anxiety and depression, which may indicate that these caregivers are used to giving help, so much so that they do not even perceive the patient's dependency. This is a "balanced typical" situation because the experience caregivers are living is congruent with their usual role.

People belonging to the second profile experienced low anxiety and depression and they did not perceive themselves as being a reference point for the others, nor for the person they assisted. This situation turns out to be totally balanced because if these people do not feel the pressure of other people's requests, they do not run the risk of fearing their inability to satisfy these requests. Moreover, this situation is consistent with their usual way of relating to others, whereby it does not allow others to rely on them. We may call them "balanced atypical" because it is atypical for caregivers who, by definition, perform a helping role, to not recognize others' dependency.

The last profile was characterized by the highest levels of anxiety and depression, and was associated with a low perception of dependency on the part of others, except on the part of the patient. To generate suffering is the weight of the dependency of the patient in an unconsolidated helping role. This profile may be called "unbalanced typical" because the typical situation of caregiving creates an unbalanced situation for these people.

Clinical Implications

It is difficult to combine the two groups of clusters to create whole profiles. Some considerations involving all the profiles deal with their common features: "typicality" and "balance". People belonging to the "balanced typical" profile experience a situation which is coherent with their usual helping role, thus they do not experience feelings of guilt because they do not experience a dislodgment of self from their core role, as the definition of guilt (Kelly, 1955) would imply. This kind of experience is reported in that literature referring to the positive aspects of caregiving in terms of love, affection, rewards, challenge, meaning, commitment, purpose in life (Nijboer, Tempelaar, Sanderman, Triemstra, Spruijt, and Van Den Bos, 1998), which reinforces the sense of personal identity of these people. They subsequently need only to be supported through having their role recognized and through being offered information on how to better care for their loved ones, but they risk experiencing guilt or being threatened if the situation changes, (e.g., if the patient died and they could no longer play their usual helping role; Schulz and Beach, 1999; Spillers, Wellisch, Kim, Matthews, and Baker, 2008). In this case they might be helped by finding an alternative way to maintain relationships and their personal identity.

The "balanced atypical" caregivers might be considered to be those who need help less because they do not experience either anxiety or depression. Probably they do not experience depression and anxiety because they do not recognize the new role that the situation they are living would imply. This constriction may be allowed by the question posed in the administration of the second grid (answering "Who would ask you for help?") that may allow the person to shift the attention from the consideration "The only person I confide in, is in danger", which arises from the first grid and which might cause higher anxiety and depression, to the consideration "I am important for many other people", which justifies the lower levels of anxiety and depression. If constriction allows them to reduce the threat of losing the person they depended on, who could be the patient him or herself, excluding this event from their perceptual field, this might become an unstable solution if a new event were to occur, like a worsening of the patient's illness or his/her death. It might be helpful in this case to foster the reconstruction of the relationship with the dependency figure that may also include the possibility of caring for him or her.

When an imbalance is experienced, usually due to experiencing a condition (caring) which is unusual for the person or which even contrasts with his or her usual role (being cared for), with subsequently greater anxiety and depression, a broader intervention is needed. It might consist of a psychotherapeutic process that would help the person reconstrue his or her role and, in so doing, face up to guilt. Anxiety might be reduced by construing what is happening, as it derives from a lack of understanding of it, and threat by reconstruing the imminent change the person is facing.

These clinical suggestions are based on a constructivist psychotherapeutic approach (Chiari and Nuzzo, 2009; Winter and Viney, 2005), but need to be tested on this population. Little research on the relationship between dependency and coping with illness has been carried out (Cipolletta, Beccarello, and Galan, 2012; Cipolletta, Consolaro, and Horvath, 2013; Talbot, Cooper, and Ellis, 1991), and none has tested the effectiveness of an intervention based on their results. Our study represents a starting point for this inquiry. We did not want to offer a taxonomy, but we had simply tried to understand caregivers' experience, respecting its uniqueness.

The profiles identified are neither good nor bad in themselves as they represent a solution, one of many possible choices, which allows the person to better anticipate events at that moment (Kelly, 1955). Furthermore, these profiles may be used for diagnostic purposes in a transitive way, namely, a way that may lead to a clinical intervention that changes as the situation changes.

Limitations and Further Directions

This was only an explorative study. Its greatest limitation was the small number of participants, which prevented us from differentiating them on the basis of the typology and the stage of cancer of the assisted person and of the kind of relationship of the caregiver to the patient, e.g., the impact of having a sick mother or father when there is a high level of dependency of the carer on the parent. This is probably different from the impact of having another person, for instance a partner, as the sick person or when the dependency is not concentrated on the patient.

As a consequence a question arises: what happens when the only figure on which the caregiver felt he or she could rely is also the one that needs to be cared for? The impact of this factor was not analysed because the numbers were not sufficient to carry out this subgroup analysis, and a different methodology would have been required to do it. In fact exploring the implications of the loss of a dependency figure implies an in-depth inquiry, which might be carried out more readily using qualitative methods.

This methodology is more appropriate to gain a deeper insight into the caregiver's role and to obtain a reconstruction of how it developed. These issues represented the point of departure for the following study.

THE SECOND STUDY

We wanted to investigate in-depth the meaning and impact of cancer in patients and caregivers' lives and relationships in order to understand the co-construction of the caring role. To this end we decided to involve both patients and their family caregivers. We hypothesized that the caregivers' roles would have been derived from their usual roles, relationship with the patient, and from the meaning the patients' illness had in their own and in patients' lives.

For caring role we meant the meaning that being cared for and caring had for patients and caregivers on the basis of their personal constructs, i.e. their personal ways of anticipating events.

In personal construct psychology a person plays a role to the extent that he or she construes the construction processes of another in a social process involving the other person (Kelly, 1955). Personal roles are construed within the interaction with others (Butt, 1998; Cipolletta, 2011; Cipolletta, in press). Thereby they are better explored within this interaction. As regard caregiving the more relevant interaction at the moment this experience is lived is the patient-caregiver relationship itself. We chose to explore it in a specific phase of the development of cancer, i.e. the chronic phase.

Three phases have been distinguished during the cancer patient's illness: acute phase, chronic phase and resolution. The acute phase is just after the diagnosis, when the family is feeling shocked and threatened. The chronic phase is when the patient is under treatment, including palliative care, and family members have to take on additional responsibility and to face different possibilities, including the possible or imminent death of the patient. In the phase of resolution the family experiences survivorship or bereavement. In the chronic phase the role of caregivers is more consolidated and we chose to explore it in the terminal condition because we wanted to homogenize the caregiving experience referring to the prognosis and the kind of care provided to the patient whereas we did not discriminate for cancer type.

Method

We involved eight patients at a hospice in Northern Italy and eight family caregivers. Six of the patients were men and two women, five were older than 65 and three younger, four were married, one unmarried and three widowed, five were retired and three worked, one had stomach, two lung, three bowel, one prostate and one pancreatic cancer. The eight caregivers were identified by the patients and these were four men and four women, five under 65 and three over 65, two were partners, four adult children, one sister and one cousin, six were married, one unmarried and one widowed, seven were working and only one retired. The final number of partakers was not predetermined.

The sample size was based on both principles of saturation, the point where variation ceases (Morse, 1993), usually when the number of interviews reaches around 15 (+/-10; Kvale, 1996), and with regard to the maximum number of people that Interpretative Phenomenological Analysis suggests, i.e. no more than 15 (Reid, Flowers, and Larkin, 2005).

Semi-structured interviews were carried out by a researcher trained in clinical interviewing and these lasted between 40 and 60 minutes. After that patients were informed on the study and gave their written consent to participate, the interviews were carried out in the patients' room with nobody else present. After a short presentation of the aim of the study, patients often spontaneously started to tell their illness story and the interviewer simply followed the free flow of the conversation. Sometimes the interviewer did ask questions regarding the self-perception of the patient before and after the diagnosis, illness experience, and the relationship with family and health care professionals. The interviews with the caregivers were carried out in a dedicated room in the hospice, where a psychologist usually meets families. After caregivers gave their informed consent, they were introduced to the theme of the meaning of illness in the lives of patients and caregivers, the communication of the diagnosis, the relationship with the patient and the health care professionals, the meaning of caregiving (self-perception before and after diagnosis, emotions and everyday life) and the meaning of the patient's imminent death.

Interview transcripts were analyzed using Interpretative Phenomenological Analysis (IPA; Smith and Osborn, 2003). The aim of this approach is to represent and understand the material as it appears, focusing on the subjective experience of participants, by identifying recurrent themes in their narratives. IPA allows for the exploration of participants' individual perspectives and for the interpretation of the meanings that their experience holds for them, offering an insider's perspective of the phenomena. In other words, it makes it possible to understand lived experience and how participants themselves make sense of their experiences.

Following the guidelines identified by Smith and Osborn (2003), we proceeded to analyze the transcripts using a bottom-up procedure, whereby the researcher generates codes from the data and not from a pre-existing theory, and includes a series of recursive steps. The first step involved a repeated, in-depth reading of the first transcript to familiarize the researcher with the patient's narrative and to get a sense of the whole. In the second step, recurrent patterns of meaning were identified and organized into potential emergent themes. In this way we sought to uncover the essence of the experience for each person as well as the common themes. Data were then organized into thematic categories, and each theme was linked to quotes that expressed the essence of their content. In the third step, I and another researcher drew links between the different themes and classified them in superordinate categories.

Finally, we re-read all interviews to verify whether the identified themes were recognizable in the transcripts and to ensure that all salient themes had been found. In accordance with a phenomenological approach we remained close to the experience as it was lived rather than trying to analyze it. We approached the material as open a mind as possible, suspending preconceptions, previous theoretical understanding, and personal beliefs. And, as van Manen (1990) has suggested, we proceeded without forgetting how life is always more complex than any description or interpretation that we may attempt.

Results

I do not report here all of the identified themes, rather I focus on just two of those relating to caregivers' experience, the meaning of caregiving and caregivers' role, and the result of the comparison of caregivers' and patients' narrations.

The Meaning of Caregiving

In caregivers' narrations, caregiving meant accepting the sacrifice of their time and resources for patients' wellbeing. Caregivers felt that they had to divide themselves between their everyday life (family and job) and the patient. This situation often allowed the caregiver to feel stronger and able to battle on, thereby catching the positive side of the situation. As the sister of a patient said:

> I always am here, I go out from work and come here. Every time I have a free moment I come here. It seems to burst to me. Life is hard, but I'm not complaining. I am a serene person, I have my family and I try not to miss anything with my daughter. [...] I am not complaining, is clear, but following G.'s cares means completely changing the rhythms of my day. At least I learnt to cope with the difficult situations head-on [...] I am combative. I was so before G. got sick and I am now. For sure such an experience puts an armor on you, this is sure! You realize that it is not all established. I have always been a hard worker, what I have I obtained through sacrifice. Thereby I have always known that it is not all established, but when you are fine you do not think about it. I am happy with my values and I am happy I bring them here with me. Making up the bottom what is right. This is what I am teaching to my daughter too.

Some people feel overwhelmed by their caregiving role. For instance, the daughter of a patient feels tired and scared and affirms that one of the most difficult things to cope with is suffering, not only one's own loved ones' suffering, but also others' suffering. She said:

> I feel a very great responsibility. It seems a thing bigger than me [...] Even if I am afraid, I am proud because death is scary, especially if it is your mother's. I only would like to see her stopping to suffer [...] Because, do you know what is the problem? It is that I have never posed any limit in caring for my mother. I have always given the maximum for her and her tumour, and I abandoned my life. Maybe I had to set some limits [...] Some days I come back from here and I am exhausted, not so much physically as mentally. I am tired, tired to run knowing that there is nothing to do [...] It changes everything, indeed, for the precision, it sucked my life! It is stealing all the energies from me. [...] It is fifteen years since I am caring for her. Always talking to physicians, going round hospitals. You cannot image what living for an illness means. Here, in this area, all know me, in all the hospitals and clinics.
>
> By the end, when you are in the waiting rooms, you are obliged to compare not only with your story, but also with others' story, and this is harmful because this obliges you to open your eyes. As part of the diagnosis [you received], you see other people suffering, other people who have their burdens to sustain, other people who accompany their loved ones to the examinations, like you do. Maybe very young children...

Responsibility is another recurrent theme associated with caregiving. It may make the person proud and often life becomes founded on it. Subsequently, when the patient dies a void is anticipated, as this narration by the son of a patient testifies.

> When you are obliged to stay in hospitals, you see suffering, illness in its pure shape, with all the consequences it implies, responsibility and void [...] accompanying my mother toward death makes me feel responsible for sure, but also proud. It is not a walk, being aware to accompany my mother toward death makes me feel very bad because she will not be here anymore, thus I'll be really alone [...] Really alone and I'll have to begin all again, without my parents [...] When you are busy as I am going from a hospital to another, you lose sight of the future. You do everything for the sick person, to make her be serene as possible. Your needs take a back seat. You see the sick person as a child to look after, to protect. And you becomes the person who has the responsibility for this serenity.
>
> I really do it willingly, but I realize now, speaking about it, that when all will be finished, I will have nothing.

Caregiving determines one's perception of oneself and one's way of being in the world. As outlined above, this experience may be construed in terms of responsibility, pride, strength, engagement and an ability to cope with suffering. But caregiving also affects interpersonal relationships, not only in terms of the loss of time and energies to invest on these relationships due to the burden of the patient's care, but also because the meanings of interpersonal relationships change. For some people caregiving ends up stifling the possibility of having other relationships, as the following quote by a patient's son testifies.

> I do not have a lunch break any more and when I finish work in the evening I come here. Thereby I have less time to do my things, less time to stay with my friends. [...] I am not looking for a woman now, I could not keep her. I would have liked to have a family, some children. But it's been so.

For someone else, caregiving allows a consolidation of their relationships giving them a new meaning, as in the case of a patient's wife, whose daughters had become emotionally closer to her since their father's illness. She said:

> Luckily there are my daughters! But it has not always gone so well. We had a lot of problems with them. When you are a parent you would like to give your children the fairer teachings and you hope they will listen you and follow your example. But it is not always like that. [...] I have a good relationship with my daughters, even if they gave me many displeasures.
>
> Anyway we remained emotionally close to each other. Especially since C. [the patient] got ill they are close to me, they help and sustain me, much more than before. Before everyone did her own life.

Sometimes caregiving allows you to compare different ways of contending with life and death, illness and care. This was the case for a patient's sister who had to compare with the patient's wife, who comes from a different culture and intends care in a different way.

> A dying person must follow the natural course of events, without force or trick. Palliation is wrong because it does not respect the divine will and is only a way to avoid seeing who is suffering. Here you are selfish because you do it only to feel better yourself. (Patient's wife)

The patient's wife would only take her husband home because if he died in a hospital, palliated and in a comatose state, his soul would not find its way to the afterlife. From these accounts caregiving appears to be a very complex role, with positive and negative aspects and a task that requires an ongoing readjustment. In what follows we will try to enter more specifically into this role.

Caregivers' Roles

A family member who becomes a caregiver often does it in accordance with his or her usual role. Many of our study participants recognized a continuity with their previous life, e.g. as regards their sense of responsibility toward the patient.

The case of a patient's son who said that he takes care of his mother because he has always done it is an example.

> I was used to manage my parents and not only for medical problems, but also in their intimate relationship. My parents, also my mother, even if more present than my father, never held the reins of the family. I have always arranged, I have always managed them, I say and said what works and what does not work. Grandparents [as he refers to his parents] must be guided as if they were children.

He built this role since childhood, when he was looking after his mother, supporting her in rebelling against his father, who he described as closed and distant. He went on to say:

> My father has never been very sympathetic. He always thought only of himself. He is a closed man, of few words, with whom it is difficult to have a relationship made of tenderness and affective exchanges. Even when I was a child I do not remember a moment when my father made me feel his presence and paternal love.

It is striking the similarity of the story of this caregiver with that of another patient's son, quoted below.

> I and my brother grew up in a family where only my father talked, only my father existed. He never listened to us, he was never a father in the real meaning of the term". Since I can remember, I do not remember even one moment when my father was affectionate and present with me. We never went out together, he never accompanied me to school or came and saw me playing football. He was always too busy doing something else.

In both cases the caregiver was freed from the constrains he felt in the family when he became an adult, rebelling, but ending up doing what he learnt for the family. In the latter case, with "sex, drugs and rock and roll" and enjoying life with friends and different women, exactly as his father did, and, in the former case, ending up taking care of his parents as he had done all his life. In these cases strong emotions are linked to the caring role. In other cases of a difficult relationship with a person being cared for, it appeals to morality that is used to justify their choice to look after a person who made them suffer. This usually occurs when the caregiver is the patient's child, e.g. the case of a patient's daughter who felt that she was abandoned when she was a child by her selfish mother, whom she cares for out of a sense of duty. Her role since she was a child was "cancelling herself" and the patient's illness confirmed this role.

> My mother has always been selfish in her life. She has always chosen only on the basis of what she desired, without thinking that there was also me. She abandoned me and when I was 18 she imposed work on me despite my dream to study. I felt I died inside. Stamping a card in a factory meant not to listen what I really wanted to do. [...] So my mother's illness changed my life: Canceling me. [...] I feel a duty to protect her, to look after her.

For others, caregiving is the only way to perpetuate a relationship that underpinned a caregiver's existence and the anticipation of the patient's death is feared because it represents the end of this relationship, as in the case of a patient's wife.

> That is why I am always here. Because I want to be here in that moment [death]. I want to stay with him until death. . [...] And I also feel the responsibility as a wife. I love my husband as the first day we married. We did a promise to ourselves and God: In health and illness until death will divide you. I do my task because I love him. [...] We have been married for forty years, we have always been together, I do not know how I'll do later.

Other times the affection that guides the caregiver is of a different kind because the relationship with the cared and the subsequent caregiver role is different, as is the case of a patient's cousin.

> Sometimes I would like not to come to avoid to see him suffering. But if I do not come, who does? We all want to die happy, do not we? I know I do the right thing. It is my task as a cousin and as a friend. [...] I lose a friend more than a cousin.

To sum up, the main reasons caregivers gave that led them to assume their caring role were: the continuity of their personal role, emotional bonds, and moral and family duty. Subsequently, different motivations and different ways of playing the caring role corresponded.

The Comparison of Caregivers' and Patients' Narrations

Taking into consideration two different points of view, the caregiver's and the patient's, allows one to observe how the life stories and experiences of each participant in the interaction meet and integrate with each other. In the caring relationship a sharing of meanings may be found between patient and caregiver. Sometimes the perceptions of the two persons differ, e.g. the perception of a physician may be different or the patient may feel too protected, treated as a child. An example of these contrasting meanings is offered by a patient and her caregiver.

> She [the caregiver] is good, but sometimes she is too protective. She always wanted it to be her to talk to the physicians, but I have always come into the clinics because I wanted to know what was happening to me.
> Thus, even if she knew it [the diagnosis] before me, I also knew it from the physician. What a ice shower! That physician did not understand really a pipe! He was not able to see my face when telling me I had a tumor. (Patient)
> I try not to make her miss anything, especially emotion. As **if she was a child** [...] Luckily there are good physicians and good nurses. They are people who do their job with an incredible passion. Also when I discovered the tumor, I remember it as if it was yesterday, in that clinic I and the physician... If you listen to my mother she says he was a very bad

physician. Instead, when he told me about the tumor, he has been very comprehensive, close to me. (Caregiver)

Being treated as a child often contrasts with the usual role of the patient and makes them feel guilty because they do not recognize themselves anymore. In fact, if the patient already feels frail and dependent due to illness and the need for care, a caring behavior that stresses this dependent position may increase these feelings. This is the case in the patient-caregiver relationship quoted above, but this complex role interplay may vary according to different patient's and caregiver's roles.

In one case the patient was used to being cared by her child, so she accepted this and the caregiver maintained his usual role. However, in another case, it was the patient who usually cared for his wife and children and he could not accept the inversion of roles brought about by the tumor. His wife also recognizes her husband as occupying this role and could not image her life without him in it. He said:

> I have always been fine: never a physician, an examination, a hospitalization. And now I am in a bad way for months. My body does what the tumor imposes! [...] **My tumor has changed not only my life but also theirs [wife's and daughters']**. It has changed the rhythms, the roles: before it was me who looked after them. Now it is them who look after me! (Patient)
>
> He [the patient] is a person of few words and introvert, but always present. He demonstrated his presence with facts more than with words. [...] **When he [the patient] will die what can I do? I am alone, I have nobody**. It will be difficult to go on without him. (Caregiver)

Finally, it may happen that both the patient and the caregiver need to affirm their autonomy. In this case the patient cannot accept the caregiver's help and the carer's solution is to keep the patient in the dark as to his condition, as in the case of this patient and his child carer.

> I am different. Everything has changed. **I am sick and I even don't know what I have!** [...] I also understand that I have something bad, even if I did not study. But nobody tell me anything. (Patient)
>
> When I was told what my father has I thought: "And now what can we do?" It has been difficult, and then I and my brother have decided to tell him nothing. (Caregiver)

Sharing and understanding were found when the patient-caregiver relationship was already based on them, as in the case of this patient and his cousin.

> Luckily my cousin has been close to me. That is why we are so linked. I worked in a factory all day long and he was the only one who came and visited me every day. (Patient)
>
> Not much has changed. I went and visited him also before [illness]. I dedicate to him the same time. But I prefer to visit him out of the hospital because here he is sad. (Caregiver)

In one case sharing in the relationship begins with the caring experience. It allows a father to reconstrue his relationship with his son and his son to accept his father and find a way to stay close to him.

I have never been an affectionate father. On the contrary I am a cumbersome father. I spoke to my sons to interrogate them. I like studying, thereby I wanted that they also studied. It was important for me. But I realized that I have been too cold with them. I have not given them many values. I have only thought them to be constant in order to obtain results. But I don't know if I was able to do it. [...] Now I notice that he [the caregiver], who is the most rebellious of my sons, the second one, stays here with me and he reach to give me affect, even if I have never established it with him. [...] When I was fine he considered me a little, now he is present, also when I am annoying, I fix on something. He demonstrate me a love I didn't think he felt. (Patient)

My father has always been selfish, he has never considered other people's feelings. It was his wife, a friend or his son, it was always him who spoke and left no space to the other to express him or herself. I know I might appear cynical, but, growing up, I understand many things on my family and on my father, that allowed me to become the man I am and to accept to live serenely this transition in his life [...] I stay close to him and try to show him that, despite everything, I love him. [...] I cuddle my father and try to stay close to him, even if he often refuses his new role, in which he is subject to others. My father does not accept that he cannot walk anymore and that he cannot live his life in autonomy, thereby the gestures of tenderness seem to annoy him. [...] I try to do with my son all what my father did not do with me. I play with him, I am present and careful to his needs. (Caregiver)

In this case the caregiver could re-construe not only his relationship with the cared, but also his role as father. Experiencing different directions of movement in his new family relationship probably helped him to cope and experience caregiving in a new way.

Discussion

Cancer represents a break in patients' and their family caregivers' lives due to the changes it implies for everyday life and the threat it represents to survival.

The experience of caregiving may also represent an interruption in a caregiver's usual role and their relationship with the patient, as in the case of the wife of a patient, whose life depended on the relationship with her husband and for whom cancer and his imminent death would mean the end of the relationship, thereby implying a deep threat. Recalling the categories of the previous study we might say that this case is an example of unbalanced atypical caregiving because the person, who is not used to confiding mainly in herself, is living a situation that obliges her to do so. Moreover, this may be considered an example of the situation where the patient is the person the caregiver depended on. His illness and imminent death provoked her anxiety because she did not know how to construe the new situation and she was also threatened by the imminent change in her life.

In most cases we found a continuity in the personal role of caregivers. In many of our study participants' stories we found recurrent experiences of rejection or distance on the part of caregivers' parents. These experiences might have led children to try to satisfy their parent's request and obtain their love through constriction, defined by Kelly (1955) as the narrowing of one's own perception field in order to avoid incompatibilities. This is evident in the patient's daughter who felt abandoned by her mother and had to stop studying, thereby feeling annihilated, or in the patient's son, who devoted his life to care for his parents renouncing his ambition to have a family of his own. In terms of Chiari et al.'s (1992) paths of dependency we can recognize in these two people the third path, characterized by a dependency mainly concentrated on oneself.

In fact, these caregivers are used to confiding in themselves and the caring experience did not change this tendency. Rather, it confirmed and reinforced it. Somebody may have reacted reaffirming this role with hostility, defined by Kelly (1955) as the effort to extort validational evidence in favor of a type of social prediction which has already been recognized as a failure, as in the case of the patient's daughter who treated her mother as a child denying her need to maintain an active role in the care of her own illness. In other cases strong emotions were linked to the caring situation and we may liken this condition to the one of the unbalanced typical caregivers who are threatened by the imminent death of the patient because this would imply a loss of their caring role. What might they do instead? This dilemma may provoke anxiety. Someone may find an alternative solution via construing a different relationship with the patient and a different role in their interpersonal relationships.

Finally we found one person who, since the very beginning, had a role relationship with the patient (and probably in his relationships in general) that was based on a reciprocal understanding rather than exclusively on the satisfaction of needs. This situation is the most promising because it offers the best chance to keep a healthy relationship with the patient that may allow both the participants in the relationship to elaborate their personal construct system. This may be helpful for the wellbeing of both. Of course it cannot keep alive the dying, but it can help the person to better cope with their illness, and allow the caregiver to accept the patient's condition, adjust to the changing situation and continually construe new roles.

Limitations and Challenges

The biggest limitation of this study was its recruitment of only caregivers of terminal patients. This means of course that it is not possible to examine some questions. These include: What is the experience of caregivers if patients are undergoing different kind of treatments and going in and out from the hospital? What are carers' expectations and how do their roles change if they anticipate they can still do something to keep the patient alive or even anticipate he or she will recover?

It is difficult to reach caregivers and to involve them in a qualitative study and this is the reason why they were not interviewed in the first study. We also had difficulty finding a location to conduct the interviews. Sometimes hospitals and other care centers do not have appropriate space for a quiet and deep encounter. In Italy hospices are considered privileged places because they offer a kind of assistance that is not only aimed at medical care, but also at guaranteeing that the dying person and family are given holistic attention (Cipolletta and Oprandi, in press).

This study was also limited by the exclusive use of the interview. The choice was due to the desire to respect and maximize the participants' freedom to choose what and how much to share, allowing them to feel comfortable. It would have been interesting to integrate interviews with dependency grids and some measures of depression and anxiety to verify if there was correspondence between the profiles identified in the first study and the experience of caregivers involved in the second.

Conclusion

The aim of this chapter was to try to understand the experience of family caregivers of patients with cancer. I tried to do this by adopting a constructivist perspective with particular reference to personal construct psychology's dimensions of dependency and transitions.

The two studies presented offered examples of ways of exploring these dimensions that may be used for research and intervention. They highlighted how being a caregiver for someone with cancer cannot be considered a unique experience because it changes according to the different personal roles of caregivers and patients and according to the different ways these roles combine in a relationship. Moreover, this relationship cannot be considered static, because it is strongly influenced by the context of peoples' everyday lives. Exploring how their roles and relationships change in different phases of a patient's or a caregiver's life represents an interesting and innovative field of investigation.

Future studies should be directed at identifying the weaknesses and the strengths of the cancer caregiving experience in order to that new possibilities may be opened up for people to play the caring role in more fruitful ways.

References

Bambauer, K. Z., Zhang, B., Maciejewski, P. K., Sahay, N., Pirl, W. F., Block, S. D., and Prigerson, H. G. (2006). Mutuality and specificity of mental disorders in advanced cancer patients and caregivers. *Social Psychiatry and Psychiatric Epidemiology*, 41, 819-824.

Beail, N., and Beail, S. (1985). Evaluating dependency. In Beail, N. (Ed.), Repertory grid technique and personal constructs: applications in clinical and educational settings (pp. 207-217). London: Croom Helm.

Beck, A. T., and Steer, R. A. (1990). *Anxiety Inventory Manual*. San Antonio, TX: Psychological Corpotation.

Beck, A. T., Steer, R. A., and Brown, G. K. (1996). Manual for the Beck Depression Inventory-II. San Antonio, TX: Psychological Corporation.

Butt, T. (1998). Sociality, role and embodiment. *Journal of Constructivist Psychology*, 11, 105-116.Fransella, F., Bell, R., and Bannister, D. (2003). A manual for repertory grid technique. Chichester: Wiley.

Chiari, G., Nuzzo, M. N. (2009). Constructivist Psychotherapy: A Narrative Hermeneutic Approach. London: Routledge, Chapman and Hall.

Chiari, G., Nuzzo, M. L., Alfano, V., Brogna, P., D'andrea, T., Di Battista, G. et al. (1994). Personal paths of dependency. *Journal of Constructivist Psychology*, 7, 17-34.

Cipolletta, S. (2011). Self construction and interpersonal distances of juveniles living in residential communities. *Journal of constructivist psychology*, 2, 122-143. doi:10.1080/10720537.2011.548218

Cipolletta, S. (in press). Construing in action: Experiencing embodiment. *Journal of constructivist psychology*.

Cipolletta, S., Beccarello, S., and Galan, A. (2012). A psychological perspective of eye floaters. *Qualitative Health Research.*, 22, 1547-155. doi: 10.1177/1049732312456604.

Cipolletta, S., Consolaro, F., and Horvath, P. (2013). When Health is an Attitudinal Matter. A Mixed-Method Research. Under submission.

Cipolletta, S., and Oprandi, N. (in press). What is a good death? Health care professionals' narrations on end-of-life care. *Death Studies*.

Cipolletta, S., Shams, M., Tonello, F. and Pruneddu, A. (2011). Caregivers of patients with cancer: anxiety, depression and distribution of dependency. Psycho-oncology. Advance online publication. doi: 10.1002/pon.2081.

Fransella, F., Bell, R., and Bannister, D. (2003). A manual for repertory grid technique. Chichester: Wiley.

Gaugler, J. E., Kane, R. L., Kane, R. A., Clay, T., and Newcomer, R. C. (2005). The Effects of duration of caregiving on institutionalization. *Gereontologist*, 45, 78-89.

Gritz, E. R., Wellish, D. K., Siau, J., and Wang, H. J. (1990). Long-term effects of testicular cancer on marital relationships. *Psychosomatics*, 31, 301–12.

Haley, W. E. (2003). The costs of family caregiving: implications for geriatric oncology. *Critical Reviews in Oncology/Hematology*. 48, 151-158.

Haley, W. E., LaMonde, L. A., Han, B., Narramore, S., and Schonwetter, R. (2001). Family caregiving in hospice: effects on psychological and health functioning among spousal caregivers of hospice patients with lung cancer or dementia. *Hospice Journal*, 15, 1–18.

Hudson, P., and Payne, S. (2008). Family Carers in Palliative Care. Oxford: Oxford University Press.

Kelly, G. A. (1955). The psychology of personal constructs (Vols. 1-2). New York: Norton.

Kvale, S. (1996). Interviews: An introduction to qualitative research interviewing. Thousand Oaks, CA: Sage.

Morasso, G., Costantini, M., Di Leo, S., Roma, S., Miccinesi, G., et al. (2008). End-of-life care in Italy: personal experience of family caregivers. A content analysis of open questions from the Italian Survey of the Dying of Cancer (ISDOC). *Psycho-Oncology*, 17, 1073-1080.

Morse, J. (1993). Drowning in data. *Qualitative Health Research*, 3, 267-9.

Nijboer, C., Tempelaar, R., Sanderman, R., Triemstra, M., Spruijt, R. J, and Van Den Bos, A. M. (1998). Cancer and caregiving: the impact on the caregiver's health. *Psycho-oncology*, 7, 3–13.

Nijboer, C., Triemstra, M., Tempelaar, R., Sanderman, R., and Van Den Bos, A. M. (1999). Determinants of Caregiving Experiences and Mental Health of Partners of Cancer Patients. *Cancer*, 86, 577-588.

Reid, K., Flowers, P., and Larkin, M. (2005). Exploring lived experience: An introduction to Interpretative Phenomenological Analysis. *The Psychologist*, 18, 20-23.

Sales, E. (1991). Psychosocial impact of the phase of cancer on the family: an updated review. *Journal of Psychosocial Oncology*, 9, 1-18.

Schulz, R., and Beach, S. R. (1999). Caregiving as a risk factor for mortality: the caregiver health effects study. *Journal of the American Medical Association*, 282, 2215-2219.

Shyu, Y. I. (2000). The needs of family caregivers of frail elders during the transition from hospital to home: A Taiwanese sample. *Journal of Advanced Nursing*, 32, 619-625.

Società Italiana di Psico-Oncologia (1998). Standard, opzioni e raccomandazioni per una buona pratica psico-oncologica. Available at: http://www.siponazionale.it/source/linee_guida.html.

Smith, J. A., and Osborn, M. (2003). Interpretative phenomenological analysis. In J.A. Smith (Ed.), *Qualitative Psychology: a Practical Guide to Methods* (pp. 51-80). London: Sage.

Spillers, R. L., Wellisch, D. K., Kim, Y., Matthews, B. A., and Baker, F. (2008). Family Caregivers and Guilt in the Context of Cancer Care. *Psychosomatics*, 49, 511–519.

Stenberg, U., Ruland, C. M., and Miaskowski, C. (2010). Review of the literature on the effects of caring for a patient with cancer. *Psycho-oncology*, 19, 1013-1025.

Talbot, R., Cooper, C. L., and Ellis, B. (1991). Uses of the dependency grid for investigating social support in stressful situations. *Stress Medicine*, 7, 171-180.

Tobacyk, J. J., and Downs, A. (1986). Personal construct threat and irrational beliefs as cognitive predictors of increases in musical performance anxiety. *Journal of Personality and Social Psychology*, 4, 779-782.

Van Manen, M. (1990). *Research lived experience*. New York: State University of New York Press.

Walker, B. M. (2005). Making sense of dependency. In Fransella, F. (Ed.), Personal construct psychology. The essential practitioner's handbook (pp. 77-86). Chichester: Wiley.

Walker, B. M. (1997). Shaking the kaleidoscope: dispersion of dependency and its relationships. *Advances in Personal Construct Psychology*, 4, 63-97.

Winter, D., and Viney, L. (2005). Personal construct psychotherapy: Advance in theory, practice and research. London and Philadelphia: Whurr Publishers.

Winter, D. A., Bell, R. C., and Watson, S. (2010). Midpoint ratings on personal constructs: constriction or the middle way? *Journal of Constructivist Psychology*, 4, 337-356.

In: Caregivers: Challenges, Practices and Cultural Influences
Editors: Adrianna Thurgood and Kasha Schuldt

ISBN: 978-1-62618-030-7
© 2013 Nova Science Publishers, Inc.

Chapter 3

ZOOMING (IN) – ZOOMING (OUT): FROM FEELING EXCLUSIVELY LIKE A CAREGIVER TO INTEGRATING CAREGIVING IN DAILY LIFE

UNDERSTANDING SUDDEN INFORMAL CAREGIVERS' PATHS

Helder Rocha Pereira[*]
Ponta Delgada Nursing School, University of the Azores, Portugal

ABSTRACT

What are the experiences faced by informal caregivers that suddenly and unexpectedly are forced to begin such a role? What are the stages of their unexpected paths? What experiences do they consider most relevant? What works or does not work for them in their interactions with professionals whose mission is to give them support in their new role?

The experiences of informal caregivers of loved ones are a widely studied topic, both in terms of assessing the caregivers' needs, of support programs available and of the implications that the responsibility of giving care (*burden*) represents to caregivers' health and well-being, amongst other things.

Nevertheless, when the unforseen focus is placed on the informal caregiver, who did not anticipate seeing him/herself as such, the available evidence is still scarce and reveals gaps that need to be addressed.

This chapter is based in the results of a phenomenological hermeneutical study (N=14 sudden informal caregivers), as well as on the integration of those results with published narratives of personal experiences of informal caregiving and relevant knowledge in this area, enabling a better understanding of the phenomenon.

---

[*] RN, Community Nurse Specialist, MEd, PhD, Ponta Delgada Nursing School – University of the Azores, UI&DE (Nursing Development & Research Unit), hpereira@uac.pt.

Pereira & Botelho (2011) have previously described the lived experience when becoming a sudden caregiver. The focus of this chapter is to globally understand the non linear path between two distinct poles, wich are characterized by unstable points of balance. There are two extremes: seeing oneself as exclusively a caregiver (Zooming (in) in the caregiver situation) and integrating caregiving in one's life (Zooming(out).

In truth, for sudden caregivers, the experience in developing their role is that of an "attack/theft" on/of their previous life. The main focus in the sudden caregiver's life becomes that of being a caregiver (giving care, worrying, feeling insecure, having to be constantly present, as well as many other aspects). Taking on that role quickly consumes the caregiver's whole life. Their focus becomes almost exclusively to develop that new role.

The unexpected, urgent and "unprepared" nature of such a situation results in focusing solely on caregiving. As time goes by and and reflecting upon the situation, the caregiver realizes that he/she cannott be comitted to a situation that limits or affects his/her wellbeing, freedom, social contacts, mental health and other responsibilities in the remaining facets of his/her life. In order to regain a sense of normality, the caregiver must detach his/herself from his/her situation and allow the role of caregiving to be harmoniously integrated along with other roles and competing needs emerging from their daily lives (Zooming (out).

This chapter (i) explores those processes based upon the experiences reported by the study participants, (ii) recalls relevant knowledge to broaden professionals' understanding of the phenomenon (for example: the transitions theory, the caregivers' career or the need of respite care) and (iii) presents a group of high clinical value indicators, identified in the research process, that may help professionals to better understand and monitor new caregivers' paths in this process of adapting themselves to suddenly becoming a caregiver.

INTRODUCTION

I honestly didn't know what I should do...
Am I prepared for this situation with my mother? I can´t say that I am prepared. I really wasn´t prepared for it. I wasn´t prepared for it (...) I don't know! Now I feel like I am obligated.. Can you understand that?
(Manuel, 29 years-old, son)

"I take care of you, of all of you and no one looks after me?" I'm taking care of them and don't look after myself. "Nobody looks after me!" I feel offended... "Nobody cares about me?!" I don't need them to do anything for me, but at least come and see me!
(Lurdes, 60 years-old, wife)

Why does Manuel feel like he is obligated? Why is Lurdes offended? The statements with which we start this chapter were taken from the experiences of two informal caregivers who had recently taken into their hands the role of careing for a loved one, without having the time to prepare or anticipate it. They are, thus, unexpected informal caregivers.

With the rise of life expectancy, the number of elderly dependent on people in society has increased, and consequently so has obligation of family members in regards to this matter. Thus, aspects related to informal caregiving have become unquestionably relevant for different professionals who have to deal with it, mainly in areas of health care and social services. Therefore, there has been a great increase in research of topics related to informal caregivers, such as: i) the characterization of the caregiver; ii) identifying training needs; iii) exploring the concept of overload (objective and subjective); iv) the impact of caregiving on daily life or on caregiver's health; v) actions aiming to minimize or ease the impact of stress; vi) the timing in which interventions should be made, amongst many other dimensions (Aneshensel, C., Pearlin, L., Mullan, J., Zarit, S., & Whitlatch, C., 1995; Ayres, 2000; Cameron & Gignac, 2008; Carretero, Garcés, Ródenas, & Sanjosé, 2009; Chappell, Reid & Dow, 2001; Crespo-López & López-Martinez, 2007; García, 2010; Hoffmann & Rodrigues, 2010; Levine, 2004a; Zarit, S. & Femia, 2008, amongst many others).

However, if we aim to understand the development of the informal caregiver's role after an unexpected and unanticipated event, the available literature on the topic is a lot less abundant (Pereira, 2006). The sudden and unexpected nature of becoming a caregiver without having had any preparation for the undertaking of that role is an experience worth understanding. Being an unexpected caregiver means having had little or no time to decide whether to assume the enormous responsibility of taking somebody else's care into one's hands.

It is likely that, in a long-term perspective, there may be no differences in the development of the caregiver's role despite its sudden or insidious begining. However, it's important to understand the challenges and particularities that taking care of someone unexpectedly may represent. Do new caregivers feel pressured to play a role that they had not previously envisioned? What stages does the caregiver go through, if the beginning of that role is not anticipated? What is the weight of unpredictability in the transition towards this new role? To what constraints and pressures is he/she exposed? What processes, values, and information support his/her decisions? What phases does he/she consider critical and essential for the development of his/her role a caregiver? What implications can be taken out of his/her experiences that may inform clinical practice?

This chapter is greatly based upon the results of a phenomenological-hermeneutical study – following Van Manen's (1990) framework – developed with 14 adult informal caregivers who embraced this responsibility unexpectedly and agreed to be interviewed in three distinct moments (two weeks, two and six months after their loved one's hospital discharge). The participants were thirteen women (seven wives, five daughters and a daughter-in-law) and a man (son). The age span ranged from 29 to 77 years of age and there was great heterogeneity in terms of socio-economic background. The study aimed (1) to clarify the meaning that the new sudden caregiver attributes to his/her transition process and (2) to understand how he/shre restructure his/her world after an unexpected and unwanted event.[1]

Four main themes were identified in the experiences of new sudden informal caregivers: "losing control over time", "feeling alone", "failing expectations", "taking over someone else's life" (Pereira & Botelho, 2011):

- *"losing control over time"* - the caregiver's daily routine becomes altered. He/She loses the ability to control time. Time suddenly feels as if it has been "stolen", and life begins to be built around schedules, over which he/she has little control.

---

[1] A detailed description of participants, recruitment procedures, the analysis' techniques, as well a comprehensive overview of the relevant themes of the lived experience of suddenly informal caregivers can be found in Pereira & Botelho (2011).

- *"feeling alone"* - feelings of lonliness and abandonment were common to the experiences of the caregiver. Even if the caregiver was not acustomed to leaving home, feeling forced to be alone reinforces the perception of lack of freedom. The caregivers can also feel alone by missing his/her old self.
- *"failing expectations"* - failing expectations are perceptual disparities between what one needs as a caregiver and what one is offered, either when the caregiver is confronted with hospital discharge or in the relationship the caregiver has with him/herslef, with his/her dependent loved ones, or with community resources available.
- *"taking over someone else's life"* - as time passes, the perception of providing care becomes more complex, acknowledging that one takes care of someone else's entire life (in terms of decisions and responsibilities) encompasses a relm far beyond the aspects related with the physical support provided to the care receivers in their daily life activities.

In this study, it was also possible to identify that the sudden caregiver's path is characterized by a movement of a non linear trajectory between two distinct poles: seeing oneself as exclusively a caregiver (Zooming in on the caregiver situation) and integrating caregiving in daily life (Zooming out).

Since the issues associated with the experience of becoming a sudden caregiver were previously described, the focus of this chapter is, thus, to understand this centering/decentering movement of caregivers in finding satisfactory balanced points when providing care to a loved one. We have chosen to present and discuss the caregiver's path in his/her first experiences of feeling overwhelmed with the demands and responsibilities of caregiving, and his/her efforts to integrate caregiving in the wider context of his/her life, based on the experience of the caregivers participating in the study as well as on other contributions of informal caregivers published in narratives (for example: Braff & Olenik, 2003; Jacobs, 2004; Levine, 2004b; Mintz, 2007; Wolpe, 2004).

This chapter (i) explores the experiences reported by sudden informal caregivers about their path in achieving balanced points, (ii) recalls prior relevant knowledge to broaden professionals' understanding of the phenomenon (for example: the transitions theory, the caregivers' career, or the need of respite care) and (iii) presents a group of high clinical value indicators, identified in the research process, that may help professionals to better understand and monitor new caregivers' paths in this process of adapting themselves to suddenly becoming a caregiver.

BEING ABSORBED BY CAREGIVING – ZOOMING IN

The commencement of caregiving after an unexpected event is characterized by a sudden immersion in the world of giving care to someone (a zooming-in movement). This caregiver involvement centers almost exclusively on the "other" that needs care, which is normally expected. It is a time of chaos, of confusion, of little reflection, of adjustments, of worrying and of feeling the need to be present at all times.

The focus of one's attention is extremely narrow and all other aspects of someone's life seem obscured when faced with this new role. The personal needs, family or demands of any other nature, if not completely ignored, are left behind, due to this new focus on almost solely the dependent person and his/her circumstances.

> I used to live to take care of my mother. I was living for her. I really was! I would leave my work, come straight home, as if she were a child that I had left home unattended for five minutes. All because I had to come home so someone else could leave. (Patrícia, 47 year-old daughter)
>
> Being dependent is precisely that, my life now develops around her needs. I am on the third, fourth or fifth level, isn't that right? Now... that's that... because... I can't really make any other plans. Anything that is out of our routine... even the slightest things... have to be quick! I have to get home immediately because... imagine on weekends – even worse! (Paula, 48 year-old daughter)

Living almost exclusively to give care to someone else leads the caregiver to identify him/herself solely as a caregiver: a role overlapping daily life. His/her worries, time, health or occupations or even still other "demands" fade away in relation to this new role that he/she has to play in the stage of life. *"If someone with whom I have emotional bonds 'really' needs me, "I will be there" for him/her (no matter what the reasons)."*

> Now it's all for him. (...) God forbid! To leave him here alone! Leaving my husband, I won't. My daughter used to say: Mom, you're ruining yourself... you don't think about yourself... only about dad. I said: "For now, there is no other way. Now I am healthy, later on, if I get sick, so be it! But as long as I can, I will help him" (...) that's my life: for him! (Olívia, 67 year-old caregiver)
>
> Nothing, nothing, whatsoever... I don't take care of myself or anything else. I used to like to (in a whisper) be well dressed, with a nice hair... with... I used to! I didn't overdress, but I was presentable! I stopped worrying about that, taking care of that. (Hirondina, 77 year-old caregiver)
>
> I think I became much more dependent on my mother than she on me, really! On my honor, I really feel that way. It's as if I had had a baby and I was totally dependent on the baby's schedule. With my mother it's similar, almost a kind of obsession! (Patrícia, 47 year-old caregiver)

Other than the dependent person, the caregiver him/herself is at risk for being "stuck" in an emotional prison, due to the quick process towards being exhausted and feeling rage, isolation and resentment. Furthermore, all these contradictory feelings are aimed towards someone that the caregiver loves (Wolpe, 2004). Caregiving can become so involving to the point that it neutralizes the caregiver's ability and availability to engage in other social interactions.

Being focused solely on caregiving may lead to the development of a bi-directional dependency between caregiver and the care receiver (Crespo-López & López-Martínez, 2007). The development of dependency processes towards the care receiver is one of the factors that may contribute to social isolation and all its repercussions. The problem arises when the dynamic of caregiver/care receiver becomes a closed system where nothing else fits, not even other family members (Crespo-López & López-Martínez, 2007).

Alongside with this pattern, there is also the emerging of "guilt". Guilt is a recurrent feeling and is present both in the narratives of the participants of this study, in published narratives of caregivers' memoires and also in empirical studies about caregivers. Guilt is a very powerful feeling.

Wolpe (2004) claims that overrating the feeling of obligation towards family leads to an attitude of self-renouncement, since the caregiver doesn't allow him/herself any time or space to engage in other activities besides caregiving (for example, to tend to his/her own needs). Reflecting upon his own experience, Wolpe considers that: "to do anything but devote oneself to a loved one's care risk condemnation from self and family" (Wolpe, 2004, p.120).

Caregivers blame themselves. There may be many sources of guilt. They blame themselves for thinking that they might not be investing 100 percent in caring for the loved one (Isabel, 65 year-old wife); they blame themselves for not being able to find time for themselves (Zélia, 27 year-old daughter); and for feeling morally forced to give care and, as such, finding time for oneself would not be appropriate (Jacobs, 2004). Caregivers also feel guilty for thinking that they might have been somehow responsible for the event that lead to the dependency (Hirondina, 77 year-old wife); for leaving things unsaid or for having wished the dependent person dead (Crespo-López & López-Martínez, 2007); for getting exasperated with the dependent person (Gabriela, 26 year-old daughter). They blame themselves when they are present and even more, when they are absent; for their actions and omissions.

Braff and Olenik (2003) also consider that guilt may be a learned response in regards to the belief that one's actions might have somehow been harmful. Dealing with one's guilt is central in the caregiver's experiences. "We feel guilty and accept that we deserve to be punished" (Braff & Olenik, 2003, p.92). This feeling doesn't help the caregiver to try to integrate caregiving in other family activities as little disruptively as possible.

The caregiver gradually realizes that keeping this pattern of focusing solely in caregiving is not sustainable or satisfactory for him/her as a person. When taking into consideration her own experience as caregiver, Mintz states: "Somewhere along the line, however, it is vitally important that you stop, take a breath, and try to gain some control over the situation, rather than letting the situation control you. It is vitally important that you choose to take charge of your life." (Mintz, 2007, p. 74)

Spreading the Center of All Attention(s) – Zooming out

The need to spread the focus of one's attention, to magnify the lenses through which caregivers face the world gradually starts to come up for several reasons: because people feel alone and tired or feel their effort is not recognized by others; because time is scarce or, on the other hand, refuses to pass; or because they realize their life has lost its meaning. Now they are permanently closed in one place and kept from having satisfying relationships. They just have routines, tasks. Deep down they have opted out of taking control over their own personal life.

The need to step away or find new horizons, means leaning towards the inclusion of caregiving in a wider array of roles.

> If she gets up to go to the bathroom to take a bath, she can also go to the table for meals and I don't have to feel guilty about it because she's lazy! She's being lazy. She just wants to

stay in bed and do nothing. And that's not good for her or is it for me. There are two other people who come home and want my attention too (the husband and the son) and besides, I'm not available anymore because I'm annoyed with having to be there every minute. That cannot be, for me to feel good… we cannot feel good on account of someone else's suffering, we must find a balance. (Zélia, 27 year-old daughter)

In order for this gradual change in one's part to occur, it's essential to "recognize the change itself" and to "realize personal needs to change". There is a gradual recognition of the overall impossibility of the situation as well as of the importance of not neglecting other needs that coexist with playing the part of caregiver: needs of professional development; of getting once again involved in prior and existing roles (such as being a mother, being a wife or husband, or even being a citizen); or simply being able to have some personal time without feeling guilty for it.

There are two processes that seem to ease the recognition of one's need to expand (and regain) one's horizons. One has to do with the degree of improvement of the dependent person's condition. Realizing that the dependent person has regained his/her autonomy, or at least can be safely home alone, serves as a certain sense of normalcy for the caregiver, in terms of getting back to his/her former reality.

And slowly she gave me reasons to trust her. So I slowly let go and didn't get angry as easily whenever I saw her trying to crawl. Slowly I stepped in less. After all, I'm not dumb. I realized she was not useless. She was a woman who needed to have her own space and it was good for her! Mostly it made her feel good because she needed it… she felt very … I'm having trouble with finding the right words… she felt oppressed, limited. She was stuck to that chair, to that corner, to people's availability. (Patrícia, 47 year-old daughter)

The second process relies more in the self-redefinition of one's part as a caregiver, of finding new priorities based on one's assessment of one's other needs as well as gaining a certain level of trust in order to include caregiving in a wider context of life, without feeling constantly tied to schedules, spaces and to the dependent person, in other words, to step back without feeling guilty.

I also need to pay attention to my wife, because if I don't, who will? At a time like this, I can't be… I'm very afraid that our relationship may suffer from it. I'm not going to say that my wife and I aren't ok, but we are starting to feel very tired, we really are. (Manuel, 29 year-old son)

Because I'm a mother, I'm a wife, but I'm also a mother. And he doesn't understand that. He wants me to put him first… the husband above everything else, and it can't be like that. My children are mine. They came out of me. Oh, my children! I've been very apart from them so he doesn't get upset. He has always been very jealous… of my dedication to them… he always wants to be first in everything. (Isabel, 65 year-old wife)

I'm going to take a trip. I was very reluctant as to whether I should go or not… but then I realized I must go because I need to take care of my mental health. (Lúcia, 65 year-old daughter-in-law)

To feel one has regained control over one's time, space or relationships are determinant factors. This in an attitude consistent with the process of re-orientation and self-redefinition that gives caregivers stability in the process of transition, which is characterized by a disruptive force that makes them need to balance changes in their daily lives (Bridges, 2001, 2004, 2009; Kralik, Visentin & Loon, 2006; Meleis et al., 2000).

Becoming a Caregiver: A Situational Transition

In transition processes, there is a basic assumption that transitions are periods of problems, of chaos and that the re-definition of self when playing new roles or when facing changes is what makes people adapt to that process of transition (Bridges, 2001, 2004, 2009). Beneath all the singularities and contexts of people going through transition processes, there are certain similarities in their experiences: there is the end of something, followed by a period of chaos and confusion and by the consciousness of that end, followed, at last, by new beginnings (Bridges, 2004). Hence, there seems to be a paradox in which in order to reach the continuity of something, one has to want to change (Bridges, 2009).

Bridges (2001, 2004, 2009) has identified three distinct phases in individuals going through transition processes, which include the consciousness, transformation and inner re-orientation: i) ending phase, ii) neutral zone phase) and iii) new beginning phase).

- ending phase – is a first phase related with feelings of loss and with the need to leave an old situation or former identity behind: "we lose or let go of our outlook, our old reality, our old attitudes, our old self-image" (Bridges, 2001, p.5);
- neutral zone phase – a period of confusion between the new and old realities in which individuals are neither playing a truly new role or are playing the previous role: "we get mixed signals some from our old way of being and some from a way of being that is still unclear to us" (Bridges, 2001, pp. 5-6). Despite being chaotic, this phase also contains a very creative potential. There are three basic dimensions of which we point out: inner disorientation (between playing a part that no longer exists and playing a new role that hasn't been set yet); experiencing feelings of having reached the end of the former world; and the birth of a neutral space which is essential to reach a questing attitude, with creative possibilities, since the previous conventional responses are no longer possible (Bridges, 2001);
- new begining phase – as certain as a transition must start with an end, it must end with a new beginning and it involves the recognition and consciousness of the two previous phases. "When we have done this, we feel that we are finally starting a new chapter in our lives (…) We have a new sense of ourselves, a new outlook, and a new sense of purpose and possibility" (Bridges, 2001, p. 6).

Transitions may be reactive, i.e. when there is a specific external change, or developmental, i.e. when it is set by natural inner aspects. Inner transformation is essential even if on the outside no changes may be identified.

Supporting individuals going through transitions cannot be solely centered on the expected result, but equally focused on understanding and helping them in the different phases of the process itself. In order to support sudden caregivers' experiences it may be clinically very useful to adopt this transitional perspective that equally takes into consideration both sides: process and outcome. According to Bridges (2004), when managing transition processes, it's extremely important to understand that one can only reach a later phase when the former is over. Thus, it may be useful to: i) consider middle steps so that people do not feel overtaken by the image of a role to play that may be very different from the one played in real life; ii) to build a system that can monitor the evolution during the transition and iii) to celebrate new beginnings (Bridges, 2004).

Transitions occur after deep changes in personal life (compulsory or chosen). They include the realization of inadequate normal behavior patterns and they imply the use of the new knowledge or changes in self-definition in a certain social context (Bridges, 2004; Kralik et al., 2006; Mu, 2004).

However, such a linear perspective of the process of transition is not consensual. Schumacher, Jones and Meleis (1999, p. 4) openly consider that "persons must go through all three stages to deal effectively with the transition. However, the stages of a transition do not necessarily occur in a linear manner. Rather, they may be sequential, parallel, or overlapping". Kralik et al. (2006), based on a previous Kralik study of women with chronic disease, have also identified a transition from a situation of *extraordinariness* – characterized by distress – and the final sense of coming back to *orderliness* – in a pattern that can be described as cyclical or recurrent. Nevertheless, different studies about transition processes have acknowledged that individuals have gone through periods similar to the phases identified by Bridges, even though in some cases, there is not a linear sequence, but rather a process characterized by advances and setbacks.

In the last decades, the concept of transition has been used both in social sciences and in health programs (Kralik et al., 2006). Research on transition processes have reinforced some aspects of great clinical use, amongst which we would like to point out: i) uncertainty as one of the most usual dimensions in transition processes – uncertainty about lack of knowledge, of information or communication with health professionals; ii) interpersonal conflict between the dynamic caregiver/care receiver; iii) and the common theme of worrying about issues ranging from the need to develop new skills or about caregiving as being incompatible with former daily tasks.

The Caregiver Career

Becoming a caregiver has been considered a process with both losses and gains throughout several stages (Cangelosi, 2009; Seltzer & Li, 2000). Once the process of becoming a caregiver has been considered a transition, it is useful to look to some frameworks that may lead to a better understanding of the phenomenon, as well as may guide research and practice. Using empirically tested frameworks may be an important tool for clinical settings by the insight they provide on the different dimensions that health professionals should assess, enabling them to review and strengthen their practice

Shyu (2000a) and Aneshensel et al. (1995)'s frameworks related to caregiving role development are useful for this purpose and parsimonious (and are similar, in several aspects) on the phases they consider.

Shyu (2000a), taking into account informal caregivers' needs during the transition from hospital to home, identifies three different phases each with particular needs: i) *role engaging* – characterized by preparing the caregiver and loved one to engage in new roles according to their needs, mostly consisting of giving information; ii) *role negotiation* – that takes place immediately after hospital discharge until reaching balance in the caregiving role, in which aspects valued have to do with the demands of tasks related with caregiving; iii) *role settling* – a process through which a stable level of caregiving is reached and in which most needs have to do with emotional support.

On the other hand, Aneshensel and colleagues (Aneshensel et al., 1995), taking into account a study developed amongst informal caregivers of Alzheimer's (n=555)[2] patients, reinforce the notion of developing a caregiver role like a career development. The main findings made it possible to identify informal caregiving as a process with different stages but with three main ones that set the *core* for what is called "caregiver's career". Those include: i) *role acquisition* - preparing oneself to assume role responsibilities; ii) *role enactment* – playing a part with all the tasks/activities related to it; and iii) *role disengagement*, a result of the mourning due to the loved one's death or due to the improvement of the loved one's condition and his/her social re-integration (Aneshensel et al., 1995).

The identification of these three wide "steps" (or phases, or stages) in the "caregiver career"[3] acknowledges different moments in the experience of caregiving. This means that interventions must consider two perspectives: according to each of the moments and as part of a changing dynamic process towards a final goal[4]. Aneshensel et al. (1995) point out that caregiving stages should not be seen as a group of rigid experiences, but rather as changing settings. Therefore, the stages previously described must be used as heuristic instruments.

The analogy of the caregiving process with the processes of career development is made due to the fact that caregiving, as with the development of a career, has normally a long timeline structure. It involves growth and implies a cumulative experience within a situation seen as a whole. However, there are differences that should be taken into account, since the timeline is undetermined; as such, this "career" is not planned and the part is (if so) only recognized within the family net (Aneshensel et al., 1995).

This idea of the caregiver career is useful, not only due to its dynamic character but also because it introduces a new perspective related to the end of the caregiving role (e.g. due to the care receiver's death). Stepping out of the role is as important as getting ready to play it or getting involved in its responsibilities. In a clinical point of view, this proposition has evident implications. Professional help cannot just consist of giving support considering a specific phase, but rather it should take into account the previous stage as well as the next one. Getting ready for "stepping out" of the role cannot start when the caregiving situation ends, for it can result in an inefficient intervention or not acting at the right time. Getting ready for "unplugging" from the part is an important goal to be addressed in an intermediate phase, when the caregiver is at the full development of his/her role. For instance, respite care programs cannot be only considered as a way of providing some pause in caregiving in order to allow informal caregivers to "get back" to the tiresome tasks with newly acquired energy. It is also a way to prepare the future, to establish social contacts and develop pleasing activities in order to prevent the consequences of solitude and social isolation. It is also an investment for the future, to ensure that once the caregiving situation is over, the caregiver's integration in society is not compromised.

---

[2] "Profiles in caregiving. The unexpected career" (Aneshensel, C., Pearlin, L., Mullan, J., Zarit, S., & Whitlatch, C.,1995).
[3] Cf. also: Cameron e Gignac (2007); Shyu (2000a).
[4] Cf. also: Bridges (2001, 2004, 2009); Meleis (2007); Meleis et al. (2000); Schumacher et al. (1999).

The experience of becoming a sudden caregiver, "falling into a part" that one did not anticipate (Figueiredo, 2007), and did not have enough time to prepare for, brings forward the need of greater professional attention to the "sudden caregiver's career". It is important to reflect upon Suzane Mintz's experience (2007): "We've «been betrayed by happenings» we couldn't control and presented with the daunting challenge of trying to re-create normalcy" (p.32).

There is a "profound injustice" in being betrayed by a story one cannot control. Thus, supporting informal caregivers should not just be limited to making caregivers competent in the care they provide. Professionals should keep in mind that that part is transitory and as such, they should ensure that, once that phase is over, the caregiver is not "stuck" in a situation of isolation of which he/she will not easily escape: that would be a double injustice.

Rethinking Respite Care

Offering respite care is not the only way to diminish the caregiver's overload perception. However, it is an important resource, functioning as a buffering factor for the consequences of stress. In fact, caregiver stress seems to be related with several aspects, such as: the time spent from the beginning of the role; the physical demands of caregiving; the level of mastery in the role; the meaning attributed to giving care to a loved one; the ability to cope with the situation; the perception of an efficient social network, amongst many others (Aneshensel et al., 1995; Ayres, 2000; Crespo-López & López-Martínez, 2007; Figueiredo, 2007). The efficiency of respite care programs may be also improved if psycho-educational dimensions are taken into account (Carretero et al., 2009; Garcés, Carretero, Ródenas & Alemán, 2010). In this wider perspective, respite care cannot mean only providing support for informal caregivers in their daily tasks, but also taking into consideration their specific needs both in terms of information and in developing coping strategies for the various demands of caregiving.

Nevertheless, the mere existence of respite care programs does not mean that caregivers will use those programs. This was one of the conclusions of Exel, Graaf, & Brouver's study (2008): no matter how many respite care programs there are, many caregivers in need of that special kind of support do not look for it. It is important to try to understand this phenomenon further because of its implications. Some of the reasons might be related with not wanting to leave care in the hands of others or thinking that the care receiver might not like being cared for by strangers (Exel et al., 2008). De La Cuesta-Benjumea (2009), in a study developed with caregivers of people with dementia, also brings some insight on this topic. In order for caregivers to rest, they need tranquility. If caregivers do not feel safe, if they are not tranquil, they will not rest, no matter what the programs available may be, because they cannot get some emotional distance, which means being tranquil about themselves and others. Jacobs (2004) points out that even if professionals, friends, and family try to force caregivers to leave home in order not to feel imprisoned, they often object to do so. He ironically points out that such an attitude may not be adequate nor the arguments that support it:

> At other times, clinicians, mistakenly assume that caregivers are downtrodden or depressed because of their self-sacrifices. For instance, we may glibly push a caregiver to «get out of the house and do something for yourself», when she feels that caring for her loved one

in their home gives her the utmost spiritual gratification. Clinicians' responses, however well-meaning or grounded in sound theories, can badly miss the mark of a given caregiver's makeup and desires" (p.112).

Such opinions and the gap between respite care programs and their actual development lead Chappell at al. (2001) to study and re-think the meaning of "respite care" for caregivers. As a result of that study, they suggest an innovative classification of "respite care", identifying six meanings of respite care according to caregivers' experiences: i) *stolen moments* – brief periods of time in which the caregiver has other activities that are not part of their caregiving routine; ii) *connections* – making contacts with people outside the caregiving context (both social support and hobbies); iii) *relief* – breaks in caregiving that allow the caregiver some distance from caregiving (body and mind), normally for holidays or longer periods, that allow them to put all their worries aside; iv) *mental or physical stimulus* – challenges from outside the caregiving situation; v) *angst-free care receiver* – caregivers mention breaks as moments when the care receiver feels fairly happy or comfortable; vi) *minimize the importance* – caregivers who don't feel a need for a break.

This new typology sets alerts for the new meanings on respite care through caregiver's eyes. The different meanings of respite care are organized in two types: i) internal respite – breaks resulting from the re-definition that caregivers make of their role or expertise as caregivers (stolen moments, minimize importance and angst-free care receiver); external respite – breaks that include using adequate support resources (relief, mental/physical boost, and connections).

Since some identified breaks occur at the caregiver's home, these breaks may not be considered important by professionals; however, they are highly valued by caregivers. Chappel et al. (2001) have reached the conclusion that caregivers are more interested in emotional aspects, rather than in the variety of respite care that is offered. Based on his personal experience, Wolpe (2004, p.42) points out that the most important challenges for caregivers have nothing to do with the number of hours they spend in caregiving, but mostly with the tremendous inner struggle: "What resentments am I allowed without being uncaring? What resistance am I allowed to her requests *(his spouse)* without being cruel? What can I demand for myself without being egocentric? What can I dream about without being unrealistic?" (p. 42). As for Mintz (2007), writing and reflecting upon her experience as a caregiver ("*A family caregiver speaks up: it doesn't have to be this hard*"), brilliantly sums up the caregiver's perspective:

> "If you lie down no one will die!" Isn´t that what we are afraid in our heart of hearts? That if we are not there, something bad will happen and we'll never be able to forgive ourselves. We imagine the worst and create a prison that locks in our body, mind, and spirit. When we don't care for ourselves we are denying the possibility that good things are more likely to be the result than bad ones. When we don't care for ourselves we are doing a disservice to those we love as well as to ourselves. It is important to give yourself the gift of permission. Ultimately that is where loving, honoring, and valuing yourself has to begin. (Mintz, 2007, p.119).

Reaching Balanced Points along the Way: Integrating Caregiving in Daily Life

The progression of the caregiving process, from its sudden beginning until reaching a possible balance, is not a linear path between total chaos and confusion towards a harmonious level of integration of caregiving with the daily life. It is rather, a path of advances and step backs in a delicate game of tentative points of balance: a path of "zooming in and zooming out" (centering/de-centering) movements, between "myself as a caregiver" (fully dedicated to the care receiver in terms of providing care but also in the time spent, the worrying, and the fears it implies) and "myself in a wider world of roles" (how "I relate to others" and allow quality time for family and friends, or whether or not "I am capable of keeping or starting new social activities").

There are other objective conditions that also interfere in reaching this balance such as: the level of dependency of the care receiver; the amount of time that is spent; the improvement or aggravation of the care receiver's condition; the access or not to support. Some of the subjective conditions that may also play an important role are coping strategies developing a resilient spirit.

There is a dynamic and changing process that leads to integrating care in daily life and it depends on finding points of balance, i.e. when caregiving is seen as satisfactory, or imbalance, i.e. when it is considered as overload (Ayres, 2000; Pereira, 2006). The sense of transformation makes the term transition applicable to such a situation – it is not just a temporary change. As a transitional situation it may be understood as: "(…) a process of convoluted passage during which people redefine their sense of self and redevelop self-agency in response to disruptive life events" (van Loon and Kralik, 2005, in Kralik, et al., 2006, p. 321). In this process or path of progressively finding balance, Ayres (2000) points out the importance of the caregiver's expectations and the strategies he/she uses in finding meaning to his/her role. The process of finding meaning in situations depends on the caregiver's present and previous experiences and his/her explanations about the specific caregiving situation based on his/her personal philosophy, moral settings, or personal evaluation about the world or him/herself. All in all, expectations and explanations influence the caregiver's range and choice of strategies. They are essential for the caregiver to evaluate his/her experiences as satisfactory or not, in order to integrate caregiving in a wider context of his/her life (Ayres, 2000). "I started to integrate … better … to accept things better and now… the same happens when my son gets home, I bathe him, do his things and do the same to my mother": that was how Zélia (27 year-old daughter) felt about her experience in our last meeting.

Shyu (2000b), taking into account the dynamic nature of this quest for reaching balance in informal caregiving, states that the active search for balanced points in a new context of life represents a coping strategy that mediates the caregiver's stress when dealing with several needs at the same time that he/she has to give care for a loved one. A dynamic strategy can be centered both in maintaining a balance that has already been achieved and in trying to find a more satisfactory balance in the event that there should be any other problematic situation during the time that caregiving occurs.

Braff and Olenik (2003) refer to this process of attributing meaning and assessment/re-assessment of self as a caregiver, saying:

> When you're able to step back and reassess your role, in order to re-gain structure and control and give yourself some respite from caregiving, your strong feelings of resentment will fade. You will discover as you prioritize that you do have choices. You don't have to put your life on hold, and you do not have to be responsible for every outcome. What a relief! (Braff & Olenik, 2003, p. 88)

In order to understand this process of finding a balance of advancements or setbacks, it may be useful to acknowledge some expressions (Figure 1) or indicators that the caregivers who participated in the present study left in their narratives and that express this movement of "de-centering" from "me as a caregiver" towards "me as also a caregiver" (Pereira & Botelho, 2011).

> - ✓ Acknowledging his/her needs as a caregiver: the necessary resources, the level of the support needed to be able to care for the dependent person.
> - ✓ Feeling comfortable in the development of new tasks (in the care given and in other responsibilities).
> - ✓ Stating the need of not living solely for the care receiver.
> - ✓ Setting limits for the development of the role.
> - ✓ Acknowledging other dimensions in need of attention: of oneself as a person/mother/father/companion; of oneself as a professional; of oneself as a citizen.
> - ✓ Re-organizing caregiving in order to integrate it harmoniously in daily life.
> - ✓ Being able to leave home feeling tranquil and safe (without being a slave of time and needing to always being present).
> - ✓ Feeling rewarded or appreciated for the quality of the care given or by the perception of the care receiver's well-being.

Figure 1. Indicators of the movement of de-centering from the caregiving situation.

Time is a necessary condition for this process but it is not enough. The mere passing of time does not ensure de-centering.

> Even today, after two and a half years have passed, I feel... I think I'm more and more lost, that's what I think. It has been two years since I've taken a holiday. Well, I do, but it doesn't feel like it, does it? (Paula, 48 year-old daughter)

The acknowledging of situations, the self-reflection about the meaning of the reason why one gives care and using respite care to manage the demands of the needs of the other without feeling guilt, are aspects to be considered.

The paths in the quest for finding transitory balances or more stable or lasting forms of balance are refracted in different ways (most of them far from an ideal or linear trajectory) depending on the contexts where caregiving occurs, as well as on the caregiver or care receiver's characteristics, i.e. the respite care they choose or support they can gather. All these variations mean that caregivers' paths are unique and are not context free.

The process is more recurring than linear. The mere existence of an ideal final goal, one of balance and integration of caregiving in daily life, allowing for the regaining of the sense of "normality" in things, doesn't make it linear. The objective and subjective conditions of the caregiver's experiences make his/her re-entry to the world inconstant, due to de-centering from their exclusive caregiving condition, (Figure 2).

For informal caregivers, this dynamic movement is lived in a net in which the knots are: "the experience of time(s) lived", "the experience of feeling alone", "the experience of taking another person into one's care", and "the experience of failled expectations" (Pereira & Botelho, 2011[5]). As the net gets tighter or looser (in the whole area or in small areas), new configurations and balances are attained between "the me as a caregiver in daily life" and "me in daily life".

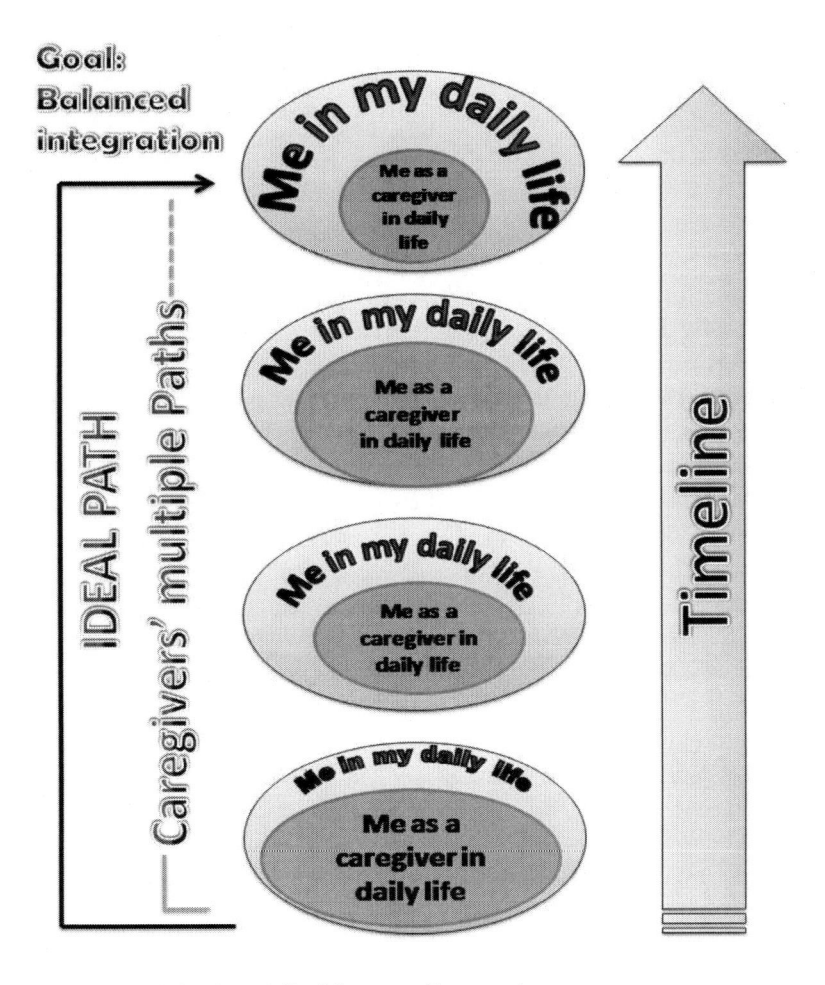

Figure 2. Integrating caregiving into daily life: a non-linear path.

CONCLUSION

Whenever people are confronted with the need to become sudden caregivers, the experience lived by them is that of an "assault" on their daily lives as they know them, due to the responsibilities of having to unexpectedly give care to someone.

---

[5] Cf. Introduction of the chapter: essential themes on the experience of suddenly becoming an informal caregiver; Cf. also (Pereira & Botelho, 2011).

The central aspect of the caregiver's life becomes his/her role as a caregiver (caregiving, worrying, insecurity, being present, identifying resources and strategies in caregiving, amongst many other aspects). Playing that new role quickly takes control of the caregiver's life. The unexpected nature and being "unprepared" for the situation requires the caregiver's almost exclusive attention to the caregiving relationship.

The caregiver often feels alone, confined to spaces and routines. He/She may feel that they lost control over time, because time is scarce or monotonous. He/she experiences overwhelming feelings due to their perception of being responsible for someone else's life and feel there is a mismatch between the available resources and their expectations. This is indeed not a little task.

As time goes by, the caregiver starts to feel that he/she cannot be caught in this situation that limits his/her well-being, freedom, social interactions, mental health and participation in the various areas in which he/she plays a part.

He/she recognizes an ideal goal for caregiving, in which he/she chooses to provide care to a dependent loved one and also expects to harmoniously integrate caregiving in the wider areas of his/her daily life. The feeling of regaining normality through the integration of caregiving in daily life, with all its other needs and demands derived from the variety of roles played (family, professional, communitarian and leisure), is an individual and gradual process that depends on the inner redefinition of the caregiver.

Can the conclusions of this study raise the voices, experiences and needs of the sudden informal caregiver? Can its participants' voices or the experiences of other caregivers who decided to share and publish their own somehow influence professionals' action when giving caregivers support in the process? We hope so. We hope the reported individual experiences may carry, as Burack-Weiss (2006) says, "informal caregivers' wisdom", so that their problems are not reduced to mere cold figures. This knowledge represents a challenge for all those who devote their work to support informal caregivers: it is a call for professional action (Munhall, 2007).

It is important to question how health professionals and social workers can give support to this movement identified in the paths of sudden informal caregivers. The one centered between "focusing oneself exclusively in caregiving" and "de-centering from caregiving", in order to integrate caregiving in a broader context of daily life. In order words, how can someone help take care of someone else's vulnerability without being completely "focused on the other" or "focused on oneself"? How can professionals help support caregivers in the progressive detachment from caregiving, monitoring their progressive balance points, and ensuring the adequate help needed in each of them? How can the uniqueness of de-centering paths be assessed; while integrating the meaning that caregivers attribute to their progressive balance steps without "pushing" them towards standard respite care that may not meet the needs of the moment they are living in?

The caregiver's path is unique, contextualized, and in need of individual assessment. In order to monitor and support the caregiver's de-centering movement, first one must recognize that there is a starting moment that is characterized by being strongly focused in the caregiving tasks and with feelings of confusion and uncertainty. Professionals should intentionally assess the duration of that period so that the caregiver may not be forever stuck in caregiving as the only activity of their life. The movement(s) and the balanced points found between "me as a caregiver" and "me in daily life" are essentially determined by the redefinition that the caregiver makes of him/herself in a particular role, in a particular time and context. Professionals need to be attentive to the de-centering signs that caregivers send. This monitoring will allow professionals to choose more accurate interventions as well as the time in which they will take place.

Obviously, it's useful to have instruments that may help to diagnose, monitor and register different responses to the caregiving situation; as are the results of this study, since they set a framework and indicators on how to understand the nature of "suddenly becoming a caregiver" through which individual experiences may be looked upon. However, we, as professionals have to be sensitive when assessing these situations, as we must ensure that caregivers have an individualized intervention matching their unique experiences. Otherwise, successful implementations will not occur, meaning that educational programs would be put into use in inadequate timings, and caregivers would be taught things they do not need and be given respite care that does not offer them relief. We will be "pushing" caregivers out of their homes, no matter how good our intentions may be, even if they are not prepared for it. We will fail to recognize that they feel alone and need "adequate dosages" of reinforcement and trust. No synergies will occur and support systems will fail, no matter how great the amount of work done.

This chapter started with the caregivers' voices. First, we presented Manuel and Lurdes' experiences as sudden caregivers, in the introduction during the chaotic phase, now we end with Gabriela's statement, showing her as having re-organized her experience, even if the objective conditions of giving care to someone have not been changed:

> From here forward my life has changed. Well, it hasn't really changed, because the routine is the same, but I've reached the conclusion that there is no use coming home in despair. There is no use in doing such a thing. It leads you nowhere and, after all, my mother had already reached that phase where she was stable… that was the time when I said not like that… you must move forward and lead your life and it was then we decided to start a business and do all this. Then, other things came up and I realized I don't need anybody else. I am not dependent on anybody else. I depend only on myself. I'm my own boss and there is no one after me telling me what I must do. That was the moment I said enough… from now on … (…) It was then I decided to make a 180 degree turn in my life and move on. (Gabriela, 26 years-old, daughter)

The Caregivers' descriptions retold an experience in transitioning towards the development of a role they had not anticipated. The experiences of the various participants claim they should be heard and remind professionals that in order for them to ease those transitions, they should keep their testimonies in mind.

REFERENCES

Aneshensel, C., Pearlin, L., Mullan, J., Zarit, S., & Whitlatch, C. (1995). *Profiles in caregiving. The unexpected carer.* San Diego: Academic Press.

Ayres, L. (2000). Narratives of family caregiving: the process of making meaning. *Research in Nursing & Health,* 23**,** 424-434.

Braff, S., & Olenik, M. (2003). *Staying connected while letting go. The paradox of Alzheimer's caregiving.* New York: M. Evans Company.

Bridges, W. (2001). *The way of transitions: embracing life's most difficult moments*. Cambridge: Da Capo Press.

Bridges, W. (2003). *Managing Transitions: making the most of change* (2th ed.). Cambridge: Da Capo Press.

Bridges, W. (2004). *Transitions: making sense of life's* (2th ed.). Cambridge: Da Capo Press.

Burack-Weiss, A. (2006). *The caregiver's tale. Loss and renewal in memoirs of family life*. New York: Columbia University Press.

Cameron, J., & Gignac, M. (2008). Timing it right: a conceptual framework for addressing the support needs of family caregivers to stroke survivors from hospital to the home. *Patient Education and Counseling*, 70(3), 305-314.

Cangelosi, P. (2009). Caregiver burden or caregiver gain? Respite for family caregivers. *Journal of Psychosocial Nursing*, 47(9), 19-22.

Carretero, S., Garcés, J., Ródenas, F., & Sanjosé, V. (2009). The informal caregiver's burden of dependent people: theory and empirical review. *Archives of Gerontology and Geriatrics*, 49(1), 74-79.

Chappell, N., Reid, R., & Dow, E. (2001). Respite reconsidered. A typology of meanings based on the caregiver's point of view. *Journal of Aging Studies*, 15, 201-216.

Crespo-López, M., & López-Martínez, J. (2007). *El estrés en cuidadores de mayors dependientes*. [Stress in dependent elderly caregivers] Madrid: Pirámide.

de la Cuesta-Benjumea, C. (2009). "Estar tranquila": la experiencia del descanso de cuidadoras de pacientes con demencia avanzada. [«Feeling tranquil»: the experience of rest among the caregivers' of relatives with advanced dementia] *Pensar Enfermagem* 13(2), 2-10.

Exel, J., Graaf, G., & Brouwer, W. (2008). Give me a break! Informal caregiver attitudes towards respite care. *Health Policy*, 88, 73-87.

Figueiredo, D. (2007) *Cuidados familiares ao idoso dependente* [Family caregiving of elderly dependet people], Lisboa: Climepsi.

Garcés, S.; Carretero, S., Ródenas, F. & Alemán, C. (2010) A review of programs to alleviate the burden of informal caregivers of dependent persons. *Archives of Gerontology and Geriatrics*, 50(3), 254-259.

García, J. (2010). *Los tiempos del cuidado: El impacto de la dependencia de los mayores en la vida cotidiana de sus cuidadores* [Timings in caregiving: the impact of elderly people in the daily lives of their caregivers], Madrid: Ministerio de Sanidad y Política Social/Instituto de Mayores y Servicios Sociales (IMSERSO).

Hoffmann, F., & Rodrigues, R. (2010). Informal carers: who takes care of them? *Policy Brief*. Viena, European Centre for Social Welfare Policy and Research. Available at http://www.euro.centre.org/detail.php?xml_id=1714 (accessed 04 August 2010)

Jacobs, B. (2004). From sadness to pride: seven common emotional experiences of caregiving. In C. Levine (ed.), *Always on call: when illness turns families into caregivers* (pp. 111-125), Nashville: Vanderbilt University Press.

Levine, C. (2004a). Introduction: The many worlds of family caregivers. In C. Levine (ed.), *Always on call: when illness turns families into caregivers* (pp.1-18), Nashville: Vanderbiltt University Press.

Levine, C. (2004b). The loneliness of the long-term caregiver. In C. Levine (ed.), *Always on call: when illness turns families into caregivers* (pp. 99-107), Nashville: Vanderbiltt University Press.

Meleis, A. (2007). *Theoretical Nursing. Development Progress* (4th ed.). Philadelphia: Lippincott Williams & Wilkins.

Meleis, A., Sawyer, L., Im, E. ,Messias, D., & Schumacher, K. (2000). Experiencing transitions: an emerging middle-range theory. *Advances in Nursing Science*, *23*(1), 12-28.

Mintz, S. (2007). *A family caregiver speaks up: "It doesn't have to be this hard"*, Sterling: Capital Books.

Mu, P. (2004). Maternal role transition experiences of women hospitalized with PROM: a phenomenological study. *International Journal of Nursing Studies, 41*, 825-832.

Munhall, P. (2007). A phenomenological Method. In P. Munhall (Ed.), *Nursing research: a qualitative perspective* (pp. 145-210). Sudbury: Jones and Bartlett.

Pereira, H. (2006). "Subitamente cuidadores informais": da incerteza ao(s) pontos de equilíbrio. Uma análise do conhecimento existente. [Suddenly informal caregivers: from uncertainty to balance. A literature review]. *Pensar Enfermagem, 10*(2), 19-31.

Pereira, H., & Botelho, M. (2011). Sudden informal caregivers: the lived experience of informal caregivers after an unexpected event, *Journal of Clinical Nursing, 20*(17-18), 2448-2457.

Schumacher, K., Jones, P., & Meleis, A. (1999). Helping elderly persons in transition: a framework for research and practice. In E. Swanson & T. Toni-Tripp-Reimer (Eds.), *Life transitions in the older adult. Issues for nurses and other health professionals* (pp. 1-26). New York: Springer Publishing Company.

Seltzer, M., & Li, L. (2000). The dynamics of caregiving: transitions during a three-year prospective study. *The Gerontologist, 40*(2),165-178.

Shyu, C.(2000a). The Needs of family caregivers of frail elders during the transition from hospital to home: a Taiwanese sample. *Journal of Advanced Nursing, 32*(1),619-625.

Shyu, Y.(2000b). Patterns of caregiving when family caregivers face competing needs. *Journal of Advanced Nursing, 31*(1), 35-43.

Van Manen, M. (1990). *Researching Lived Experience. Human Science for an Action Sensitive Pedagogy.* New York: SUNY.

Wolpe, G. (2004) A crisis of caregiving, a crisis of faith. In C. Levine (Ed.) *Always on call: when illness turns families into caregivers* (pp. 34-44). Nashville: Vanderbilt University Press.

Zarit, S. & Femia, E. (2008). Behavioral and psychosocial interventions for family caregivers, *Journal of Social Work Education*, 44(3), Supplement, 49-57.

In: Caregivers: Challenges, Practices and Cultural Influences
Editors: Adrianna Thurgood and Kasha Schuldt

ISBN: 978-1-62618-030-7
© 2013 Nova Science Publishers, Inc.

Chapter 4

PARENTAL AND EDUCATORS' JUDGMENTS AND ATTITUDES TOWARD LIFE CHALLENGES OF PEOPLE WITH INTELLECTUAL DISABILITIES: FUNCTIONAL MEASUREMENT CONTRIBUTIONS TO SPECIAL EDUCATION FROM A COGNITIVE ALGEBRA APPROACH

Guadalupe Elizabeth Morales, Ernesto Octavio Lopez, David Jose Charles, Claudia Castro Campos and Martha Patricia Sanchez
Cognitive Science Laboratory, Psychology Department,
Universidad Autonoma de Nuevo Leon, Mexico

ABSTRACT

For a long time, a person with an intellectual disability (ID) was ignored as a human being. Their interests, aspirations and needs were not contemplated as a priority. Fortunately, in many societies this inappropriate and deep-rooted vision seems to be changing. New efforts coming from parents, teachers and carriers to promote the human rights of this population have had a direct effect on improving the quality of their lives. For example, nowadays a more open attitude can be identified. ID individuals may be included in regular school and work.Their right to exercise a sexual life is considered. In this chapter, we argue that comprehending the cognitive nature of parents and caregivers´ beliefs, attitudes and judgments toward persons with ID, will provide significant life improvements in this population. Specifically, the Information Integration Theory (IIT) research approach will be introduced. It allows scientific scrutiny about how contextual and human factors of a society are integrated into systematic thinking (cognitive algebra). We discuss how the IIT approach can be used whenever improvement of life conditions of people with ID is considered. Emerging research studies in this direction are discussed next.

1. LIFE CHALLENGES FOR PEOPLE WITH INTELLECTUAL DISABILITY

"I believe that life has plenty of challenges and these are even bigger for a person with Down syndrome ...."

Pablo Pineda

Through our lives we face endless challenges that frequently become opportunities to improve our own emotional, intellectual and social development. This is especially true for people with intellectual disabilities (ID) where accessibility to resources and social support allow them to cope with the circumstances of daily life. For instance, people with Down syndrome (DS)(at least a considerable number of members from this population), if provided with appropriate conditions, can achieve an independent life with challenges as well as satisfactions,similar to anyone else´s life.

Unfortunately, since ancient times people with ID have suffered enormous discrimination due to their atypical intellectual condition and this stigma imposes adouble challenge for them every day. One challenge relates exclusively to their own disability and another one to stereotypes and ignorance about their intellectual condition.

As we will discuss next, a well-established system of beliefs about people with ID rules over the minds of many people and this has limited human rights and sustained the discriminatory position over this population. The best scenario for this appointed system of beliefs mistakenly visualized people with ID in the past as divine manifestations and because of this they were treated well. However, on the other side of the coin, due to their physical attributes and atypical behavior they were used for circus entertainment. Even more, some people believed they were possessed and sometimes they were condemned to death (Schleichkorn, 1981).

Nowadays a brighter future is currently being developed over populations with ID since professional caregivers, teachers, groups of parents and institutions are organizing themselves to promote systematic efforts to change life conditions (e,g, educational, social accessibility, labor rights, etc.) and this includes efforts to transform the current conceptualization that society has about ID into a new one based on academic scrutiny. As a direct consequence of this renewed view a distinction has emerged to distinguish a person from her/his disability and consequently to recognize people with ID as persons and not as objects named "disability". To provide a wider view on these changes, let us first introduce a brief background on how society has considered ID.

2. INTELLECTUAL DISABILITY CONCEPTUALIZATIONS AND ITS DEFINITION THROUGHOUT HISTORY

There are not many systematic records on populations with ID (North Dakota Center for Persons with Disabilities, 2009). Perhaps the oldest record on ID relates to a single 1552 B.C. Egyptian document entitled "The therapeutic Papyrus of Thebes" (Harris 2006), which describes medical considerations and treatment for physical and intellectual disability due to brain damage (Schleichkorn, 1981). Better known records come from ancient Greece where

ID was attributed to gods' divine interventions, and Greek council meetings were convened to "evaluate" and intervene to stop offending them more. This is especially true for the Spartan Greek civilization, where neonates with some kind of disability were thrown away into a deep pit (Biasini, Grupe, Huffman & Bray, 1999). Additional stigma over this vulnerable population can be seen in the second century A.D., during the peak of the Roman Empire. This was a dark time for plenty of misfortunate people with ID. The best thing that could happen to a member of this population was to be sold for entertainment.

This attitude regarding people with ID diminished little in the Middle Ages (s.V-XVA.D) and new ways to take care of them were introduced. For instance, they could be put into jail cages (idiot cages) to avoid they caused any problems. Frequently, these cages were allocated to a city's downtown area so people could have some free entertainment by watching them. Renaissance brought improved conditions for this population by introducing a more constructive conceptualization about ID based on academic considerations. It is precisely in this time context that John Locke (1690) published his famous document "An Essay Concerning Human Understanding" where the concept of mental retardation is distinguished from mental sickness. In his own words: "Herein seems to lie the difference between idiots and madmen, that madmen put wrong ideas together and reason from them, but idiots make very few or no propositions and reason scarce at all (see Locke, 1690, p. 94)".

Now, Locke was a believer that individuals are born as "tabula rasa" and this led some people to promote the idea that people with ID are capable of learning how to change toward an optimal mental development. In this spirit, Jean Marc Gaspard Itard presented the first systematic treatment on children with ID (see Itard, 1801-1806). He showed that by using a sensitive human approach as well as specialized educative strategies, members of this group could achieve learning goals. Following these efforts Seguin (1866), under Itard´s supervision, documented some causes and treatments related to ID, which by that time was labeled as "idiocy". From this approach Seguin developed the "Physiology Method" to educate children with ID. Mostly, this training program considered that physiological and moral aspects as well as senses should be educated in order to have an impact over cognitive development. This rationale followed, and a direct relationship between sensorial information like vision, hearing and cognition was assumed. Without any doubt, physical training and individualized training programs were revolutionary ideas during Itard times and these ideas were the foundation bricks of special education.

Later, at the beginning of the eighteenth century, a new concern emerged about how to identify children who really needed special education. To this respect, Alfred Binet and Theodore Simon (1905) developed a test (Binet-Simon Individual Tests of Intelligence) that allowed detection of children in need of special attention (also see Binet& Simon, 1904a, 1904b). Here, the original first version of the test introduced the subnormal and normal categories to assess children's intellectual capacities. The subnormal category in turn used different levels: 1) idiocia, 2) imbecility, 3) moronity (Sheerenberger, 1983).

Even when the birth of psychometric tests of intelligence represented a landmark to the advancement of psychology, it also lead to the renewal of the old dark Eugenic tradition derived from the ancient Greek civilization to look towards human perfection. Take for instance, the case of the Eugenic psychologist Henry Herbert Goddard who believed that "feeble-mindedness" was hereditary (see Goddard, 1912: *The Kallikak Family: A Study in the Heredity of Feeble-Mindedness*). According to this author it was necessary to use intelligence tests to detect what he called "defectives" to avoid their offspring since avoiding their reproduction implied that the mental deficiency chain would end. These Eugenic ideas brought severe consequences to persons with ID and during the first half of the twenty century more than 42,000 members of this population were submitted to sterilization procedures in the USA (Radford, 1991). These ideas expanded across the world (e.g., Germany) having devastating consequences over the ID population. Fortunately, discovering multiple etiologies for ID discredited the single idea that the intellectual disability was hereditary. This academic progress, paralleled by social events like a new consciousness and sensitivity to others' suffering coming from the World War II holocaust, helped to stop Eugenic approaches toward these vulnerable populations.

Thus, approaching people with ID as human beings requires understanding not only a strong historically established system of beliefs but changes the nature of thought toward new concepts that allow them improved life conditions. Academic approaches have begun to achieve this goal by changing the ID nomenclature and definition. Specifically, a conceptual change was made over the initial ID definition terms as inherent, inseparable and permanent (e.g., retards) towards a definition that envisions intellectual disability as a person's life condition (e.g., as a person with intellectual disability). This view is reflected in current ID definitions where it is understood to be a condition consisting of limitations on intellectual performance (IQ coefficient), communication abilities, personal care and social abilities (adaptive behavior or adaptive functioning) (National Dissemination Center for children with disabilities, NICHCY, 2010).

Note from this definition the adaptive behavior consideration. This not only relates to biological aspects but social and environmental concerns. Here it is assumed that the perception and attitude that society has towards this population, impinges constrained social and environmental contexts over them (The World Health Organization, WHO, 2001). These perceptions derive from protocols that demand specific behavior from them in all aspects of their daily life, like labor rights and labor scenarios or educational rights.

3. SOME GENERAL REMARKS ON INTELLECTUAL DISABILITY AND ATTITUDES TOWARD MEMBERS OF THIS POPULATION

> "Disability need not be an obstacle to success... In fact we have a moral duty to remove the barriers to participation, and to invest sufficient funding and expertise to unlock the vast potential of people with disabilities."
>
> Professor Stephen W. Hawking (2011)

Disability is part of human life. Many people during their development will experience some kind of transitory or permanent disability. According to the World Health Organization (WHO, 2011), more than one billion people in the worldlive with some kind of disability (15 % of world population) and around 200 million people have considerable functional problems. This is relevant since people with disabilities are one of the most marginalized groups in the world. Shedding more light on this, the WHO's *World Report on Disability* 2011 indicates high health vulnerability in this population that can be prevented, and that members of this population have less economic participation and have the highest poverty indexes. Discrimination against members of this population varies depending on personal and contextual factors. For example, in terms of labor opportunities people with intellectual disabilities have low probabilities of getting a job and educational opportunities favor people with physical disabilities rather than people with ID. Thus, not only do biological constraints impose a heavy weight on these people but there are also contextual factors, like limited political regulations that maintain discriminatory attitudes towards this population.

As will be devised through this chapter, our main concern is to propose new academic ways to understand the attitude processes toward the ID population since they basically determine political regulations to build social environments where people with this condition will live (see Hahn, 1985). As we have thoroughly expressed before, negative attitudes maintain discrimination and blocks their way to better living conditions (Corrigan, 2000; Corrigan & Watson, 2002) but new positive attitudes toward this population have emerged (Florez, Aguado&Alcedo, 2009). This attitude change is not as simple as it might look. For example, Hernandez, Keys and Balcazar (2000) reported in a study that whereas employers showed a general positive attitude in offering work opportunities to people with ID they had the same negative attitudes toward the specific attributes of these possible workers. The same phenomenon was reported for regular school inclusion where teachers were in favor of including children with disabilities but they were not so willing to have them in their own classroom. Only a small minority of teachers were willing to do so (Scruggs &Mastropieri, 1996).

The discrepancy between general and specific attitudes is the tip of the iceberg of a more complex psychological phenomenon. For instance, defining what an attitude is, is not always an easy task. Attitude definitions are under heated academic debates, and some definitions demand consideration of mental states that rule and guide goal oriented behavior, others consider the dimensional emotional aspects with respect to an object (e.g. one dimension: pleasure vs. unpleasant) or the behavioral component where a person has a learned preference to react in a positive or negative way towards an event. Also, there are attitude definitions that emphasize the cognitive appraisal process (Oskamp& Schultz, 2005).

These appraisals, tendencies, mental states and emotional moods toward objects or events can be expressed voluntarily in a controlled fashion and because of this they are known as explicit attitudes (Ottaway, Hay den, & Oakes, 2001). In contrast, automatic reactions, sometimes not accessible to consciousness, have been termed as implicit attitudes (Banaji&Bhaskar, 2000). It has been suggested however, that both kinds of attitude are composed at least by three general main components: A behavioral one, a cognitive component and an emotional component (Barriga, 1998) (see Figure 1).

Measurement techniques for each attitude component have been proposed depending on the intrinsic nature of the component. Take the case of explicit attitudes, where in spite of strong criticism to the use of self reports, questionnaires, scales, and other items to measure attitudes (Petty &Briñol, 2010), they constitute the main measurement tools.Implicit and automatic processing attitude measurement indirect methods, like affective priming (Fazio, 1995; Oskamp& Schultz, 2005) or implicit association tests (IAT) (Greenwald, Banaji, Rudman, Farnham, Nosek&Mellot, 2002; Greenwald, Nosek&Banaji, 2003) are among the most used measurement tools. These and other methods have been used to study attitudes toward ID in a variety of fields (e.g. education, sexuality, etc.) and they have provided in valuable information on how people perceive people with intellectual disabilities. Recently a new approach has been introduced in this area, namely, the Information Integration Theory

(IIT). This approach has also successfully begun to provide insightful information about cognitive processing underlying attitudes toward ID. Since the goal of this chapter is to show the benefits of this approach inside special education research, let us provide some background on it next.

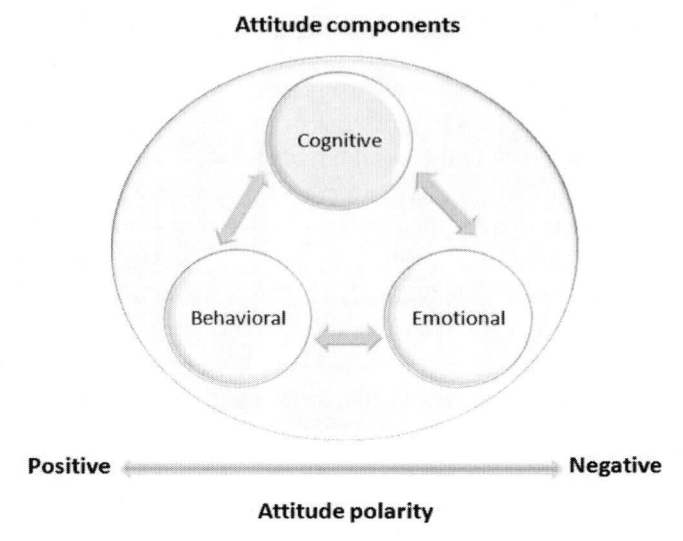

Figure 1. A simple graphic description of attitude components that lead to positive and negative evaluations toward events or persons.

4. FUNCTIONAL MEASUREMENT CONTRIBUTIONS TO SPECIAL EDUCATION FROM A COGNITIVE ALGEBRA APPROACH

All of us throughout our entire development are confronted with situations demanding decision making that usually has profound implications in our life. In order to achieve successful decision making, our brains depend on carefully evaluating and integrating relevant information. This complex behavior frequently seems to obey systematic ruled cognitive processing that can be analyzed using an IIT approach.

The IIT theoretical approach assumes that human behavior is functionally goal oriented. Take, for example, parents looking for useful information to help their children under special education or requiring institutional assistance whenever their expectations of their children's development are not met. The opposite also happens, that is, some parents abandon the idea of helping their children if their expectations are not achieved. In both cases, approaching helping behavior (positive connotation) or avoiding behavior (negative connotation), it is possible to observe the parents functional goal oriented behavior (expectations). This intentionality axiom allows quantification and empowers IIT to measure multi-causal mental processes previously considered inaccessible (e.g. emotions, moral judgment, etc., Anderson, 1982).

This multi-causal measurement approach visualizes humans as biological and psychological organisms that not only process different relevant pieces of information but ntegrates them in a systematic way. This idea is graphically illustrated in Figure 2 (Anderson, 1982).

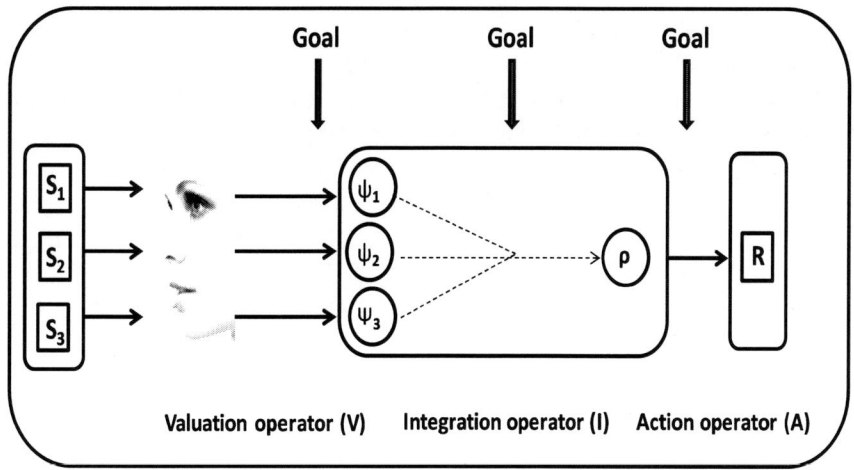

[Figure: diagram with S₁, S₂, S₃ → Valuation operator (V) → ψ₁, ψ₂, ψ₃ (Integration operator (I)) → ρ → R (Action operator (A)), with three "Goal" arrows above.]

Modified of Anderson, 1982.

Figure 2. Integration Information Theory diagram shows how relevant stimuli (S_i) are extracted from an environment and psychologically represented through a valuation process (V) with cognitive coefficients (ψ_i). All of these different variables will be systematically integrated (I) to form a unified implicit response (ρ) that will produce an explicit response (R) through an action operator (A). Note that all feed forward phase processing is mediated by a goal.

As we can observe from Figure 1, a person is considered to be submerged inside a sea of information variables (S_i). Then the person needs to select those most meaningful variables to evaluate them psychologically. After this valuation process has taken place (V), the psychological values (ψ_i) are systematically integrated (Integration operator I) throughout a cognitive rule in order to produce a unified psychological response (ρ). Then, this integration processing may lead to a transformed physical manifestation (R) by an action operator (A).

These cognitive concepts of valuation, integration and action can be used to understand and explore cognitive judgments to school inclusion. This is so since teachers, caregivers and parents related to ID frequently enroll themselves in decision making concerning their children's educational or clinical status. Take, for instance, a possible special education scenario where an imaginary child with ID named "Juan" has improved his behavior after he regularly attended a special education school and language proficiency courses. His parents think that he is now capable of attending a regular school program and they chose a nearby school for this purpose since they heard this school has a good reputation and flexible teachers. However, Juan´s psychologist believes he is not ready yet because he has some problems in controlling his sphincter and his personal care is not up to a normal standard. Moreover, the aforementioned school seems not to be ready to receive children with ID since their teachers have no experience on teaching children with special needs.

The above scenario is perfect to illustrate the IIT analytical capacity over possible cognitive processing (e.g. main character inferential processing, acceptability judgment, etc.) used to undertake a decision on school inclusion. The functional measurement graph from Figure 3 shows the different possible factors to be evaluated (by the psychologists and the parents) and systematically integrated them into a goal-oriented response (making a decision) to either accept or reject school inclusion.

Here, language proficiency, sphincter control, teachers´ experience, and other factors are the observable pieces of information (S_i). Then, these variables are psychologically valuated (valuation operator V; ψ_i) by the involved protagonists. It is important to mention that this valuation process depends on the person´s motivation to promote the child into the regular school program. By a systematic combination of valuated factors (integration operator; I) the parents and the psychologist converge to judgment formation (perhaps an implicit response ρ) that will be translated into an explicit response (R) through an action operation (A). In this case the explicit response implies to reject or promote Juan into a regular school program.

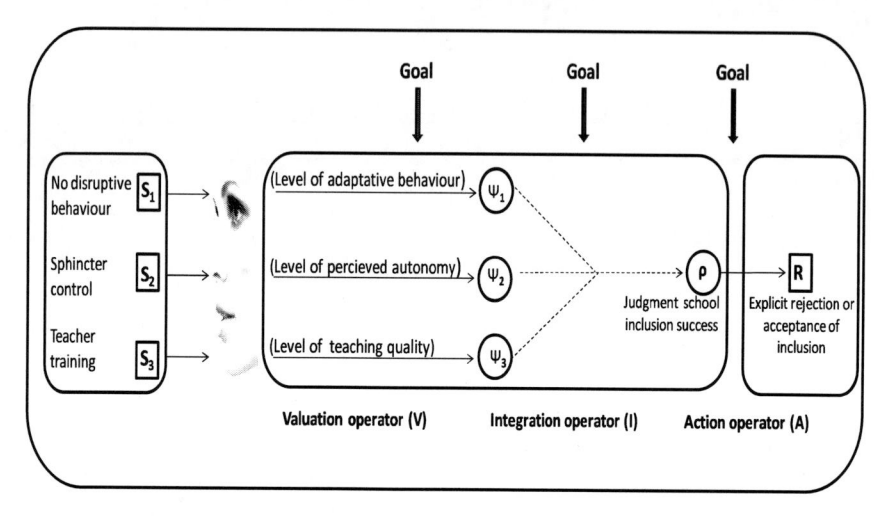

Figure 3. The diagram shows the IIT schema extrapolation over a school inclusion scenario. The feed forward diagram shows the three processes V-I-A going from observable pieces of information (S) up to an observable response (R).

The IIT approach allows us to translate all of the above systematic cognitive functioning into mathematical representations in such a way that a significant response depends on a mathematical rule integration of valuated factors. That is:

$$\rho = I(s_1, s_2, s_3)$$

where ρ is a response determined by an integration function (I) of observable factors (S_1, S_2, etc.). The graphic data pattern produced by the above function is an important element inside the IIT approach since it visually allows us to identify if an algebraic ruled behavior underlies cognitive judgment. According to Anderson (1991, 1996, 2008), visualization of IIT data patterns reveal integration schemas (additive, multiplicative or average) of non-observable cognitive processing (V-I-A) that leads to implicit and explicit responses (ρ - R). Thus, the cognitive algebraic behavior of a mental process reveals meaningful invariance through systematic information integration.

Overall, IIT methods to visual data patterns have empowered cognitive research to identify the universal principles of cognitive behavior through several cognitive domains (nomothetic approach). Also, this approach allows identification of this cognitive ruled behavior on a single case basis, that is, individual or personal analysis (idiographic approach).

The current empirical support seems to suggest that valuation processes are more of a personal matter whereas integration rules better describe general cognitive group behavior. Then, even when personal valuation may relate to cultural or social constraints, the integration rules apply to a variety of domains (see Anderson, 1982; Guillet, Hermand & Mullet, 2002).

Algebraic cognitive patterns can be identified through visual inspection of factorial design interaction graphs (Morales, 2012; Anderson, 1996; 2008). Typical patterns revealing systematic cognitive behavior are additive, multiplicative or average rules (Guedj, Muñoz-Sastre, Mullet & Sorum, 2009; Falconi & Mullet, 2003). Specifically, data patterns showing parallel lines in a factorial interaction graph reveal a summative rule whereas multiplicative cognitive ruling behavior is characterized by data forming a fan pattern of lines in an interaction graph. Average rules are characterized by crossover patterns (see Anderson, 1982, 1996; also see Neto & Mullet, 1998; Farkas, 1991; Guillet et al., 2002; Lazreg & Mullet, 2001).

A wide empirical data base providing evidence for these cognitive ruled behaviors has been obtained from IIT researchers on several behavior fields (Mullet, Morales, Makris, Rogé & Muñoz-Sastre, 2012, also e.g., love, Falconi & Mullet, 2003; sexuality, Esterle, Muñoz-Sastre & Mullet, 2008; Morales, Lopez, Esterle, Muñoz-Sastre & Mullet, 2010; medical concerns, Hervé, Mullet & Sorum, 2004, Frileux, Muñoz-Sastre & Antonini, 2004; Guedj, Gibert, Maudet, Muñoz-Sastre, Mullet & Sorum, 2005; Guedj et al., 2009; interpersonal relationships: Farkas, 1991; pleasure related to visual and auditory stimuli: Lazreg & Mullet, 2001; Makri & Mullet, 2003; Health: Hermand, Mullet & Lavieville, 1997; Muñoz-Sastre, Mullet, & Sorum, 1999; Simeone, Hermand & Mullet, 2002, bioethics, Mullet, Sorum, Teysseire, Nann, Morales Ahmed, Kamble, Olivari, & Munoz-Sastre, 2012), including no conscious cognitive processing.

Now, let us consider some remarks about IIT and attitudes toward ID. Some years ago the IIT approach was used to explore this topic regarding the general population (see Esterle et al., 2008; Morales et al., 2010) and over parents or caregivers´ judgment related to ID and sexuality (Morales, Lopez & Mullet, 2011). Moreover, additional seminal research on love and ID research (Morales, 2012) and blame and forgiveness (Morales & Lopez, in press) has been produced using an IIT approach. From this initial research it can be derived that other areas of research related to the way people perceive ID can provide valuable information by using this theoretical approach. This is the case for studying attitudes toward school inclusion and ID that is discussed next.

4.1. A General Overview of Attitudes and Judgments toward the Challenge of Including People with Intellectual Disabilities into Regular School Programs

Education is a fundamental right to all of us. However, compared to the general population, people with ID are significantly less likely to enroll in educational programs. This is so because school inclusion of this population into regular school programs demands a new school system. To achieve such a change it is necessary to have a renewed commitment from government institutions to carefully analyze academic findings in order to improve current educative laws and renew educational infrastructure settings (WHO, 2011).

Related to this, recently, educational systems of several countries have shown a more open position to embrace people with ID in their regular education programs. As a result of this change of view, there has been an increased interest in studying attitudes toward school inclusion (e.g., USA: Gao & Mager, 2011, Russia: Oreshkina, 2009, India: Raver, 2001). Mainly, this research enhances the understanding of the principal actors' attitudes regarding school inclusion (Gaad & Khan, 2007).

Because of this, a new field of research in special education has emerged regarding the study of the perception and attitudes toward regular school inclusion, and by different methods (qualitative and quantitative), instruments (e.g., see scales, Alahababi, 2009; Ross-Hill, 2009; questionnaires, Kalyva, Gojkovic & Tsakiris, 2007; interviews, Gaad, 2004) samples (special education teachers: Alahababi, 2009; regular school teacher, Mahat, 2008; parents of persons with ID, Waddington & Reed, 2006, students, Malinen & Savolainen, 2008) across several countries (e.g., EE. UU., Ross-Hill, 2009, Jordania, Al-Zyoudi, 2006; Serbia, Kalyva et al., 2007; Australia, Westwood, 2001; Pakistan, Fontana & Lari, 2001).

International research on attitudes toward inclusion of people with special education needs can vary throughout countries (Leyser, Kepperman & Keller, 1994) and samples (e.g., teachers: Ross-Hill, 2009; Kalyva et al., 2007). For example, in the USA Ross-Hill (2009) found that most teachers supported the inclusion practice in regular classrooms or they showed a neutral consensus as it relates to their teaching assignment. In contrast, a Serbian study Kalyva et al. (2007) found that teachers expressed slightly negative attitudes towards the inclusion of children with special education needs.

Furthermore, available evidence suggests that several contextual variables influence attitudes towards school inclusion (e.g., the teaching level, Leyser et al., 1994; the education system kind, Alahbabi, 2009). Moreover, it has been observed that particular teaching variables (e.g., teachers' beliefs, training and experience, Kalyva et al., 2007, Al-Zyoudi, 2006, Leyser et al., 1994) have a strong effect on the attitudes toward school inclusion. For instance, Kalyva et al. (2007) observed that Serbian teachers who had special education teaching experience were more open and had a positive attitude towards school inclusion compared to those teachers with no special education teaching experience. Another study from Jordania Al-Zyoudi (2006), observed that the teaching experience and teachers´ type of training of affected their attitudes towards inclusion. In the United Arab Emirats (Alahbabi, 2009) it was observed that the type of education system (regular or special) and the teaching grade (Kindergarten, elementary, high school and preparatory) also affected teachers´ attitudes.

It has been also observed that other factors, related to the nature of the disability, influence teachers' attitudes toward school inclusion (e.g., nature of disability, demographic variables, etc.). This is the case for Jordania where Al-Zyoudi (2006) reported that teachers´ attitudes towards ID school inclusion were strongly influenced by the type of disability and its severity. Convergent evidence reported by Cook (2001) showed that the teacher's expectations vary depending on the severity of the disability. Furthermore, Leyser et al. (1994) noticed that school inclusion criterions seem to be affected by sample factors such as demographic status. Complementing this evidence, Alahbabi (2009) reported that group membership seems have an effect on attitudes.

Overall, these findings are valuable information describing the type of attitudes, the acceptability level of acceptability, and factors that influence attitudes toward ID school inclusion. Now let us explore how people cognitively use or combine these attitude factors to elaborate acceptability judgments toward regular school inclusion and ID. In order to achieve this goal we will introduce the previously described IIT inside the field of school inclusion.

4.2. Cognitive Algebra and the Case of Attitudes toward School Inclusion and Intellectual Disability

In a typical IIT study, the experiment participants are presented with written scenarios that describe situations that are representative of their daily lives. That is IIT studies intend to capture the social aspect of the phenomena under study (multi-causal complexity) and because of this the IIT has some ecological validity. These experimental design-based scenarios consider that the cognitive task required of participants (e.g. make a judgment) may activate different cognitive processing levels (controlled, automatic, non-conscious, etc.), to induce or activate a different range of behavior (general principles - single case valuation) and evoke cognitive parallel processing of factors (multi-causal).

To download the above IIT remarks into the special education field let us consider school inclusion and ID. Here, institutional factors (e.g. political considerations, accessibility to services), contextual variables (e.g. group size, school grade, etc.), social interaction conditions (familiarity with ID groups, frequency of interaction, etc.), population characteristics (e.g. severity of disability) and personal variables (like personal belief on success) can be considered as factors framing special education teachers´ judgment and attitudes toward ID and school inclusion. An IIT model of a special education teacher considering school inclusion would visualize her/him as first evaluating accessible information factors about context, ID type, etc. Then she/he will systematically integrate this information to make a judgment to support or reject the possibility of including a person with ID into a regular school program. This probability of successfully school integration judgment is a direct result of a cognitive algebraic function combining relevant factors (e.g., Gender, type of disability, severity of disability, social environment, educational settings, etc.). That is, the Probability of Success Index (PSI) is a cognitive variable that linearly depends on the integration of contextual and personal factors, such that:

$$PSI= f(w_G \text{ Gender} * w_D \text{ Disability} * w_{Se} \text{ Severity} * w_{SE} \text{ Social Environment} * w_{SchE} \text{ School Environment}).$$

This equation implies a cognitive integration function that combines weighted (W_j) factors.

To illustrate the implication of the previous cognitive algebraic equation let us consider a pilot study that was carried by our cognitive science lab. Here, a sample of 30 special education teachers were required to read 32 cards, each describing in a few lines a brief story (vignette) about the process of integrating a student with ID or a physical disability (PD), into a regular school environment. Below each printed scenario, a question about the probability of success for achieving school integration was introduced. Then, below the question, a 10-point scale response with a left hand anchor label saying "Nothing successful" and as a right hand anchor label "Completely successful" was presented. For example:

Rosa has a mild intellectual disability. She has Down syndrome. Rosa´s family supports her. She lives in a very favorable social environment. This year she will be enrolled to attend regular school. The institution has trained professionals as well as devices and tools needed to provide an appropriate service to people as in the case of Rosa.

To what extent do you consider that Rosa´s regular school inclusion process will be successful?

Nothing o-----o-----o-----o-----o-----o-----o-----o-----o-----o Completely
Successful   successful

The 32 vignettes were designed by considering a 2x2x2x2x2 within subject factorial design. That is, Gender (Female/Male) x Severity of Disability (Low/High) x Kind of Disability (Physical: Neuromotor disability/Intellectual disability: Down syndrome) x Social Environment (Favorable/Unfavorable) x School Environment (with/without adaptation).

The obtained data was analyzed having in mind a cognitive algebra processing view. Remember that this approach assumes that if two or more factors are psychologically integrated by a mathematical rule then the interaction graph obtained from an experimental design visually shows systematic data organization in a two-dimensional space (Morales, 2012; Anderson, 1996, 2008). Then, a 2x2x2x2x2 within subjects ANOVA procedure was carried over the participant's raw data (see Table 1). Data analysis was carried on considering Gender x Disability x Severity x Social environment x School environment. This design was chosen after establishing that participants´ gender had no effect and it was not involved in any interaction term. The significance criterion was set at p <.001.

In general, as it can be observed from the table 1, participants showed a moderate perceived probability of success (M = 5.6) for school inclusion of persons with disabilities (either Intellectual or Physical). This perception was strongly influenced by the contribution of school environment (η^2_p = .86), social environment (η^2_p = .78), and the severity of the disability factor (η^2_p = .46). Here, contextual factors (School environment and Social environment) appeared to have higher weighting than individual factors (Severity of disability). Gender and type of disability showed no main effect. This means that participants considered the same probability of success to achieve school inclusion for men and women with ID or PD.

On the other hand, no significant interactions were observed among the most relevant factors by using the significance criterion p<.001 (see Table 1). The interaction graph data pattern suggests that participants integrate Severity, Social Environment and School Environment through using an additive cognitive algebraic rule. This can be observed from data performance shown in Figure 4.

These contextual factors (school environment and social environment) seemed to be more relevant for school inclusion than individual factors (disability kind and disability severity). This finding was interesting since this information could be used as an indicator of locus of control mechanisms inside a school inclusion process.

This is important if we consider that now we can measure perceived locus of control changes throughout time in persons related to ID education. Specifically, we would be able to have an index describing how expectations of professors, parents, etc. change whenever environmental school factors can or cannot be controlled.

Table 1. ANOVA for attitudes toward school inclusion study

Source	df	MS	df	MS	F	p	η^2
Gender (G)	1	0.01	29	2.76	0.006	ns	.0002
Disability (D)	1	9.60	29	4.67	2.05	ns	.06
Severity (S)	1	207.20	29	8.40	24.64	0.001	.46
Social environment (SE)	1	1450.41	29	13.56	106.95	0.001	.78
School environment (ScE)	1	2362.53	29	12.89	183.24	0.001	.86
G*D	1	6.33	29	1.52	4.14	ns	.12
G*S	1	3.26	29	1.37	2.37	ns	.07
D*S	1	1.06	29	2.18	0.48	ns	.01
G*SE	1	3.50	29	2.131	1.64	ns	.05
D*SE	1	2.60	29	3.77	0.69	ns	.02
S*SE	1	8.06	29	1.90	4.22	ns	.12
G*ScE	1	1.06	29	2.36	0.45	*ns*	.01
D*ScE	1	2.39	29	1.67	1.43	*ns*	.04
S*ScE	1	8.43	29	1.75	4.82	*ns*	.14
SE*ScE	1	4.26	29	1.76	2.42	ns	.07

Thus the Probability of Success Index of (PSI) is a linear function (summative) of combining weighted factors as follows:

PSI = $f(w_{SchE}$ School environment + w_{SE} Social environment + w_{SevE} Severity)

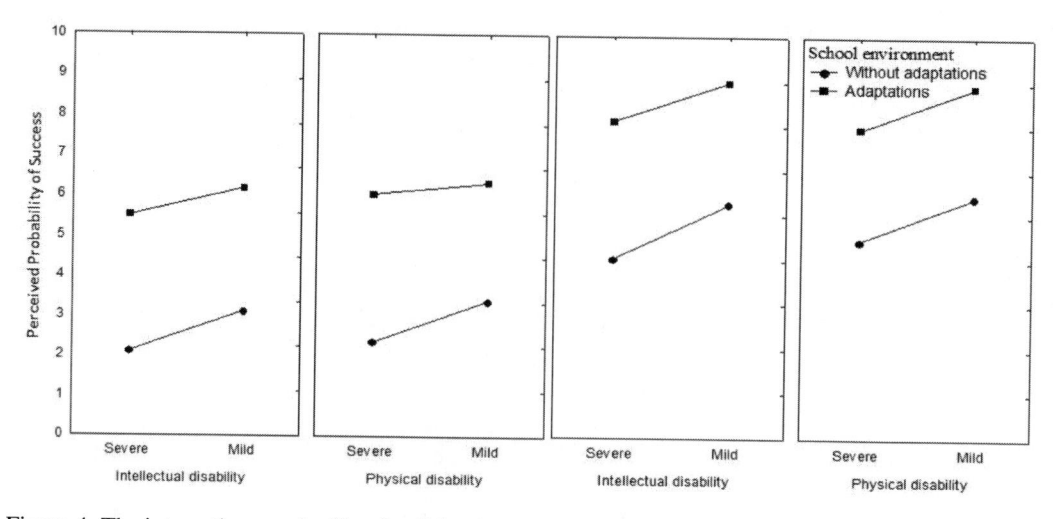

Figure 4. The interaction graph effect for School environment, Disability Level, Kind of Disability, and Social environment having perceived probability of success judgments of school inclusion as the dependent variable.

Considering these results, another study was designed to explore in more detail how factors related to school environment affect the perceived probability to achieve a successful inclusion process. As in the first study, the objective of the experiment was to estimate factor weights from participants' performance as well as to determine the information integration cognitive rule underlying the perceived probability of success judgment (PSI), such that:

$$PSI = f(w_G \text{ Gender} * w_{Se} \text{ Severity} * w_{SL} * \text{ School level} * w_{TE} \text{ Teaching experience})$$

In this study 104 special education students were required to read 36 cards, each describing a short story of a school inclusion process of one young person with ID (vignette). At the end of each scenario a question appeared requiring the participant´s probability of success judgment to the described situation. Below the scenario question, a 10-point response scale having a "No successful" left hand anchor and a "Completely successful" as a right hand anchor was presented. For example:

Maria has an intellectual disability. She has mild mental retardation. Now, she is enrolled in a special education institute. In short time, she will be attending kindergarten with a regular school program. Although, the future Maria´s teacher is trained to attend students with a disability, Rosa will be her first student with intellectual disability.

To what extent do you consider that Maria´s regular school inclusion process will be successful?

Nothing o-----o-----o-----o-----o-----o------o-----o-----o *Completely*
Successful   *successful*

Again, the 36 vignettes were obtained having in mind a repeated measure factorial design that combined four factor levels (2x3x3x2). That is, Gender (Female/Male) x Severity of Disability (mild/moderate/severe) x Social Level (Kindergarten/Primary/High school) x Teaching Experience (with experience/without experience). Then, an ANOVA 2x3x3x2 was carried over the participant's raw data (see Table 2). Data analysis was carried on by considering Gender x Severity x School level x Teaching experience. This design was chosen after establishing that participants´ Gender had no significant effect and was not involved in any interaction term. The significance criterion was set at p <.001.

Results indicated a high perceived probability of success (M = 6.8) to achieve regular school inclusion of persons with intellectual disabilities. This perception was strongly regulated by the contribution of teaching experience (η^2_p =0.73), severity of the disability factor (η^2_p = 0.66) and school level (η^2_p = 0.17) as it can be seen from Table 2. It is clearly observed that factors related to school environment (teaching experience and school level) and individual factors (severity of disability) contribute in a relevant way to the school inclusion prognostic provided by participants to each case.

Table 2. ANOVA for study of attitude toward school inclusion considering school factors

Source	df	MS	df	MS	F	p	η^2
Gender (G)	1	0.006	103	0.74	0.009	0.92	0.00008
Severity (S)	2	1033.54	206	5.1	202.68	0.001	0.66
School Level (SL)	2	66.14	206	3.0	22.32	0.001	0.17
Teaching experience (TE)	1	81.55	103	11.0	281.55	0.001	0.73
G*S	2	0.13	206	0.9	0.15	ns	0.001
G*SL	2	2.32	206	0.8	2.93	ns	0.02
S*SL	4	1.07	412	1.12	0.95	ns	0.009
G*TE	1	0.5	103	0.8	0.64	ns	0.006
S*TE	2	4.68	206	1.845	2.54	ns	0.024
SL*TE	2	0.46	206	1.1	0.42	ns	0.00

Moreover, participants showed a higher perceived probability of success index when a teacher had experience (M = 7.74) compared to a teacher that has no real teaching experience even if he was theoretically trained (M = 5.918). Furthermore, prediction of success varied according to the severity of disability: Mild disability M= 7.67, Moderate disability M= 6.94 and Severe Disability M= 5.86.

There was a slight school level effect over the judgments of perceived success. Specifically, it was observed that whenever the school year was more basic, the study participants perceived more chances for a successful school inclusion of a person with ID (M = 7.07 for kindergarten, versus 6.78 for primary school and 6.62 for high school). As in the first study, Gender tested as non-significant. This means that participants consider the same probability of success for school inclusion for men and women with ID. No significant interaction was observed among the most relevant factors considering a criterion of p<.001. This implies that participants integrated Teaching experience, Severity of disability and School Level factors in an additive way. It can be observed from Figure 5, once more that the perceived Probability of Success Index (PSI) is a summative linear function such that:

$$PSI = f(w_{TE} \text{ Teaching experience} + w_{SD} \text{ Severity of disability} + w_{SL} \text{ School level}).$$

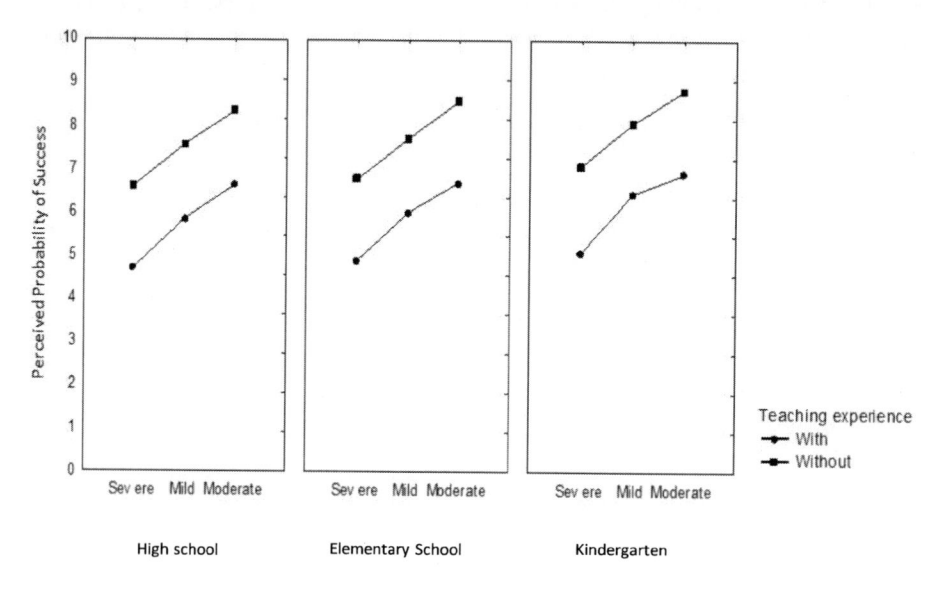

Figure 5. The graph shows the obtained interaction effect among the teaching experience, Disability Level, School level over perceived success of probability judgments.

Overall, participants showed an optimistic view regarding the possibility of successful school inclusion of ID cases. Here, three factors were considered to be essential in achieving a successful inclusion process (teaching experience, severity disability and school level). The teaching experience emerged as the more relevant factor. This perception was dependent on an additive combination of the most relevant study factors (school environment, social environment and severity of disability).

A more thoroughly analysis of these results allows two concluding remarks. First, the study data analysis revealed that participants had a moderate perceived success of probable school inclusion of persons with any kind of disability (physical or intellectual). Second, in both studies, participants' judgments were based on cognitive integration rules where relevant factors were combined using a cognitive additive rule. It would be interesting to observe if this rule, as well as the valuation of factors, can be maintained through samples of another nature (e.g., psychologist with experience in regular school integration, special education teachers, etc.). In fact, in two new studies, special education teachers provided similar results regarding the use of cognitive rules, although variations in factor valuation were observed (see Morales, Bautista, Charles & Lopez, 2012). More research including the experience factor is needed to explore these differences.

4.3. Concluding Remarks on Studying School Inclusion and ID from an Integration Information Theory Approach.

Anderson´s idea about the mathematical nature of our cognitive mind can be useful for exploring several fields inside ID and in any other kind of disability. Due to its methodlogical flexibility and ecological considerations the IIT approach seems to be very suitable to explore ID topics as it has been previously shown.

Moreover, information about cognitive integration rules not only allows one to make behavioral predictions but to put under academic scrutiny how people may vary their perceptions about ID whenever some factors related to this population are not considered or missing.

Different uses of this approach can be currently observed inside the ID field. For instance, Morales et al. (2010, 2011) carried on an IIT comparative study on how a French sample and a Mexican sample perceived sexuality among ID persons. Valuation processes as well as integration rules could be obtained to typify systematic cognitive behavior to both samples. Another study (only in a Mexican sample) showed that is possible to typify differences inside the same culture. Here, even when the same integration rule can be observed to judge sexuality and ID, the valuation process varied depending on the group a person belongs (caregiver, teacher, etc.). Other area to apply IIT research could be labor inclusion and ID, for example initial and exploratory research in this field from the present authors suggests that common people and students of special education perceive people with ID as having more probability of success if they get enrolled in artistic or manual activities than if they are involved in public services or technology. Indeed, in the Mexican society most special programs favor craft abilities, carpentry, etc.

As a final concluding remark on IIT and ID we would like to emphasize the empowerment offered by a deeper analysis of cognitive systematic behavior underlying perceptions and attitudes of vulnerable populations. Academic scrutiny in this direction will lead to better life conditions for this population and academic guidance can be provided to require modifications to institutions whenever school inclusion and ID are to be considered.

REFERENCES

Alahbabi, A. (2009). K-12 Special and general education teacher´s attitudes toward the inclusion of students with special needs in general education classes in the United Arab Emirates (UAE). *International Journal of Special Education, 24*(2), 42-54.

Al-Zyoudi, M. (2006). Teachers' attitudes towards inclusive education in Jordanian schools. *International Journal of Special Education, 21*(2), 55-62.

Anderson, N. H. (1982). *Methods of information integration theory.* New York: Academic Press.

Anderson, N. H. (1991). *Contributions to information integration theory.* Hillsdale, NJ: Erlbaum.

Anderson, N. H. (1996). *A functional theory of cognition.* Mahwah, NJ: Erlbaum.

Anderson, N. H. (2008). *Unified social cognition.* USA: Taylor & Francis Group, L.L.

Banaji, M. R., & Bhaskar, R. (2000). Implicit stereotypes and memory: The bounded rationality of social beliefs. In D. L. Schacter & E. Scarry (Eds.), *Memory, brain, and belief* (pp. 139-175). Cambridge, MA: Harvard University Press

Barriga, S. (1998). *Psicología Social* [Social psychology] Ed. Mc GrawHill. España.

Biasini, F. J., Grupe, L., Huffman, L., & Bray, N. W. (1999). Mental retardation: A symptom and a syndrome. In S. D. Netherton & D. Holmes (Eds.), *Child and adolescent psychological disorders: A comprehensive textbook* (pp. 6-23). New York: Oxford University.

Binet, A. & Simon, T. (1904a). Méthodes nouvelles pour le diagnostic du niveau intellectuel des anormaux [Electronic version]. *L'année psychologique. 11*, 191-244.doi : 10.3406/psy.1904.3675. Retrieved November 20, 2012, from http://www.persee.fr/web/revues/home/prescript/article/psy_0003-5033_1904_num_11_1_3675

Binet, A. & Simon, T. (1904b).Application des méthodes nouvelles au diagnostic du niveau intellectuel chez des enfants normaux et anormaux d'hospice et d'école primair [Electronic version]. *L'année psychologique. 11*, 245-336. doi : 10.3406/psy.1904.3676. Retrieved November 20, 2012, from http://www.persee.fr/web/revues/home /prescript /article/psy_0003-5033_1904_num_11_1_3676

Binet, A. & Simon, T. (1905, April 28). New Methods for Diagnosing Idiocy, Imbecility, and Moron Status. Paper presented in the International Congress of Psychology in Rome.

Cook, B. (2001). A comparison of teachers' attitudes toward their included students with mild and severe disabilities. *Journal of Special Education, 34*(4), 203-213.

Corrigan, P. & Watson, A. M. (2002). Understanding the impact of stigma on people with mental illness. *World Psychiatry,* 1(1), 16–20.

Corrigan, P. W. (2000). Mental health stigma a social attribution: Implications for research methods and attitude change. *Clinical PsychologySciencePractice,*7(1), 48–67. doi: 10.1093/clipsy.7.1.48

Esterle, M., Muñoz-Sastre, M. T., & Mullet, E. (2008). Judging the acceptability of sexual intercourse among persons with learning disabilities: French lay people's viewpoint. *Sexuality & Disability, 26*(4), 219-227. doi: 10.1007/s11195-008-9093-9.

Falconi, A. & Mullet, E. (2003). Cognitive algebra of love through the adult life. *The International Journal of Aging & Human Development, 57*(3), 275-290. doi: 10.2190/NPQH-MDLX-F48U-AA35

Farkas, A. J. (1991). Cognitive algebra of interpersonal relationship. In N. H. Anderson (Ed.), *Contributions to information integration theory* (Vol. 2, pp. 43-99). Hillsdale, NJ: Erlbaum.

Fazio, R. H. (1995). Attitudes as object-evaluation associations: Determinants, consequences, and correlates of attitude accessibility. En R. E. Petty & J. A. Krosnick (Eds.), *Attitude strength: Antecedents and consequences* (pp. 247–282). Hillsdale, NJ: Erlbaum.

Florez, G. M. A., Aguado, D. A. L. & Alcedo, R. M. A. (2009). A review and analysis of programmes promoting changes in attitudes towards people with intellectual disability. *Annuary of Clinical and Health Psychology, 5*, 81-94.

Fontana, D. & Lari, Z. (2001). The Curriculum in Special Needs Education in Pakistani schools. *International Journal of Special Education, 16*(1), 21-41.

Frileux, S., Muñoz-Sastre, M. & Antonini, A, S. (2004). Acceptability for French people of physician-assisted suicide. *Death Studies, 28*(10), 941-53. doi:10.1080/ 07481180490512028

Gaad, E. & Khan, L. (2007). Primary mainstream teacher´s attitudes towards inclusion of students with special education needs in the private sector: A perspective from Dubai. *International Journal of Special Education, 22*(2), 95-109.

Gaad, E. (2004). Cross-cultural perspectives on the effect of cultural attitudes towards inclusion for children with intellectual disabilities. *International Journal of Inclusive Education, 8*(3), 311-328, 18. doi: 10.1080/13603110420000194645.

Gao, W. & Mager, G. (2011). Enhancing preservice teachers' sense of efficacy and attitudes toward school diversity through preparation: a case of one U.S. Inclusive teacher education program. *International Journal of Special Education, 26*(2), 92-107.

Goddard, H. H. (1912). *The Kallikak family: A study in the heredity of feeble-mindedness.* New York: Macmillan. [Electronic version]. Retrieved November 20, 2012, from http://digitalarchive.gsu.edu/col_facpub/7

Greenwald, A. G., Rudman, L. A., Nosek, B. A., Banaji, M. R., Farnham, S. D. & Mellott, D. S. (2002). A Unified Theory of Implicit Attitudes, Stereotypes, Self-Esteem, and Self-Concept. *Psychological Review, 109*(1), 3–25.

Greenwald, A., Nosek, B. & Banaji, M. (2003). Understanding and using the implicit association test: I. An improved scoring algorithm. *Journal of Personality and Social Psychology, 85*(2), 197-216.

Guedj, M., Gibert, M., Maudet, M., Muñoz-Sastre, M. T., Mullet, E. & Sorum, P. C. (2005). The acceptability of ending a patient´s life. *J. Med. Ethics, 31*(6), 311-317.

Guedj, M., Muñoz-Sastre, M. T., Mullet, E. & Sorum, P. C. (2009). Is it acceptable for a psychiatrist to break confidentiality to prevent spousal violence? *International Journal of Law and Psychiatry, 32* (2), 108–114.

Guillet, L., Hermand, D. & Mullet, E. (2002). Cognitive processes involved in the appraisal of stress. *Stress and Health, 18*(2), 91–102.

Hahn, H. (1985). Disability policy and the problem of discrimination. *American Behavioral Scientist, 28*(3), 293 – 318.

Harris J. C. (2006). *Intellectual disability: understanding its development, causes, classification, evaluation, and treatment.* New York: Oxford University Press.

Hawking, S. (2011). Prologue. In World Health Organization: WHO (2011). *World report on disability.* Retrieved November 20, 2012, from http://www.who.int/disabilities/ world_report/2011/en/

Hermand, D., Mullet, E., & Lavieville, S. (1997). Perception of the combined effects of smoking and alcohol on cancer risks in never smokers and heavy smokers. *Journal of Health Psychology, 2*(4), 481–491.

Hernandez, B., Keys, C., & Balcazar, F. (2000). Employer attitudes toward workers with disabilities and their ADA employment rights: A Literature Review. *Journal of Rehabilitation, 66*(4) 4-16.

Hervé, C., Mullet, E., & Sorum, P. C. (2004). Age and medication acceptance. *Experimental Againg Research, 30*(3), 253-273.

Itard, J. M. G. (1801 et 1806). Mémoire et Rapport sur Victor de l'Aveyron (1801 et 1806) [Electronic version by Palpant, P.]. In Collection « Les auteur(e)s classiques » Paris: Bibliothèque 10-18. Retrieved November 20, 2012, from http://classiques.uqac.ca/classiques/itard_jean/victor_de_l_Aveyron/itard_victor_aveyron.pdf

Kalyva, E., Gojkovic, D. & Tsakiris, V. (2007). Serbian teachers' attitudes towards inclusion. *International Journal of Special Education, 22*(3), 31-35.

Lazreg, C. K. & Mullet, E. (2001). Judging the pleasantness of form–color combinations. *The American Journal of Psychology, 114*(4), 511–533.

Leyser, Y., Kepperman, G., & Keller, R. (1994). Teacher attitudes toward s mainstreaming: A cross-cultural study in six nations. *European Journal of Special Needs Education, 98*(1), 1-15.

Locke, J. (1690). *An essay concerning: Human understanding* (25th Ed). London: Thomas Tegg. Retrieved November 20, 2012, from http://archive.org/details/ human under standi00lockuoft

Mahat, M. (2008). The development of a psychometrically-sound instrument to measure teachers' multidimensional attitudes toward inclusive education. *International Journal of Special Education, 23*(1), 82-92.

Makri, I. & Mullet, E. (2003). Judging the pleasantness of contour–rhythm–pitch–timbre musical combinations. *The American Journal of Psychology, 116*(4), 581-611

Malinen, O. & Savolainen, H. (2008). Inclusion in the east: chinese students' attitudes towards inclusive education. *International Journal of Special Education, 23*(3), 101-109.

Morales, G. E. & Lopez, E. O. (in press). *Down syndrome, beyond the intellectual disability: persons with their own emotional world.* Nova Publisher.

Morales, G. E. (2012). Functional measurement to cognitive mechanisms underlying attitudes toward sexuality and intellectual disability: New empirical directions. In Nicholas E. Peterson & Whitney Campbell (Eds.), *Sexuality: Perspectives, Issues and Role in Society* (pp. 29- 54). N.Y. USA: Nova Science Publishers, Inc.

Morales, G. E., Bautista, A. K., Charles, D. J. & Lopez, E. O. (2012). *Cognitive algebra as a new measurement perspective on the special education teacher´s attitudes toward regular school inclusion of persons with intellectual disability.* Unpublished manuscript.

Morales, G. E., Lopez, E. O. & Mullet, E. (2011). Acceptability of sexual relationships among people with learning disabilities: family and professional caregivers´ views in Mexico. *Sexuality and Disability Journal, 29*(2), 165-174.

Morales, M. G. E., López, R. E. O., Esterle, M., Muñoz Sastre, M. T. & Mullet, E. (2010). Judging the acceptability of sexual intercourse among people with learning disabilities: A Mexico-France comparison. *Sexuality and Disability Journal, 28*(2), 81-91.

Mullet, E., Morales M. G. E., Makris, I., Rogé, B. & Munoz-Sastre, M. (2012). Functional Measurement: An Incredibly Flexible Tool. *Psicologica, 33*, 631-654.

Mullet, E., Sorum, P. C., Teysseire, N. Nann, S., Morales M. G. E., Ahmed, R., Kamble, S., Olivari, C. & Munoz-Sastre, M. (2012). Functional Measurement in the Ficld of Empirical Bioethics. *Psicologica, 33*, 665-681.

Muñoz-Sastre, M.T., Mullet, E., & Sorum, P.C. (1999). Relationship between cigarette dose and perceived risk of lung cancer. *Preventive Medicine, 28*(6), 566–571.

National Dissemination Center for Children with Disabilities(2010). *Discapacidades Intelectuales* [Intellectual disabilities]. Retrieved November 20, 2012, from http://nichcy.org/wp-content/uploads/docs/spanish/fs8sp.pdf

Neto, F., & Mullet, E. (1998). Decision making as regards migration: Wage differential, job opportunities and the network effect. *Acta Psychologica, 98*(1), 57-66.

North Dakota Center for Persons with Disabilities (2009). *Mythbusters disability datebook: disability historical accomplishments.* Retrieved November 20, 2012, from http://www.ndcpd.org/resources/perceptions/2010%20disability%20final.pdf

Oreseshkina, M. (2009). Education of children with disabilities in Russia: on the way to integration and inclusion. *International Journal of Special Education, 24*(3), 110-120.

Oskamp, S., & Schultz, W. (2005). *Attitude and opinions* (3a. Ed.). New Jersey: Lawrence Erlbaum Associates, Publishers.

Ottaway, S. A., Hayden, D. C., & Oakes, M. A. (2001). Implicit attitudes and racism: Effects of word familiarity and frequency on the Implicit Association Test. *Social Cognition, 19*(2), 97-144.

Pineda, P. (n/d). *Pablo Pineda concienciando sobre el síndrome de Down. Parte II* [Make aware on Down syndrome. Part II][Video file]. Retrieved November 20, 2012, from http://www.youtube.com/watch?v=zTFT2jibkEo&feature=relmfu

Petty, R.E. & Briñol, P. (2010). Attitude structure and change: Implications for implicit measures. In: Bertram Gawrosky & B. Keith Payne (Eds.), *Social cognition: Measurement, theory, and applications.* New York: Guilford Press.

Radford, J. P. (1991). Sterilization versus segregation: Control of the 'feebleminded', 1900-1938. *Social Science and Medicine, 33*(4), 449-458.

Raver, S. A. (2001). India: training teachers for children with Mental retardation. *International Journal of Special Education, 16*(1), 54-67.

Ross-Hill, R. (2009). Teacher attitude towards inclusion practices and special needs students. *Journal of Research in Special Educational Needs, 9*(3), 188–198.

Scruggs, T. E. & Mastropieri, M. A. (1996). Teacher perceptions of mainstreaming/inclusion 1958-1995: A research synthesis. *Exceptional Children, 63*(1), 59-74.

Schleichkorn, J. (1981). Deinstitutionalization and Normalization of Persons with Mental Retardation: The Role of a Physical Therapist in Community Placement. *Journal of the American Physical Therapy Association. 61*(10), 1438-1441.

Seguin, E. (1866). *Idiocy: and its treatment by the physiological method.* New York: W. Wood & co. Retrieved November 20, 2012, from Ebook and Texts ArchiveCornell University Library http://archive.org/details/cu31924012161810

Sheerenberger, R. C. (1983). *A history of mental retardation.* Baltimore: Brookes Publishing Co.

Simeone, A., Hermand, D., & Mullet, E. (2002). Judging the probability to be infected through sexual contact. Risk: Health, Safety and Environment, (in press).

Waddington, E. M. & Reed, P. (2006). Parents' and local education authority officers' perceptions of the factors affecting the success of inclusion of pupils with autistic spectrum disorders. *International Journal of Special Education, 21*(3), 151-164.

Westwood, P. S. (2001). Making special schools ordinary: is this inspirational or confused thinking? *International Journal of Special Education, 16*(1), 7-21.

World Health Organization (2001). *International classification of functioning, disability, and health (ICF).* Geneva: Author. Retrieved November 20, 2012, from http://www.disabilitaincifre.it/documenti/ICF_18.pdf

World Health Organization (2011). *World report on disability.* Retrieved November 20, 2012, from http://www.who.int/disabilities/world_report/2011/en/.

In: Caregivers: Challenges, Practices and Cultural Influences ISBN: 978-1-62618-030-7
Editors: Adrianna Thurgood and Kasha Schuldt © 2013 Nova Science Publishers, Inc.

Chapter 5

THE EXPERIENCE OF CAREGIVING ACROSS MYTHS AND CULTURES

Camilla Pietrantonio,[1] Francesco Pagnini,[1,2] Paolo Banfi,[3] Gianluca Castelnuovo[1,4] and Enrico Molinari[1,4]

[1]Department of Psychology, Catholic University of Milan, Milan, Italy
[2]Niguarda Ca' Granda Hospital, Milan, Italy
[3]Department of Neuromuscular Disease,
Fondazione Don Gnocchi, Milan, Italy
[4]Istituto Auxologico Italiano Istituto di Ricovero e Cura a Carattere Scientifico (IRCCS),
Psychology Research Laboratory, San Giuseppe Hospital, Verbania, Italy

ABSTRACT

The person who gives care, the caregiver, must be aware of the disease, should be taught by qualified staff about strategies and optimal techniques to be applied on behalf of the care receiver to deal with the difficulties of everyday life.

The vast literature on the subject has now shown that caregiving cannot be reduced to a simple phenomenon that is attuned only to the fulfillment of a patient's needs. The question of assistance is very complex because it involves many aspects of health and the level of support necessary to the individual in need, but also to the organization of social care, to the policies that manage and ensure its delivery. The notion of assistance regards all those cultural elements and values that relate to field of ethics, justice and social equality, individual well-being and community.

Culture gives meaning to the events that occur in our lives, by ascribing to each one different values and emotions so the importance of cultural influences is essential in caregiving too. A broad range of literature has investigated the relationship among the characteristics of caregivers' culture, the role of the emotions and the mode of action of caregivers.

In the present and, even more so, in the future, it appears that daily confrontation with illness, disability, non-self-sufficiency will be a continuing challenge to our civilization, social welfare systems and health systems so a new vision of the "economy of care" is warranted.

"Real generosity dispenses more aid than recommendations."

Gustave Flaubert

1. FROM THE MYTH OF CURA TO THE FIGURE OF CAREGIVER

Once, when *Cura* (a Roman divinity whose name means "Care") was crossing a river, she picked up a bit of muddy clay and began to give it a form. Then she saw Jupiter and asked him to instill spirit into this clay form. Jupiter agreed. But when the goddess wanted to give her name to it, Jupiter objected and insisted that it be given his name instead. While the two gods quarreled, Tellus (goddess of Earth) intervened, demanding that the form be given her name. The disputants chose Saturn as judge, who announced his decision: "Jove, you will receive the spirit at death. Tellus, you will receive the body at death because you gave your own body for its creation. But Cura, who first gave shape to it, will care for this being during its life. To settle the dispute, Saturn called the creature homo because it was made from humus" [Igino, C.G., 1933].

Cura struggled to keep her creatures alive while the other gods, since they could not destroy what time had established, decided that half of the beings would be enough for Cura, while they took charge of the other half. Thus *homo* was divided into two parts: male and female. From that time on, Cura stopped following the follies of the other gods; where they wanted to divide, she wove relationships; where they created injuries, she took care of the wounded, and for every death, she brought forth a new life.

The myth of *Cura* emphasizes three aspects: humans are born from the earth and thus express its fragility; human transience rises with the survival of the soul after death; and humans need care for the duration of life.

This myth shows our human vulnerability: we need to be supported by care and need a prompt and constant presence in our personal lives and in our community. The relational structure of a person allows us to define ourselves as "human" through the ability to take care of someone or something. Caring becomes a way of being in the world. In the same way that the mythological figure of Cura shaped humans with tenderness, devotion and feeling, and assumed the burden of responsibility, staying with the person throughout life, so these dimensions have become integral to the definition of the human being.From myth to reality, care is a matter of great importance in the lives of human beings.

Today, the person who gives care, is literally called "caregiver": someone who continuously attends to the needs of a person who is not self-sufficient. The caregiver may be a relative or someone close, who looks after the sick or disabled person at home, or in other structures. One who takes on this role must be aware of the disease, should be taught by qualified staff about strategies and optimal techniques to be applied on behalf of the care receiver in order to deal with the difficulties of everyday life.

1.1. The New Approach to Disease and Caregiving

The need for a "helper" role arises from the search for support when a family member is faced with disease or disability. The occurrence of disease is always an event fraught with emotion that obliges us to redefine our future prospects , our relations with others, how we "make sense" of what is happening, and often leads to the necessity of accepting the support and help of someone. The description/meaning of illness brings into play several aspects, including the relationship between the human being and nature, with oneself and with others. Physicians and care professionals must be aware of the variability of the situation, using an idiographic approach [Pagnini, Gibbons and Castelnuovo, 2012].

Today the concept of disease is changing, and there is increasing focus on the patient as a person in his totality. Given this new focus, the role of caregiver is becoming more important.

An key aspect of this new approach has been brought to light by the observations of Kleinman (1980) who points out a fundamental distinction between the two English words: *disease* and *illness*. In this distinction *disease* means illness understood in biomedical terms, such as organic lesion or aggression of external agents, an event that is defined and measured through a series of organic parameters of physical or chemical nature; whereas *illness*, in contrast, is understood as the subjective experience of being ill that is experienced by the person and culturally mediated. In addition to these two terms, he also introduced the concept of *sickness* indicating a disorder in its general meaning in a population, in relation to macro-forces such as economic, political, institutional [Kleinman, A., 1980].

This new approach has been accompanied by an increasing attention to the concept of Quality of Life (QoL). According to the World Health Organization, this is defined as *"an individual's perception of his/her position in life in the context of the culture and value systems in which he/she lives, and in relation to his/her goals, expectations, standards and concerns. It is a broad-ranging concept, incorporating in a complex way the person's physical health, psychological state, level of independence, social relationships, and their relationship to salient features of their environment"* [The WHOQoL Group, 1994]. For some authors [Apolone, Ballatori, Mosconi and Roila 1997], the QoL concept covers a broad spectrum, which can be modified in a complex way by the perception of their health in bio-psycho-social terms, by the level of independence and by social interaction with their specific environment.

This new vision of the sick person has led to several changes in approach: first, to the idea of disease itself; second to the person with a disease, and third, to the care and rescue procedures. The United Nations Convention on the rights of persons with disabilities, starting from this concept, has established as *"States Parties to this Convention recognize the equal right of all persons with disabilities to live in the community, with choices equal of others, and they adopt proceedings adequate and appropriate to facilitate full enjoyment by persons with disabilities of this right and their full inclusion and participation in society "*[1].

---

[1] On 19 December 2001, when the work on the elaboration of an international document officially started, the General Assembly, at the request of the Commission on Human Rights and Social Development, in Resolution 56/168, established the "Ad hoc Committe ". It consists of about half of the 191 UN members, representing all continents, of different ethnic, religious and political inspiration.
Also members without the right to vote as the Vatican State, the European Commission, the Arab League, ONU, World Health Organization (WHO), the World Bank and the International Labour Organization (ILO) participate with full rights.
From 2001 to 2006, there were eight sessions of the "Ad Hoc Committee", during which they discussed the issues on individual articles and some other problems. An innovative aspect that characterized the birth of the Convention is the presence of civil society: the United States requested the participation of the "experts" on disability policies, that is, persons with disabilities. It is an unprecedented event that representatives of civil society (through organizations and associations of persons with disabilities) are be recognized as full members of a Committee of the General Assembly.

This definition helps us to deal with disability and illness according to all the factors, thus overcoming the strictly medical approach that normally marks the policies regarding people with disabilities and inevitably, their families.

The need for this approach was also emphasized by the introduction in 2001 of the International Classification of Functioning, Disability and Health (ICF), by the World Health Organization, which requires a methodology for analysis and identification the person with disabilities aimed at building a profile of functioning based on the bio-psycho-social model [Engel, G., 1977]. This approach has focuses on the sick person as the center of a system and an environment in which different exogenous variables affect the condition of the patient.

The recognition of the dignity of every person must be the starting point and reference for a society that defends the value of equality and for a society that makes a commitment to the principle that illness and disability do not constitute criteria for social discrimination.The problem does not lie in cancelling the difference or the limitations, but in recognizing the potential for expansion and enrichment of the quality of life.

2. PRACTICES AND CHALLENGES OF CAREGIVERS

The onset of disease is marked by moments of potential difficulty concerning the first communication of the diagnosis, the impact with the health care and medical staff, and the uncertainty of the diagnosis. In this period, hopes and fears can alternate, and there might be a search for experimental therapies. The relationship with the body and dignity are both "wounded" and the sudden imbalance arises in personal and family life as well as in social and economic terms. Other factors and critical moments can be identified in the continuation of the disease, in the process of communication between doctors and recipients of care, regarding the body that changes, in relationship problems. The family especially faces a change of dynamics that governed the family unit up to that point. The social and economic problems that they may have to face during the disease are numerous:, making choices in determining the course of treatment, during the end of life, and in the process of mourning after death.

In the presence of disease, it is essential that the person recognizes his or her condition and agrees to take charge, but it is also necessary that the caregiver teach the patient how to do it, by promoting *"empowerment"* [Aujoulat, I., Deccache, A., 2002] and increasing the capacity to make choices and transform those choices into desired actions and outcomes. Empowerment is a multi-dimensional social process that helps people gain control over their own lives. It is a process that fosters power in people for use in their own lives, their communities and in their society, by acting on issues they define as important.

Central to empowerment arc actions that build individual and collective assets, and improve the efficiency and fairness of the organizational and institutional context which govern the use of these assets.

Between patients and caregivers it is important to establish an effective *partnership*, based on good therapeutic training that establishes the precise division of tasks and areas of responsibility of each.

2.1. The Role of the Caregiver and Regulatory Protection

It is up to the caregiver to provide proper and dignified management of the assisted person, respecting that person's wishes. In addition the caregiver must make proper use of benefits in compliance with regulations and maintain a relationship with institutional services and to provide, at different levels of intensity, for all the daily needs of the patient (personal hygiene, nutrition, health care...).

Good communication in the patient's family helps to avoid many problems or at least, help to deal with them with greater confidence [Watzlawick, P., Beavin, J.H., Jackson, D.D., 1967]. For this reason, the caregiver's task is to use clear and correct language that is reassuring but does not encourage unreal hopes in the sick person. It is important to understand exactly what the patient is asking and to respond specifically to his or her requests without projecting the caregiver's own anxieties [Sandrin, L., Brusco, A., Policante, G., 1989].

The ill are often highly dependent on their caregivers, without whom they could not carry out basic bodily care such as feeding, bathing, getting up, moving etc. The extensive spread of home care by informal caregivers occurs for different reasons, including the reassurance of the patient of remaining at home, feelings of shame and rejection for receiving assistance from strangers and the high cost of a "formal" caregiver or of the structures involved in intensive care.

The vast literature on the subject has now shown that *caregiving* can not be reduced to a simple phenomenon that is attuned only to the fulfillment of a patient's needs by a care provider.

Rather, it is a complex interaction in which both the caregiver that the patient are closely interdependent and take care of each other, often within a pre-existing relationship.Interaction may even include negotiating the process of care that is likely to increase in intensity as the disease progresses [Taccani, P., Tognetti, A., De Bernardinis, S., Florea, A., Credendino, E., 1999]. We observe a profound change of role that brings with it not only a series of challenges and difficult tasks, but also a new self-image and several rewards.

The question of assistance is very complex because it involves many aspects of health and the level of support necessary to the individual in need, but also to the organization of social care, to the policies that manage and ensure its delivery. In short, the notion of assistance regards all those cultural elements and values that relate to field of ethics, justice and social equality, individual well-being and community. Thus, regulatory protection of the caregiving role differs according to the country in question.

The category Long Term Care (LTC) covers all projects of health care or medical care for elderly or disabled persons who are not able to regularly carry out everyday activities without outside help (Economic Policy Committee - European Commission). Spending on LTC can be broken down into macrofunctions, which distinguish among home care and semi residential *(at home)*, residential care *(institutions)* and monetary assistance *(cash benefits)* [Coleman, B. J.,1995].

In Italy, for example, various laws have been introduced in the last decade to protect the caregiver [Mauri, L., Pozzi, A., 2007]. Since 1978, the Ministry of Health has regulated this discipline with increasing precision and there have been many investigations to define and update the Essential Care Levels. They are the crucial levels of health care, the set of activities and services that must be provided and uniformly guaranteed by the National Health

Service over the whole national territory and in the community. Its guiding principles are inspired by the notion of human dignity and to the need for solidarity, effectiveness and appropriateness of intervention, efficiency and equity. Unfortunately, even today the role of the family caregiver does not have a financial reward, so that remuneration, security protection and pensions are not expected.

In contrast, other European countries provide remuneration for this role. In Germany, for example, the state provides the patient with an amount of money that allows the patient to choose whether to buy services on the market or to pay a family member who acts as caregiver.

In any case, all the available international experience shows that defining service levels is a very complex goal, both socially and technically. In addition, this question is constantly evolving, and must take into account any scientific and technological innovations that influence assessments of effectiveness and appropriateness of performance.

There is substantial literature on the role of caregiver (more than 15 000 publications on PubMed). In the future it will be necessary to study, predict and standardize economic and regulatory recognition for the position of caregivers in all countries because they are critical partners in the health system. A new perspective on informal and family caregiving is needed, to recognize their value and contribution, as well as their emerging challenges.

Government, experts, patient advocates, service providers, caregivers, neighbors, business and the community, with all the bridging social networks, should all have a stake in sustaining informal caregivers and caregiving.

Social networking, a resource yet to be tapped to its full potential, is a source that can positively impact informal caregiving within the economic reality of health care system.

"The challenge for policy makers is to determine how best to meet the range of needs, insure that families are not overburdened and, at the same time, control publicly funded costs" [Health Canada, 1997-98].

3. CARING FOR PEOPLE WITH DEMENTIA, NEURODEGENERATIVE AND NEUROMUSCULAR DISORDERS

The involvement and the care burden of caregivers varies according to the type of disease, its gravity, and of the support network.

The relationship between a caregiver and an Alzheimer's patient can be profoundly altered, since this type of dementia can change the personality characteristics of the patient, thus requiring a progressive transformation of roles and affective interactions. The level of help changes with the evolution of the disease; in the early stages, the caregiver must help the senior in the tasks that can no longer be coped alone, such as the management of household activities, the maintenance of role and social contacts.

With the progression of symptoms, the assisted person becomes increasingly dependent even for basic daily activities such as hygiene, nutrition and so on. The caregiver must become increasingly aware of all potentially dangerous situations for the patient [Haley W.E., 1997]. The family is very important for care and assistance to the person with dementia. The caregiver is often chosen directly by the patient, on the basis of relational and behavioral dynamics that elect one member of the household as a person closely involved in decision-making and in taking charge of the range of growing and changing needs.

The effects of dementia on the family are clearly highlighted by studies, carried out in various social welfare contexts; these studies evaluated the effects of symptoms, the different stages of the disease and the consequences of stressful and emotional care for a long time care of patients with senile dementia [Zarit, SH, Reever KE, Bach-Peterson, J., 1980; Raina, P., O 'Donnell, M., Schwellnus, H., Rosenbaum, P., King, G., Brehaut, J., Russell, D., Swinton, M., King, S., Wong, M., Walter, SD, Wood, E., 2004].

The "negative" symptoms of mood of the patient elicit a greater level of stress, especially apathy, indifference, depression, irritability and the patient's "refusal" to cooperate or to get help.

These factors are the main causes that lead to the institutionalization of the patient. It is interesting to note that aspects regarding the quality of the caregiver-patient relationship prior to the onset of the disease can, in some way, influence the tasks of caregiving and thus have a more or less negative impact on stress and burden of care [Vellone, E., Piras, G., Sansoni, J., 2002].

Family involvement is also very high in the case of neuromuscular diseases; however, the integrated intervention of care organizations, schools and public administrations local is equally necessary. Building (or perhaps "re-building") the quality of a person's life is based on multifunctional and multidisciplinary cooperation. It must be designed, organized and checked on a regular basis, often re- orienting goals or strategies as required. Each socio - environment in which the person interacts or is located is affected by this participation and collaboration.

The approach to neuromuscular and neurodegenerative disease, that often appears during the patient's growth must be "ecological"; it must be based on the principle that therapy, whether physical, psychological or social should be targeted appropriately to situations of a growing child (home, school, friendships). It should also be integrated, so that it evolves along with the development of the young patient and his/her family and all those who are involved in the life of the sick child. Due to the complexity of these type of diseases, the care network requires a high level of expertise that is constantly updated, each in relation to its functional role.

The psychological consequences of the diagnosis of ALS on caregivers, for example, has become essential object of study of psychological research; in the period following diagnosis, the most common feelings are: disorientation, guilt and anger. For this reason it is useful to provide contacts for services to support families and patients. In the case of people suffering from ALS, the patient-caregiver relationship is very special because there is deep involvement and substantial mutual interdependence between the two [Wasner, M., 2008].

The majority of studies on patients with ALS has focused almost exclusively on the construct of caregiver burden and the effects this has in terms of quality of life of both caregivers and patients [Dow, B., Haralambous, B., Giunmarra, M., Vrantsidis, F., 2004; Raina et al., 2004; Hauser et al., 2006].

Caregivers are required to support the patient in progressive loss of physical abilities and to meet the emotional impact on themselves and on their afflicted family member. These persons often feel an overwhelming sense of uncertainty and helplessness due to the lack of knowledge of the symptoms of the disease as it evolves, and the solitude in which many caregivers find themselves. It often has a strong influence on the wellbeing of the caregiver, and also indirectly on the patient.

4. PSYCHOLOGICAL ASPECTS IN CAREGIVERS

In addition to the physical problems of a disease, psychological ones arise both for patients and their families. The disease is a critical event that affects not only the one who bears the physical signs, but the entire family is forced to face a number of uncomfortable personal, relational and organizational effects. As a result of the change and the redistribution of roles, the whole family must undergo reorganization and rehabilitation in both concrete and symbolic ways. One person in the family, usually female, often ends up totally involved in the new situation and takes charge of first-person patient care, assuming the role of the caregiver, usually identified in the spouse (or partner) or, in the case of an elderly parent, the son or daughter.

The main risk is that the caregiver takes on a role of guardian-prisoner. In dealing with both the burden and the desire to take care of the sick, the caregiver sometimes tends to overshadow the patient's needs. There is a vast amount of literature on this subject, especially in the last few years, that takes into account the stressful and emotional consequences of caring for a disabled person for a long time and that points out the impact of caregiving on the mental health of the caregiver [Knight, B.G., Fox, L.S., Chou, C.P., 2000].

Research on this issue has found that the distress of the caregiver is positively correlated to the patient; that is, psychological distress increases with the growing intensity of care, consequently resulting in a worsening of the patient's condition [Rabkin et al., 2005]. In parallel with the progression of the disease and the consequent increase in the burden of care, levels of anxiety and depression often increase while the quality of life worsens for both patient and caregiver [Pagnini et al., 2010; Pagnini et al., 2011; Pagnini, et al., 2012a; Pagnini, et al., 2012b; Pagnini, et al., 2012c; Pagnini, in press]..
Restrictions on personal and social life and physical problems and emotional stress, consequent to taking on the role of caregiver, are the most critical factors. For these reasons, several studies have called attention to the vital importance of access to clear and accurate information from qualified and reliable persons, relevant to each stage of the disease [Buckman, R. (1992).; Lerman, C., Daly, M., 1993; Gattellari, M., Butow, P.N., Tattersall, M.H.N., *et al.* 1999;]

Johnson and Marsh [Marsh, D., Johnson, D., 1997] have argued that there is a need to pay greater attention to the difficulties that caregivers face when dealing with the health care system, because even the best efforts of caregivers put them under enormous pressure and have a major impact on their quality of life.

4.1. Caregiver Burden

In the relationship between caregiver and patient, the very important concept of *caregiver burden*; that is, *"the set of physical, psychological or emotional, social and economic factors that may be experienced by those members of the family who are in charge of an elderly invalid"* [Ankri et al., 2005] has gained increasing attention. It is defined as "*burden of assistance"* perceived by the caregiver, resulting in psychological disorder, characterized by anxiety, depression and physical malaise. It was found that the caregiver burden is positively correlated with depression and QoL in caregivers. The intensity of care and the number of hours spent in home assistance are the two factors that influence the increase in perceived levels of burden and are independently correlated with higher levels of depression [Chiò et al., 2005; Pagnini et al., 2010].

According to White et al. [White et al., 2001] the burden perceived by caregivers varies according to gender, age, socio-economic conditions, the presence and quality of a support network, financial circumstances, the presence or absence of social support, expectations and strategies to cope with stress. Determinants also include environmental factors such as support of family and friends, the support of the health care system, availability and satisfaction of environmental resources.

The presence of anxiety, depression and high stress can impair the caregiver's performance in important areas of daily life, such as work, relationships and family and can give rise to symptoms of physical distress. To assist the patient, the caregiver often reduces the time that is available for himself/herself and the other members of his or her own family. Personality characteristics, severity of illness and physical quality of interpersonal relationships seem to have a prominent role in the assessment of quality of life.

An important source of support can come from associations of people with the same problems and from specialized professionals. Talking about common problems, listening to the experiences of others can be very useful to relieve the burden of care for caregivers.

5. CULTURAL INFLUENCES

Recent history clearly shows that the life of an individual can be affected by events and processes taking place thousands of miles away. Worldwide awareness of global change implies greater international cooperation and further studies about cultural influences. Therefore greater knowledge of different cultures has become essential in a globalized world.. While this presents a considerable challenge, at the same time, it allows us to get in touch with individuals, cultures, economies and different languages. Information now moves quickly due to economic, geopolitical and social relationships in the media, modern technology and transport In addition, people and goods are the source and manifestation of globalization as a process that leads to global interdependence. Today it is known as "*glocalization*". It is a neologism introduced by the Polish sociologist Zygmunt Bauman, to adjust the view of globalization to local realities and to study better relations with the international area. The term "*globalization*" is considered ambiguous and contradictory in its semantic universe; for this reason Bauman wanted to introduce the new word to indicate the economic behavior in the context of a certain place, to suggest the respect for the land, its customs and traditions, enhancing the uniqueness and pushing traditional businesses, large or small, to the development of markets [Bauman, Z., 2005].

Intercultural education is the concept that underlies this perspective. The 'General Assembly of the United Nations (also known as UNGA, United Nations General Assembly), the largest and most representative institutional organ of the United Nations (New York, September 8, 2008 www.un.org / millenniumgoals) has stated that *"the most important challenge that we collect now is to ensure that globalization becomes a positive force for all mankind"*. It is composed of representatives of all the member States of the United Nations, with the exception of Taiwan, Northern Cyprus and Palestine.

There is a need for a transition from a model of contemporary culture, supported by *scientistic* ideology (which sees unlimited progress of medical knowledge and technology as the solution for all problems), to a model based on the notion of sustainable medicine centered on the person; it must give greater emphasis to the concept of assistance rather the concept of care. It is no longer considered sufficient to cure the disease; now it is necessary to cure the sick person, in a more holistic sense. The notion has shifted from "curing" to "taking care" of the other. In this perspective, the importance of cultural influences is essential.

Culture gives meaning to the events that occur in our lives, by ascribing different values and emotions to each one. Differences in emotional expressions, for example, are produced because members of different cultures learn to have different emotional reactions to events [Camras et al., 1992].

The culture of an individual isn't a diagnostic category and cannot fully explain how an individual will think and act, but it can help health care providers to anticipate and better understand how and why families make decisions and deal with events in a certain way. Emotions and the approach to a disease, or a patient, the type of aid given and the mode of support may well be related the culture of origin and consequently, these factors should be paid careful attention.

Three key issues play a major role in regard to the social implications of chronic disease and disability:

1. The culturally perceived cause of a chronic illness or disability is significant in all cultures. The perceived reason that an illness or disability have occurred in a particular individual and/or a particular family will have a significant role in determining the attitude of the family and the community to the individual and the disease [Lock, 1993].
2. The outlook for survival (usually conceptualized in terms of actual physical survival), affect both the immediate care as well as the amount of effort in planning for the future care and education.
3. The social role that is considered appropriate for disabled or chronically ill will help to determine the amount of resources that a family and the community will invest in the individual. This includes issues of education and training, participation in family and social life of the community, individual autonomy and long-term planning. In some societies the social role related to gender can influence the care provided depending on whether the patient is a male or a female [Augè, M., Herzlich, C., 1986].

For different cultures, chronic disease and disability are seen as a form of punishment. In some countries in Africa, in the Caribbean, in some Pacific Rim countries and in some Native American tribes, witchcraft is strongly related to health and disability. An individual who has been bewitched is assumed to be a victim, but is not necessarily seen as innocent. Among the Lugbara of Uganda some illnesses are perceived as a curse of ancestral spirits, for negative behavior that an individual has adopted towards the elders of their family group [Middleton, J.F.M., 1960]. In the past, in Western France, when misfortune and disease affected a man, his family and his property, it was interpreted and treated not as a single event but as the result of an attack of witchcraft [Favret-Saada, J., 1977]. Among the Wolof of Senegal, some symptoms are considered the sign of possession [Zempléni, A., 2005],.

In other societies where the belief in reincarnation is strong, such as in Southeast Asia or in diverse Indian societies, a disability is often seen as direct evidence of a transgression in a previous life. Disabled persons are often avoided by others and exhorted to lead virtuous lives to atone for the sins of their past lives.

In all these cases the disabled person is considered to some extent responsible for their own problems and as a result, the members of a particular community may be reluctant to respond to requests for assistance or to social integration.

In some ethnic groups, parents of children with disabilities may be reluctant to ask for help or advice in an attempt to hide the sick child. This may be done for several reasons: shame or embarrassment about the condition of a child, an attempt to protect it from outside society, difficulty in accepting the disease. Even when families are aware of the need of special services, they may be reluctant to participate in aid programs, fearing that it would call attention to the physical or intellectual limitations of their family members.

This is of particular interest in the care of pre-school children with chronic illness or disability who still need to be enrolled in educational programs. Often, parents of these children may hesitate or refuse to participate in aid programs if their child does not need immediate medical attention.

In ancient times, the Chinese, for example, believed that the causes of the disease were established by an evil spirit which crept into the body thereby altering its vital rhythms [Caruso, P., 1974] A doctor's explanation of how a genetic disease spreads through a family can be readily accepted; nevertheless, the earlier belief in a curse, or bad blood may persist.

5.1. Caregiver, Emotions and Culture

A broad range of literature has investigated the relationship among the cultural characteristics of caregivers,, the role of their emotions and their mode of action.. Several studies have found differences between Eastern and the Western caregivers, in dealing with the disease and modes of providing care.

Mothers in collective societies such as those in East Asia, evaluate the affective skills of the children and respond to their emotions differently than Western mothers [Markus and Kitayama, 1991]these latter tend to apply a cognitive approach with children [Wang, 2006] or give causal explanations [Wang, 2001] to explain to their children what they feel.

The approach of caregivers from Oriental cultures is different. Studies show that Chinese parents, for example, following the principles of Confucianism and Taoism, believe that the education of children rests primarily with mothers [Ho, 1986] even at the cost of many sacrifices [Chao, 1994]. Confucianism and Taoism hold that the emotions are harmful to the body, for the soul and for interpersonal relationships; for this reason the Chinese emphasize the importance of self-control and serenity. They believe that love is expressed through solid discipline and children must be obedient and observe filial piety.

Following these principles, Oriental parents adopt a moralistic approach to the education of children [Ekblad, 1984] and the technique adopted is educational training [Bowes, Chen, Li, & Li, 2004], teaching lessons and rules directly, giving their children moral explanations, thereby encouraging emotional control in children [Ho, 1986]. Adults rarely engage in obvious exchanges of affection with their children [Chen et al., 1998].

Among these studies carried out by the Institute of Education in Hong Kong [Siu Mui Chan, 2012] has shown that there is a connection between the beliefs of the Chinese mothers and negative expressions of the emotions of children.

. Park and Cheah (2005) found that Korean mothers tended to use their beliefs about children's development, and to use their thoughts to decide when they felt the children were ready to control their negative emotions.

However studies have revealed that despite significant differences between East and West, there is evidence of a reciprocal cultural influence between Western and Oriental [Luk-Fong, 2006] that is reflected in many areas.

When speaking of caregivers, it is important to address the issue of independence and dependence and related cultural influences. Some studies have shown that the society also influences the way in which autonomy is defined and manifested. The experience of independence is related to the social composition of the population, and to diverse cultural, social and economic issues that may increase or decrease the probability to experiment with either state [Walker, 1982]..

In contrast, other studies, such as those carried out by Secker (2003), have also demonstrated the ability to combine high levels of dependence with the experience of independence.

If disability and disease are present, thus requiring the assistance of a caregiver, the sick person inevitably faces some losses, such as total autonomy, and the diminishing of horizons of possibility. Despite this, it is possible to remain relatively active in the world by finding new conditions and defining new horizons [Benner, 2001]. Physical accessibility, that is the possibility of physical access to public and private places of daily life, is very important for the self-realization of independence in patients who require treatment and is in line with the results that have been obtained through studies on the life experiences of people with a neurological disease [Finlayson et al, 2004; LaDonna, 2011]. A recent study by LaDonna (2011) found that the inability to participate in spontaneous activities, resulting from limited mobility due to diseases also restricted the patient's experience of freedom.

The relationship between patient and caregiver is mediated also by emotional expressions and these, in turn, are influenced by each one's own culture. Research suggests that human beings are born with an innate ability to spontaneously produce the same facial configurations when their emotions are aroused; however, it is equally clear that there are cultural differences in such displays. One of the most popular ways to characterize the differences in cultural events is through the mechanism of emotional display rules learned at a young age [Ekman and Friesen, 1969].

Several cross-cultural studies have shown that collectivist cultures approve of the expression of positive emotions because they promote the harmony of the group (eg, Matsumoto, 1991), while individualistic cultures are more open to expressions of conflict [Triandis et al., 1988]. Matsumoto and Kupperbusch (2001) showed that the participants in their study, belonging to a collectivist culture, masked more of their negative feelings from the investigator, whereas individuals belonging to an individualistic culture did not demonstrate the same results.

Ekman (1972) has reproduced and extended previous findings and showed that "collectivist" participants also masked positive feelings from the experimenter, suggesting the existence of display rules that prescribed the suppression of all emotions and not just the negative ones. The most recent studies [Matsumoto et al., in press] have mapped display rules in more than 30 cultures of the world and revealed the same results. This result is commensurate with the results from both Ekman (1972) that Kupperbusch and Matsumoto (2001).

CONCLUSION

In the present and, even more so, in the future, it appears that daily confrontation with illness, disability, non-self-sufficiency will be a continuing challenge to our civilization, social welfare systems and health systems. All over the world, disability and illness will face the inevitable scarcity of economic resources. At the same time, the need will grow for proper planning social care in public systems that already grapple with the issue of streamlining budgets and prioritizing the allocation of funds.

Family caregivers need to be recognized in their role by health care professionals with whom they come into contact. They need to receive information about the disease, on practical caregiving activities and available services, in particular, with respect to psychological issues [Banfi et al., 2009]. Furthermore, they must be helped to understand how their role may extend beyond the "usual" tasks. They must be educated, receive support and psychological care [Pagnini, Simmons at al., 2012], through innovative psychological consultation services [Molinari et al., 2012].

What seems to unite the results obtained in different studies is the essential importance of supporting carers. Caregivers often get sick themselves if they do not receive adequate support during the illness of their family member. This fact invites a critical cause for reflection since there are considerable economic savings if caregiving is entrusted to a family member; however, for this solution to be feasible *over the long term*, it is vital that the caregiver in turn be supported by sources in the broader community and society itself. Developing this potential alliance between the family caregiver and external sources of support implies mutual benefit for all parties.

The maintenance of social support, of training activities *before* assuming the role of family caregiver may decrease the chances of a caregiver developing health problems due to long hours spent in taking care of a sick person. A qualified external person can coordinate the assistance and serve as a valuable liason to those internal and external resources that allow for greater long-term sustainability of the caregiver's role and also in terms of practical and emotional support to the caregiver after the death of the patient.

With a new vision of the "economy of care", it is possible to find more virtuous ways to govern public spending than those currently in place. It is also feasible to more accurately describe caregiving requirements and, in particular, the effectiveness of available caregiving resources (such as family members). However, to do this, it is vital to focus careful attention on the *conditions* for maintaining such effectiveness. Through a sound cost/benefit analysis, it is conceivable to imagine a significant leap in the quality, effectiveness and solidarity in response to this growing need.

ACKNOWLEDGMENT

The authors would like to thank Janice Giffin for her valuable assistance in the correction of the final manuscript

REFERENCES

Ankri, J., Andrieu, S., Beaufils, B., Grand, A., & Henrard, J. C. (2005). Beyond the global score of the Zarit Burden Interview: useful dimensions for clinicians. *International Journal of Geriatric Psychiatry,. 20*, p. 254-260.

Apolone, G., Ballatori, E., Mosconi, P., & Roila, F. (1997). Misurare la qualità di vita in oncologia., Roma: Il Pensiero Scientifico Editore.

Augè, M., & Herzlich, C. (1986). *Il senso del male. Antropologia, storia e sociologia della malattia.*, Milano: Il Saggiatore Editore.

Aujoulat, I., Deccache, A., Patient education and empowerment. *A review of the literature.* 10th International Conference on Health Prompting Hospitals, Bratislava, 2002.

Buckman, R. (1992). *How to break a bad news: a guide for healthcare professionals.* Baltimore: John Hopkins Press .

Banfi, P., Rossi, G., Pagnini, F., Cellotto, N., Gorni, K. O. T., Lunetta, C., & Corbo, M. (2009). Towards a multi-step informed consent: Considerations and proposals for a good practice. [Verso un consenso informato a più fasi: Considerazioni e proposte per una buona prassi] *Clinica Terapeutica, 160(6)*,p.425-426.

Bauman, Z., (2005). *Globalizzazione e glocalizzazione*, Roma: Armando editore, ,.

Benner, P. (2001). The phenomenon of care. In: S. Toombs (Ed.), *Handbook of phenomenology and medicine,*. Dordrecht, The Netherlands: Kluwer Academic Publishers, p. 351Y369.

Bowes, J. M., Chen, M., Li, S. Q., & Li, Y., (2004). Reasoning and negotiation about child responsibility in urban Chinese families: Reports from mothers, fathers and children. *International Journal of Behavioral Development,. 28*, p. 48–58.

Camras, L. A., Oster, H., Campos, J. J., Miyake, K., & Bradshaw, D. (1992). Japanese and American infants responses to arm restraint. *Developmental Psychology,. 28(4)*, p. 578-583.

Caruso, P. (1974). *Il pensiero selvaggio.*, Milano: Il Saggiatore, p. 378.

Chao, R. K., (1994). Beyond parental control and authoritarian parenting style: Understanding Chinese parenting through the cultural notion of training. *Child Development,. 65*, p. 1111–1119.

Chen, X., Hastings, P. D., Rubin, K. H., Chen, H., Cen, G., & Stewart, S. L. (1998). Child-rearing attitude and behavioral inhibition in Chinese and Canadian toddlers: A cross-cultural study. *Developmental Psychology,. 34*, p. 677–686.

Chiò, A., Gauthier, A., Calvo, A., Ghiglione, P., & Mutani, R. (2005). Caregiver burden and patients' perception of being a burden in ALS. *Brief Communications,. Neurology, 64*: p. 1780-1782.

Coleman, B. J. (1995). European models of long-term care in the home and community. *Int. J. Health Serv*, *25(3)*, p. 455-74.

Dow, B., Haralambous, B., Giunmarra, M., & Vrantsidis, F. (2004). What Carers Value. *Review of Carer Literature and Practice*. Melbourne Victoria Australia: Rural and Regional Health and Aged Services Division Victorian Government Department of Human Services,.

Engel, G. *(1977)*. The need for a new medical model: a challenge for biomedicine. *Science*, *196, 129–136.*

Ekblad, S. (1984). Children's thoughts and attitudes in China and Sweden: Impacts of a restrictive versus a permissive environment. *Acta Psychiatrica Scandinavica,.* 70, p. 578–590.

Ekman, P. & Friesen, W. V. (1969). *The repertoire of nonverbal behavior: Categories, origins, usage, and coding..*

Ekman, P. (1972). Universals and Cultural Differences in Facial Expressions of Emotion. In Cole J. (Ed.), Nebraska Symposium on Motivation (Vol. 19, pp.207-282). University of Nebraska Press.

Favret-Saada J. (1977). *Les mots, la mort, les sorts*. Paris: Gallimard.

Finlayson, M., Van Denend, T. & Hudson, E. (2004). Aging with multiple sclerosis. *Journal of Neuroscience Nursing,. 36(5)*, p. 245Y251, 259.

Gattellari, M., Butow, P. N., Tattersall, M. H. N., *et al.* (1999). Misunderstanding in cancer patients: why shoot the messenger ? *Ann Oncol, 10*, 39-46.

Haley W. E. (1997). The family caregiver's role in Alzheimer's disease. *Neurology 48 (Suppl 6),* S25-S29.

Hauser, J. M., Chang, C., Alpert, H., Baldwin, D., Emanuel, E. J., & Emanuel, L. (2006). Who's caring for whom? Differing perspectives between seriously ill patients and their family caregivers. *American Journal of Hospice and Palliative Medicine,. 23*, p. 105-112.

Health Canada (1997-98). The Future of Caregiving. *Seniors Info Exchange*, Winter, p6.

Ho, D. Y. F., (1986). Chinese patterns of socialization: A critical review. In: M. Bond (Ed.), *The psychology of the Chinese people*. New York: Oxford University Press,. p. 1–31.

Igino, C. G., (1933). *Hygini Fabulae*. (a cura di), Rose H. I., Siathoff, Lione,.

Kleinman, A., (1980). *Patients and healers in the context of culture*. Berkeley: University of California Press .

Knight, B. G., Fox, L. S., & Chou, C. P. (2000). Factor Structure of the Burden Interview. *Journal of Clinical Geropsychology,. 6(4)*, p. 249-258.

LaDonna, K. (2011). A literature review of studies using qualitative research to explore chronic neuromuscular disease. *Journal of Neuroscience Nursing,. 43(3)*, p. 172Y182.

Lerman, C., Daly, M. (1993). Walsh WP, *et al*. Communication between patients with breast cancer and health care providers. *Cancer, 72 (9),* 2612-20.

Lock, M. (1993). Cultivating the body, *"Annual Review of Anthropology",. 23*, p. 133-55

Luk-Fong, Y. Y. P., (2006). Hybridity in a guidance curriculum in Hong Kong. *International Journal for Advancement of Counselling,. 28*, p. 331–342.

Lunghi, M. (1992). *Le espressioni spirituali dei popoli primitivi*., Brescia: Università Cattolica.

Mauri, L., & Pozzi, A. (2007). Le politiche di long-term care in Italia. I principali nodi del dibattito. *Mutamento sociale, 17*, p. 1-19.

Markus, H. R. & Kitayama, S. (1991). Culture and the self: Implications for cognition, emotion, and motivation. *Psychological Review,. 98*, p. 224-53.

Marsh, D., & Johnson, D. (1997). The family experience of mental illness: Implications for intervention. *Profess. Psychol. Res. Pract.,. 28*, p. 229-237.

Matsumoto, D. R. (1991). Culture and self: An empirical assessment of Markus and Kitayama's theory of independent and interdependednt self-construal. *Asian Journal of Social Psychology, 2*, p. 289-310.

Matsumoto, D. & Kupperbusch, C. (2001). Idiocentric and allocentric differences in emotional expression and experience. *Asian Journal of Social Psychology,. 4*, p. 113–131.

Middleton, J. F. M., (1960). *Lugbara Religion: Ritual and Authority among an East African People*. London: Oxford University Press for the International African Institute,.

Molinari, E., Pagnini, F., Castelnuovo, G., Lozza, E., & Bosio, C. A. (2012). A new approach for psychological consultation: The psychologist at the chemist's. *BMC Public Health, 12(1.).*

Oster, C. and Pagnini, F. (2012). Resentment, hate, and hope in amyotrophic lateral sclerosis. *Frontiers in Psychology,* 3(Nov).

Pagnini, F. (in press). Psychological well-being and quality of life in Amyotrophic Lateral Sclerosis: a review. *International Journal of Psychology,* DOI: 10.1080 /00207594. 2012.691977.

Pagnini, F., Banfi, P., Lunetta, C., Rossi, G., Castelnuovo, G., Marconi, A., Fossati, F., Corbo, M., & Molinari, E. (2012a). Respiratory function of people with amyotrophic lateral sclerosis and caregiver distress level: a correlational study. *BioPsychoSocial Medicine, 6(14).*

Pagnini, F., Gibbons, C. J., & Castelnuovo, G. (2012). The importance of an idiographic approach for the severe chronic disorders-the case of the amyotrophic lateral sclerosis patient. *Frontiers in Psychology,* 3(Nov).

Pagnini, F., Lunetta, C., Rossi, G., Banfi, P., Gorni, K., Cellotto, N., & Corbo, M. (2011). Existential well-being and spirituality of individuals with amyotrophic lateral sclerosis is related to psychological well-being of their caregivers. *Amyotrophic Lateral Sclerosis, 12(2),* p. 105-108.

Pagnini, F., Lunetta, C., Banfi, P., Rossi, G., Fossati, F., Marconi, A., ... Molinari, E. (2012b). Pain in amyotrophic lateral sclerosis: A psychological perspective. *Neurological Sciences,* 33(5), p.1193-1196.

Pagnini, F., Lunetta, C., Banfi, P., Rossi, G., Gorni, K., Castelnuovo, G., ... Molinari, E. (2012b). Anxiety and depression in patients with amyotrophic lateral sclerosis and their caregivers. *Current Psychology, 31(1),* p. 79-87.

Pagnini, F., Manzoni, G. M. & Castelnuovo, G. (2009). Emotional intelligence training and evaluation in physicians. *JAMA - Journal of the American Medical Association, 301(6),* p. 600.

Pagnini, F., Rossi, G., Lunetta, C., Banfi, P., Castelnuovo, G., Corbo, M., & Molinari, E. (2010). Burden, depression, and anxiety in caregivers of people with amyotrophic lateral sclerosis. *Psychology, Health and Medicine*, *15(6)*, p. 685-693.

Pagnini, F., Simmons, Z., Corbo, M., & Molinari, E. (2012). Amyotrophic lateral sclerosis: Time for research on psychological intervention? *Amyotrophic Lateral Sclerosis, 13(5)*, p. 416-417.

Park, S. & Cheah, C. S. L., (2005). Korean mothers' proactive socialization beliefs regarding preschoolers' social skills. *International Journal of Behavioral Development,. 29*, p. 24–34.

Rabkin, J. L., Albert, S. M., Del Bene, M. L., O'Sullivan, I., Tider, T., Rowland, L. P., & Mitsumoto, H. (2005). Prevalence of depressive disorders and change over time in late-stage ALS. *Neurology,. 65(1)*, p. 62-67.

Raina, P., O'Donnel, M., Schwellnus, H., Rosenbaum, P., King, G., Brehaut, J., Russel, D., Swinton, M., King, S., Wong, M., Walter, S. D., & Wood, E., (2004). *Caregiving process and caregiver burden: conceptual models to guide research and practice,.* BMC Pediatrics.

Sandrin, L., Brusco, A., & Policante, G. (1989). *Capire e aiutare il malato.* Torino: Edizioni Camilliane,.

Secker, J. (2003). *Promoting independence: But promoting what and how? Ageing and Society,. 23*, p. 375Y391.

Simpson, E. P. & Appel, S. H. (2005). Editorial. Individual and health-related quality of life assessment in amyotrophic lateral sclerosis patients and their caregivers by Lo Coco, G., Lo Coco, D., Cicero, V., Oliveri, A., Lo Verso, G., Piccolo, F., La Bella, V. *Journal of the Neurological Sciences,. 238*, p. 1-2.

Siu Mui Chan (2012). Links between Chinese mothers' parental beliefs and responses to children's expression of negative emotions. *Early Child Development and Care,. 182:6*, p. 723-739.

Taccani, P., Tognetti, A., De Bernardinis, S., Florea, A., & Credendino, E. (1999). *Curare e prendersi cura.* Roma: Carocci.

The WHOQoL Group (1994). The development of the World Health Organization Quality of Life Assessment Instrument (the WHOQoL). In: J. Orley and W. Kuyken (Eds). *Quality of Life Assessment: International Perspectives.* Heidelberg: Springer-Verlag.

Triandis, H. C., Bontempo, R., Villareal, M. J., Asai, M., & Lucca (1988). Individualism and collectivism: Cross-cultural perspectives on selfngroup relationships. *Journal of Personality and Social Psychology,. 54*, p. 323-338.

Vellone, E., Piras, G., & Sansoni, J. (2002). *Stress, ansia e depressione delle caregiver di pazienti affetti da malattia d'Alzheimer,. 14.* p. 223-32.

Voltaggio, P. (1992). *La catena migratoria.*, Bologna: Il Mulino, p. 103-107.

Walker, A. (1982). Dependency and old age. *Social Policy and Administration,. 16(2)*, p. 115Y135.

Wang, Q. (2001). Did you have fun?. American and Chinese mother–child conversations about shared emotional experiences. *Cognitive Development,. 16*, p. 693–715.

Wang, Q. (2006). Developing emotion knowledge in cultural contexts. *International Society for the Study of Behavioral Development Newsletter,. 1(49)*, p. 8–12.

Wasner, M. (2008). Resilience among patients with amyotrophic lateral sclerosis (ALS) and their caregivers. *Schweizer Archiv für Neurologie und Psychiatrie,. 159(8)*, p. 500-505.

Watzlawick, P., Beavin, J. H., & Jackson, D. D. (1967). *Pragmatica della comunicazione umana*. Roma: Astrolabio.

White, C. L., Lauzon, S., Yaffe, M. J., & Wood-Dauphinee, S. (2001). Toward a model of quality of life for family caregivers of stroke survivors. *Quality of Life Research,. 13*, p. 625-638.

WHO, *ICF. International Classification of Functioning, Disability and Health*, Geneva 2001.

Zarit, S. H., Reever, K. E., & Bach-Peterson, J. (1980). Relatives of the impaired elderly: correlates of feelings of burden. *Gerontologist,. 26*, p. 649-655.

Zempleni A. (2005). Elementi di psicopatologia wolof-lebou: disturbi mentali e stregoneria, In: Attenasio, L., Casadei, F., Inglese, S., e Ugolini, O. (a cura di), La cura degli altri. *Seminari di etnopsichiatria.*, Roma: Armando editore. p. 179-197.

In: Caregivers: Challenges, Practices and Cultural Influences ISBN: 978-1-62618-030-7
Editors: Adrianna Thurgood and Kasha Schuldt © 2013 Nova Science Publishers, Inc.

Chapter 6

RESILIENCE IN CAREGIVERS

Violeta Fernández-Lansac[*] and María Crespo[†]
Department of Clinical Psychology - Complutense University, Madrid, Spain

ABSTRACT

Caring for a dependent relative is a major source of stress and it is common to consequently suffer emotional issues, such as depression or anxiety symptoms. However, a large number of caregivers perceive their situation as a positive experience, and feel uplifts or satisfaction at times. Hence, why do some caregivers adapt to this situation while others do not? This study of resilience aims to answer this question.

Resilience in caregivers refers to the overall capacity of individuals to face caregiving without having their mental health severely compromised, or their usual functioning altered. According to Connor and Davidson's approach (2003), this capacity comprises a number of resources and individual skills, among which the following can be found: **competence, tenacity, trust** in one's **instincts, tolerance to negative affect, strengthening effects, positive acceptance to change, secure relationships, control,** and **spiritual influences.** Research has shown that the sum of these subcapacities acts as an important protective factor that attenuates the impact of objective stressors on mental health. Elucidating the variables **that determine the development of caregivers' resilience** is therefore a major step forward to identify how individuals overcome chronic stress situations.

Bearing this in mind, the study at hand has been conducted with a sample of 111 Spanish non-professional caregivers of elderly relatives. Its aim was to analyze the connection between resilience, as a mediator factor, with different variables regarding: care context, primary and secondary stressors, appraisals, other mediator variables (social support, intrapsychic resources and personality characteristics), together with the emotional status of caregivers. The outcomes of this study will be integrated into a conceptual model of **caregivers'** resilience. The implications of this work in clinical practice will be discussed in this chapter.

Keywords: Resilience; caregiver; adaptation; chronic stress; burden

---

[*] Email: violetaf@pdi.ucm.es, Phone: (34) 913942984
[†] Corresponding author : Email: mcrespo@psi.ucm.es, Phone: (34) 913943122.

1. INTRODUCTION

Current research has consistently shown that informal or non-professional caregivers of elderly relatives are exposed to chronic stress, which negatively affects their physical and psychological state. Caregivers have consequently been found to suffer high levels of depression, anxiety, anger and burden, as well as different health problems and difficulties to handle everyday life activities. In addition, they show low scores in general wellbeing (see Pinquart & Sörensen, 2003a; Vitaliano, Zhang & Scalan, 2003).

However, it has also been documented that, even if their emotional state is affected, a large number of individuals are able to successfully carry out their new role as caregivers and even extract positive aspects, or gains, from their experience. Along this line, Cohen, Colantonio and Vernich (2002) found, in a study that comprised 289 informal caregivers, that 73% of them reported at least one positive aspect of caregiving. The most frequent aspects identified by participants were those related to feelings of companionship, fulfillment/reward or enjoyment, among others. Additionally, some authors have highlighted the presence of satisfaction levels in caregivers (e.g. Lawton, Moss, Kleban, Glicksman & Rovine, 1991), associated to their personal characteristics and individual resources (i.e. maintaining leisure time and abstaining from using emotional ventilation as a coping strategy), as well as to the nature of the previous affective bond between the caregivers and their relative (López, López-Arrieta & Crespo, 2005).

Both concepts, positive aspects, or gains, and caregiving satisfaction, are denominated in general terms as *uplifts*, which have been described as small satisfactions (Kinney & Parris-Stephens, 1989) or as "a source of positive affect, such as feeling useful, appreciating closeness to the care recipient, and experiencing pride in one's own abilities to handle crises" (Pinquart & Sörensen, 2003b, pp. 114). These uplifts are connected to low levels of burden and depression in the caregiver (Pinquart & Sörensen, 2003b), as well as high life satisfaction (Morano, 2003). This data suggests that appreciating the positive aspects of caregiving plays an important role in the caregivers' emotional state, and therefore it deserves attention.

Combining these findings, two principal lines of caregiving research can be distinguished. On the one hand, an extended one that focuses on the negative impact of the care situation (emphasizing the development of symptoms) and that is useful to develop therapeutic interventions; on the other hand, one focused on the identification of positive effects of caregiving that could prevent caregiver distress and contribute to health promotion if applied clinically. These two lines of work are complementary, and a comprehensive approach to caregiving should take both into consideration.

The use of the *resilience* concept regarding the caregiver population is an important advancement in the way to integrate different caregiving approaches. Resilience study therefore provides a good opportunity to analyze the factors that are involved in how some caregivers adapt to this situation, and extract positive experiences from it, while others do not. Knowing the factors that determine caregiver's resilience is essential to predict the different patterns of evolution in caregivers.

1.1. The Resilience Concept

The study of resilience has a long tradition in psychology, closely linked to the research of protective factors in risk populations. Originally, the word *"resilience"* was used to refer to the unexpected, successful, and positive development of children in adverse contexts, as shown by Werner and Smith's famous experiments, in 1982. *Resilience* has gradually been applied to all sorts of populations, specially those regarding traumatic events (e.g. Bonanno, Galea, Bucciarelli & Vlahov, 2007; Hoge, Austin & Pollack, 2007) or bereaved individuals (e.g. Bonanno, Moskowitz, Papa & Folkman, 2005), and it has proven to be useful to illustrate how humans cope with difficult situations.

Despite its widespread diffusion, the definition of resilience is still controversial and different authors understand it in a variety of ways. Resilience has been defined as "a dynamic process encompassing positive adaptation within the context of significant adversity" (Luthar, Cicchetti & Becker, 2000, p. 543) or "(...) a stable trajectory of healthy functioning across time, as well as the capacity for generative experiences and positive emotions" (Bonanno, 2004, p. 21).

Despite the ambiguity in both definitions, some authors have progressed in the operationalization of the concept. Along this line, Connor and Davidson (2003) conceive resilience as a global capacity to cope with adversity. It combines specific individual skills such as the notion of personal competence, trust in one's instincts, tolerance to negative affect, positive acceptance of change or sense of control. Resilience is therefore understood as a multidimensional construct that incorporates the three dimensions (control, commitment and change) considered by Kobasa (1979) in his definition of hardiness.

Conceptualization of resilience as an individual capacity has allowed the development of several instruments to measure it (e.g. **Block & Kremen, 1996; Jew**, Green & Kroger, 1999; Wagnild & Young, 1993). These aim to assess a variety of personal attributes or sub-capacities that contribute to the adaptation of individuals when facing unfavorable situations. Connor and Davidson (2003) have also created their own resilience scale: the well-known *CD-RISC* scale, which is considered one of most useful measuring instruments to date for this purpose (e.g.White, Driver & Warren, 2008).

It has been applied to patients suffering posttraumatic stress disorder (PTSD), community samples, primary-care outpatients, psychiatric inpatients, and generalized anxiety disorder patients (GAD) (Connor & Davidson, 2003). Other authors have expanded the use of the scale, thus adapting it to different sociocultural contexts, such as China or Iran (e.g. Khoshouei, 2009; Yu & Zhang, 2007), and populations, for example, patients of chronic illnesses (e.g. Vinaccia, Quiceno & Remor, 2012).

1.2. The Study of Caregiver's Resilience

Although resilience has been studied in several populations, its use regarding chronic stress situations, as caregiving, is more restricted. Unfortunately, very few papers have addressed resilience in caregivers and those that do, show significant limitations, namely the absence of a solid and integrated theoretical framework (Fernández-Lansac & Crespo, 2011).

Generally, caregiver' resilience concerns the overall capacity of an individual to face caregiving without severely compromising his psychological health, or altering his usual functioning (Fernández-Lansac, Crespo, Cáceres & Rodríguez-Poyo, 2012). Research shows that this capacity is common among informal caregivers, who tend to show moderate or high resilience levels (e.g. Garity, 1997; Wilks & Croom, 2008). Resilience has also been studied in formal caregiving contexts.

In a study carried out with caregivers who work in Spanish residential homes, high scores in CD-RISC were found among participants (Menezes de Lucena, Fernández, Hernández, Ramos & Contador, 2006).

On analyzing the factors that can make an impact on the development of caregiver's resilience, authors have put an emphasis on the role of both external and internal variables. Among these, it is worth mentioning those aspects regarding the care context and the status of the care recipient (such as aggressive behaviors), use of formal resources, social support, appraisals and coping styles (Gaugler, Kane & Newcomer, 2007; Wilks & Croom, 2008; Wilks, Little, Gough & Spurlock, 2011).

For example, resilient caregivers tend to use problem-focused or task-focused coping strategies (Garity, 1997; Wilks et al., 2011) and private prayer (Wilks & Vonk, 2008) more often than non-resilient ones. The role of appraisal is even clearer, so much so that Gaugler et al. (2007) include it in their own definition of resilience, where it is considered as lower perceived burden when caregiving becomes highly demanding. Similarly, Braithwaite (2000) talks about "resilience appraisals".

In the above mentioned works, resilience emerges as an important predictor of the caregiver's emotional status because it presents a strong inverse association to the development of emotional distress. High levels of resilience are therefore associated to low burden, low levels of psychiatric symptoms (anxiety and depression) and high levels of wellbeing in caregivers (Braithwaite, 2000; O'Rourke et al., 2010). In addition, Gaugler et al., (2007) explain that resilience makes it easier to predict the adaptation to transitions in dementia caregiving (i.e. institutionalization or death of care recipient). Resilience can thus protect caregivers from symptoms, and it contributes to maintain their wellbeing. At the same time, the mental health of caregivers has an impact on the care recipient situation and, consequently, in their mental status.

Outcomes from the study carried out with formal caregivers suggest that the connection between resilience and burnout (which would be considered the equivalent to burden on job) can be mediated by engagement (vigor, dedication and absorption) (Menezes de Lucena, et al. 2006). In the same way, resilience in nonprofessional caregivers is likely to interact with other mediating factors, such as appraisal, coping or social support; and as a result of this interaction the likelihood of suffering the negative effects of caregiving is either increased or decreased.

However since research about resilience in caregivers is still scarce, conclusions must be drawn cautiously. The specific factors that predict the development of different resilience levels are little known; and their relationship with other variables is far from being clear. The present study aims to contribute in this direction.

1.3. Aim of the Current Study

The current study investigates resilience in Spanish caregivers of elderly relatives, stemming from Connor and Davidson's (2003) definition of resilience as a global capacity, composed by different specific subcapacities. The aim of this research is to assess caregivers' resilience and to analyze its relationship to a great number of variables, which, following the caregiving stress model outlined by Pearlin, Mullan, Semple, and Skaff (1990), will be clustered in the following categories: (a) *caregiving context*; (b) *primary and secondary stressors*; (c) *appraisals*; (d) *mediator variables*; and (e) *consequences* or *emotional state of caregiver*.

This paper has been preceded by a preliminary study carried out by the same authors, in which 53 caregivers of patients with dementia were included (see Fernández-Lansac et al., 2012). In this study, resilience was associated with better mental health, positive appraisals, effective coping strategies, personality traits and several individual resources.

The present work is therefore an extension of this previous research, where the sample is extended to improve the scope of the conclusions. The goal of the study is to measure the impact of resilience on the emotional status of caregivers, in order to elucidate if it acts as an individual protective factor in situations of chronic stress, such as caregiving. A theoretical model of caregiving resilience will be outlined below.

2. DESIGN AND METHODS

2.1. Participants

Participants were recruited from different Spanish centers and associations of patients with dementia or other age-related diseases. To be eligible for this study, caregivers had to meet the following criteria: (a) to be providing care for a dependent older patient in the community (aged over 60); (b) to be the principal caregiver of patient; (c) to permanently live with the patient; (d) to have been caring for the patient for at least 6 months; (e) for the patient to require extended supervision and assistance with everyday activities. Dependence was established by using the activities of the daily living (ADL) index (Katz, Ford, Moskowitz, Jackson & Jaffe, 1963), where limitation in one or more items indicates the presence of disability. 129 participants were initially included in the study, but 18 of them did not complete the evaluation. The overall sample therefore consisted of 111 caregivers.

Caregivers were individually assessed. Their participation in the study was voluntary. In addition, they were informed of the goals of the study, they were guaranteed the confidentiality of the information provided, and they signed a consent form before taking part in the study.

2.2. Variables and Measures

Data collection was carried out through two assessment batteries: an interview and a self-rating assessment survey to complete at home and then give back personally or by post. The measures that each battery comprises are described below and are summarized in Table 1.

Table 1. Variables and measures

Variables		Measure
Caregiving context	Characteristics of caregiver, care recipient and relationship between caregiver and elderly	Structured personal interview
Stressors (primaries and secondaries)	Care recipient status	GDS, ADL and interview
	Problems of care recipient	RMBPC (frequency scale), and interview
	Characteristics of caregiving	Interview
Appraisals	Burden	CBI
	Reaction to care recipient's problems	RMBPC (reaction scale)
	Caregiving satisfaction	CSS
Mediator variables	Social support	SSQSR
	Neuroticism and extraversion	NEO-FFI
	Self-esteem	Rosenberg Scale
	Self-care	Interview
	Self-efficacy	Revised Scale for Caregiving Self-Efficacy
	Coping	Brief COPE
	Resilience	CD-RISC
Emotional state	Depression	BDI-II
	Anxiety	HAD-A
	Maladaptation	MS

2.2.1. Interview Instruments

- *Semistructured personal interview:* It was designed *ad hoc* to assess characteristics of the caregivers (e.g. age, sex...), patient features (e.g. age, diagnosis...), and care characteristics (e.g. duration of caregiving, daily schedule as caregiver...). It included a specific item that assesses the caregiver's self-care habits.
- *Global Deterioration Scale (GDS)* (Reisberg, Ferris, de Leon & Crook, 1982; Spanish adaptation by Cacabelos, 1990): It assesses the global cognitive level or functional capacity of the care recipient. It shows a high inter-rater reliability (.82, .92) and it correlates with other instruments, as MMSE (Cacabelos, 1990).
- *Activities of Daily Living (ADL) Index* (Katz et al., 1963; Spanish adaptation by Cruz, 1991): It is used to measure the functioning of the care recipient on six sociobiological functions. It has an appropriate validity, as well as a high internal consistency and inter-rater reliability (Beckett et al., 1996).
- *Social Support Questionnaire, Short form Revised (SSQSR)* (Saranson, Saranson, Shearin & Pierce, 1987; Spanish adaptation by Saranson, 1999): It measures the number of people supplying support and the caregivers' satisfaction with this support. It shows an appropriate internal consistency and it has a proper inter-rater reliability (Crespo & López, 2007; Saranson et al. 1987).
- *Revised Scale for Caregiving Self-Efficacy* (Steffen, McKIbbin, Zeiss, Gallagher-Thompson & Bandura, 2002; *ad hoc* Spanish adaptation): It measures caregiving self-efficacy covering three domains: obtaining respite, responding to disruptive patient behaviors and controlling upsetting thoughts. It has a adequate internal consistency and inter-rater realiability (Steffen et al., 2002).

2.2.2. Self-rating instruments

- *Connor-Davidson Resilience Scale (CD-RISC)* (Connor & Davidson, 2003; ad hoc Spanish adaptation): It values individual perception of resilience in the previous month. It has high internal consistency (alpha=.89) and test-retest reliability (.87) (Connor & Davidson, 2003; Menezes de Lucena et al., 2006).
- *Revised Memory and Behavior Problems Checklist (RMBPC)* (Teri et al., 1992; ad hoc Spanish adaptation): It focuses on the behavior and memory problems of the dependent person (frequency) and the impact that they have on the caregiver (reaction). It has an alpha of .84 for frequency, and alpha of .90 for reaction scale (Teri et al., 1992).
- *Caregiver Burden Interview (CBI)* (Zarit, Reever, & Bach-Peterson, 1980; Spanish adaptation by Martín et al., 1996): It measures the subjetive burden of the caregiver. The CBI has a fair test-retest reliability and an adequate internal consistency (Vitaliano, Young & Russo, 1991).
- *Caregiving Satisfaction Scale (CSS)* (Lawton, Kleban, Moss, Rovine & Glicksman, 1989; Spanish adaptation by López & Crespo, 2003): It is the most frequently used scale to measure the positive aspects of caring. It shows a good internal consistency and reliability (Lawton et al., 1989; Brody, Litvin, Hoffman & Kleban, 1992).
- *NEO-FFI Personality Inventory* (N and E Scales) (Costa & McCrae, 1999; Spanish adaptation by TEA Editions, 1999): It is a shortened version of NEO PI-R that assesses the big five personality traits. In this study, only the Neuroticism (N) and Extraversion (E) scales were selected, which in the original version have an alpha of .90 and .84 respectively (Costa & McCrae, 1999).
- *Rosenberg Self-Esteem Scale* (Rosenberg, 1965; Spanish adaptation by Echeburúa & Corral, 1998): It assesses self-satisfaction. It shows an adequate internal consistency and a good test-retest reliability (Fleming & Courtney, 1984).
- *Brief COPE Inventory* (Carver, 1997; Spanish adaptation by Crespo & López, 2003): It assesses the use of different coping strategies. Total strategies have been classified under three factors: problem-focused coping, emotion-focused coping, and transcendence search (López, Crespo, Arinero, Gómez & Francisco, 2004).
- *Beck Depression Inventory-II (BDI-II)* (Beck, Steer & Brown, 1996; Spanish adaptation by Sanz, Navarro &Vázquez, 2003): It is the most commonly used depression questionnaire. The internal consistency of this version reaches a Cronbach's alpha of .90 in subclinical samples (Sanz et al., 2003).
- *Anxiety subscale of the Hospital Anxiety and Depression Scale (HAD-A)* (Zigmond & Snaith, 1983; Spanish adaptation by Caro & Ibáñez, 1992): It detects anxiety arising from the physical symptoms caused by the illness; with appropriate psychometric properties (Bjelland, Dahl, Haug & Neckelmann, 2002).
- *Maladaptation Scale* (MS; in Spanish, Escala de Inadaptación; see Echeburúa, Corral & Fernández-Montalvo, 2000): It assesses the extent to which caregivers' current problems affect various areas of their everyday lives, thus differentiating between adaptation and maladaptation (Echeburúa et al., 2000).

2.3. Data Analysis

When missing data did not exceed 15% of the total data of each test, these data were replaced with the mean value in the remaining items of test. Participants exceeding this percentage of missing data were not included in the analysis. In order to calculate internal consistency for the CD-RISC and the other measures, the Cronbach's alpha internal consistency coefficient was computed.

As can be seen in Table 2., alpha coefficients found for all instruments ranged between .753 and .952, which is considered an acceptable internal consistency (i.e. alpha >.70). Only one subscale (transcendence search of brief COPE) had a value below .70.

Table 2. Internal consistency of measures (n=111)

Measures	Cronbach' alpha (α)
Activities of Daily Living (IADL)	.753
Satisfaction with social Support (SSQSR)	.854
Scale for Caregiving Self-Efficacy	.867
Connor-Davidson Resilience Scale (CD-RISC)	.897
Memory and Behavior Problems Checklist (RMBPC)	
Frequency Scale	.927
Reaction Scale	.952
Caregiver Burden Interview (CBI)	.910
Caregiving Satisfaction Scale (CSS)	.842
NEO-FFI Personality Inventory	
Extraversion Scale	.840
Neuroticism Scale	.827
Rosenberg Self-Esteem Scale	.854
Brief COPE Inventory	
Problem-focused coping	.841
Emotion-focused coping	.828
Transcendence search	.605
Beck Depression Inventory (BDI-II)	.905
Anxiety subescale of HAD	.849
Maladaptation Scale	.879

Descriptive statistics (means, standard deviations and percentages) were used to characterize the sample, as well as aspects of the care recipient and the caregiving context. Since there is no normative data to interpret resilience levels, results in this variable were compared to the data reported by Connor and Davidson (2003) and Menezes de Lucena et al. (2006) using t tests, after checking the adjustment of the variable to normal distribution, using Kolgomorov-Smirnov test.

Correlations between resilience and the different variables included were analyzed. Pearson correlation was used (r_{xy}) for quantitative variables, while Spearman correlations (r_s) were used for ordinal variables.

For dichotomous variables, point-biserials correlations were established (r_{pb}). Qualitative variables with more than two possible values (i.e. marital status, kinship) were dichotomized. To prevent Type I errors, Bonferroni adjustment for multiple comparison was used (p <.002).

3. RESULTS

3.1. Sample Characteristics

There was a predominance of women among the participants (73.9%); most were middle age (M=62.36 years old; S.D.=12.23), and married or living with their partner (71.2%). Over half of the caregivers (68.5%) did not work at the time of assessment: they were retired (62.3%), unemployed (18.2%), housewives (18.2%) or students (1.3%). Though there were differences in their education level, most had finished high school, 36% of the participants had a university degree.

The care recipient's children and spouses were predominant among the caregivers (50.5% and 41.4%, respectively). Similarly, most of the care recipients were women (72.1%); their mean age was 80.96 (S.D.=9.78) years old. They mostly presented a diagnosis of dementia (86.5%), mainly Alzheimer type (84.4%); and they needed assistance for an average of 3.44 (S.D.=1.80) activities of their daily living. Care recipients had a moderate-high cognitive impairment, with a mean of 4.76 (S.D.=1.63) in GDS.

Concerning the history and characteristics of the support provided, the caregivers had been taking care of their relatives for a mean of 55.15 (S.D.=44.47) months (about 4.5 years). They spent a weekly average of 110.27 (S.D.=46.72) hours attending their relatives. Most of them received some sort of familiar help (68.2%) and used some kind of formal service (94.4%).

3.2. Caregivers' Resilience

The mean resilience score in the CD-RISC was 64.04 (S.D.=14.64; Median=63; Q1=54; Q4=73), and the values obtained, adjusted to normal distribution (z=0.76, p=.618). When compared to Connor and Davidson's data (see Table 3), significant differences (p<.001) were found among all the different groups, with the exception of Generalized Anxiety Disorder (GAD) patients.

Specifically, caregivers' resilience scores were higher than Posttraumatic Stress Disorder (PTSD) patients' ones, but lower than the scores found in the general population, primary care, and also psychiatric outpatients.

Additionally, resilience in informal caregivers was significantly lower than resilience among the professional caregivers of older patients in Menezes de Lucena et al.'s study (2006) where the CD-RISC was also applied.

Table 3. Comparison of CD-RISC scores in caregivers of elderly dependent relatives and other groups

Group	N	Mean (SD)	Median (1st, 4th Q)	t df=110	p
Caregivers	111	64.04 (14.64)	63 (54, 73)	---	---
General population [1]	577	80.4 (12.8)	82 (73,90)	-11.77	<.001
Primary care [1]	139	71.8 (18.4)	75 (60,86)	-5.58	<.001
Psychiatric outpatients [1]	43	68.0 (15.3)	69 (57, 79)	-2.85	.005
GAD patients [1]	24	62.4 (10,7)	64.5 (53, 71)	1.18	.239
PTSD patients (group 1) [1]	22	47.8 (19.5)	47 (31, 61)	11.69	<.001
PTSD patients (group 2) [1]	22	52.8 (20.4)	56 (39, 61)	8.09	<.001
Professional caregivers of elderly people [2]	265	70.0 (13.57)	---	-4.28	<.001

GAD = Generalized Anxiety Disorder; PTSD = Posttraumatic Stress Disorder
[1] Connor & Davidson (2003); [2] Menezes de Lucena et al. (2006)

Table 4. Scores of the different variables and correlates with resilience (n=111)

Variables	Mean (SD)/%	r_{xy}	p
Caregiving context			
Age	62.36 (12.23)	.002	.981
Sex			
Women (vs. men)	73.9	-.091	.344
Marital status			
No partner (vs. with partner)	28.8	-.008	.936
Educational level			
Low level studies or compulsory education (vs. high level studies)	38.7	.103	.284
Job			
Inactive (vs. active)	68.5	-.076	.430
Kinship with the care recipient			
Children (vs. spouse)	50.5	.065	.496
Stressors			
Care recipient' diagnosis			
Dementia (vs. other disease)	86.5	-.206	.030
Months as caregiver	55.15 (44.47)	-.034	.731
Hours per week as caregiver	110.27 (46.72)	-.055	.578
Cognitive impairment of care recipient (1-7)	4.76 (1.63)	-.334	<.001
Dependence in activities of daily living (0-6)	3.44 (1.80)	-.165	.086
Cognitive or behavioral problems of care recipient (0-96)	30.12 (16.77)	-.307	.001
Appraisals			
Burden (22-110)	13.87 (9.75)	-.334	<.001
Reaction to cognitive or behavioral problems (0-96)	23.00 (18.16)	-.383	<.001
Caregiving satisfaction (6-30)	23.68 (4.82)	.278	.003
Mediator variables			
Perceived social support (0-54)	17.89 (13.48)	.203	.033
Satisfaction with social support (6-36)	31.61 (5.03)	.273	.004
Neuroticism (0-48)	19.97 (8.55)	-.632	<.001
Extraversion (0-48)	27.69 (8.24)	.557	<.001
Self-esteem (10-40)	31.12 (4.62)	.624	<.001
Adequate self-care (vs. poor)	54.5	.349	<.001
Self-efficacy (0-100)	68.96 (19.68)	.426	<.001
Coping strategies (1-4)			
Problem-focused coping	2.35 (.57)	-.102	.294
Emotion-focused coping	2.97 (1.57)	-.306	.001
Transcendence search	1.77 (.63)	.104	.286
Emotional state			
Depression (0-63)	13.87 (9.75)	-.585	<.001
Anxiety (0-21)	7.62 (4.30)	-.508	<.001
Maladaptation (0-30)	14.95 (6.89)	-.349	<.001

3.3. Resilience Correlates

Table 4 shows the scores obtained by participants in all variables considered, grouped following the categories of caregivers' stress proposed by Pearlin et al. (1990): (a) caregiving context; (b) primary and secondary stressors; (c) appraisals; (d) mediator variables; and (e) emotional state of caregiver. In this table, the correlation between the different variables and resilience scores can also be observed.

Firstly, it can be seen that resilience is not significantly associated with any aspect of the *caregiving context*. Resilience is not related to age, sex, marital status, educational level, or kinship between caregivers and care recipients.

Furthermore, few *caregiving stressors* were associated to caregivers' resilience. The only two stressors that showed significant correlations to the main variable were cognitive impairment of care recipient, and frequency of behavioral and memory problems. Specifically, higher caregivers' resilience was associated to lower cognitive impairment ($r_{xy}=-.334$, $p <.001$) and to fewer behavioral and memory problems in elderly dependents ($r_{xy}=-.307$, $p=.001$). Care recipient's diagnosis and level of dependence for daily living activities did not present significant correlations with CD-RISC. The amount of time that caregivers spent on assistance tasks was not associated to their resilience either.

Regarding *caregiver appraisal*, the outcomes prove that higher scores in caregivers' resilience were associated with a lower subjective burden ($r_{xy}=-.334$, $p <.001$), and less concern regarding behavioral and memory problems manifested by care recipients ($r_{xy}=-.383$, $p <.001$). However, caregiving satisfaction did not reach the required value when Bonferroni's adjustment was applied.

The most relevant associations were those between resilience and the so called *mediator variables*, regarding coping, resources and individual characteristics of caregivers. Specifically, resilience showed a significant direct correlation with extraversion ($r_{xy}=.557$, $p <.001$), self-esteem ($r_{xy}=.624$, $p <.001$), self-efficacy ($r_{xy}=.426$, $p <.001$), and self-care ($r_{xy}=.349$, $p <.001$); and there was a significant inverse correlation between resilience and neuroticism ($r_{xy}=-.632$, $p <.001$) and the use of emotion-focused coping by caregivers ($r_{xy}=-.306$, $p=.001$). Other strategies of coping were not associated to resilience, neither social support nor satisfaction with it. However, if a significant level of $p <.05$ would have been established, satisfaction with social support would be significantly associated to resilience.

Finally, resilience was highly correlated with caregivers' *emotional state*. Consequently, higher resilience scores were associated to lower levels of depression ($r_{xy}=-.585$, $p <.001$), less anxiety symptoms ($r_{xy}=-.508$, $p <.001$), and less adaptation problems ($r_{xy}=-.349$, $p <.001$).

CONCLUSION

This study analyzes resilience in long-lasting stress situations, thus changing the focus of caregiving research from pathology and symptoms to health and wellbeing promotion, and protective factors. When analyzing resilience in this population, the first finding is that resilience is influenced by the caregiving situation. According to Connor and Davidson (2003), resilience is quantifiable and influenced by health status, with individuals with mental illnesses showing lower levels of resilience than the general population. In this line, the level of resilience found in caregivers was significantly lower than that found in the overall population and even other risk populations, exceeding only the level of resilience in PTSD patients, and at similar levels to that of GAD patients (Connor & Davidson, 2003). Actually GAD and caregiving have in common the pervasive nature of anxiety. Furthermore, participants of this study scored lower in resilience than those found in professional caregivers (Menezes de Lucena et al., 2006). These results support the well-established negative effect of caregiving in the emotional status and also in the individuals' personal resources, with a greater impact when the care is carried out by a relative, rather than a professional caregiver.

Nonetheless, data showed important differences among caregivers in their resilience capacity: 19% of the caregivers scored equal or higher than the mean value in general population (i.e. 80.4), in the reference study by Connor and Davidson (2003). When analyzing the variables that can influence the development of different resilience levels, the first thing that is observed is that aspects related to the caregiving context were not associated to caregiver's resilience. So, it seems that resilience depends neither on sociodemographic characteristics of the caregiver (i.e. sex, age, marital status), nor on his kinship with the care recipient (children or spouse). In addition, the majority of stressors (i.e. time spent in caregiving or dependency level of elderly) and diagnosis were not associated with resilience. These data do not correspond to the results obtained by others authors, who argue that resilience is related to care demands (e.g. Gaugler et al., 2007), and that these demands increase when the person assists an elderly with dementia (e.g. Pinquart & Sörensen, 2003a). In this work the impairment of care recipients, together with the memory and behavioral problems that they manifested were the only two stressors that had a significant impact on caregiver's resilience. In fact, the aspects with a greater weight in the outcomes were those concerning subjective aspects related to the caregiver. In this sense, the way in which participants assessed the stressors (burden and reaction to care recipient problems, but not caregiving satisfaction) was correlated to their resilience, rather than to the stressors.

Major associations were found in regard to mediator variables. High resilience scores were related to higher extraversion, self-esteem, self-efficacy, and self-care; as well as lower neuroticism and less use of emotion-focused coping. Resilience consequently seems to be mainly influenced by internal resources and aspects of the caregivers' personality. This is not surprising because it is well documented that resilient people tend to meet a number of individual characteristics, which include positive temperamental and dispositional qualities, perceived competence, intelligence, positive self-worth, interest in social relationships, solid problem-solving skills or sense of optimist; and they tend to experience more positive emotions (Ong, Bergeman, Bisconti & Wallace, 2006; Tedeschi & Kilmer, 2005; Werner, 1995). On the other hand, and contrary to all expectations, resilience was not significantly associated with social support, being this one of the mediator factors that has received more attention (e.g. Wilks & Croom, 2008). However, although it failed to be significant, a direct relationship between satisfaction with social support and resilience was observed. This finding shows once again the importance of subjective, more than objective, aspects. The number of people that help caregivers has therefore less impact on their resilience than the way in which these people are valued.

Another issue that was raised by this study is whether those caregivers with high resilience are also less prone to develop emotional problems. Knowing that mental health influences resilience, the question is: does this relationship occur conversely too? In other words, is resilience a protective factor in chronic stress situations such as caregiving? Results of this study showed that resilience was significantly and inversely related to emotional symptoms (anxiety, depression) and adaptation problems. Therefore, resilience levels could act as an indicator for the development of emotional problems, as is suggested by some authors (e.g. O'Rourke et al., 2010). Unfortunately, this study provides cross-sectional data, and it therefore does not inform of the directionality of the connection between variables. This is the major limitation of this research. The most plausible hypothesis would contemplate bidirectional influences, so that resilience capacity would allow people to successfully cope with stress; but conversely, it would also be influenced by the successful and unsuccessful adaptation to previous stressors and by health status. Resilience could thus be conceived as an interactive factor that enables individuals to successfully cope with adverse situations; and that is conversely determined by the individual's current emotional state, as well as by how he/she has coped with past experiences.

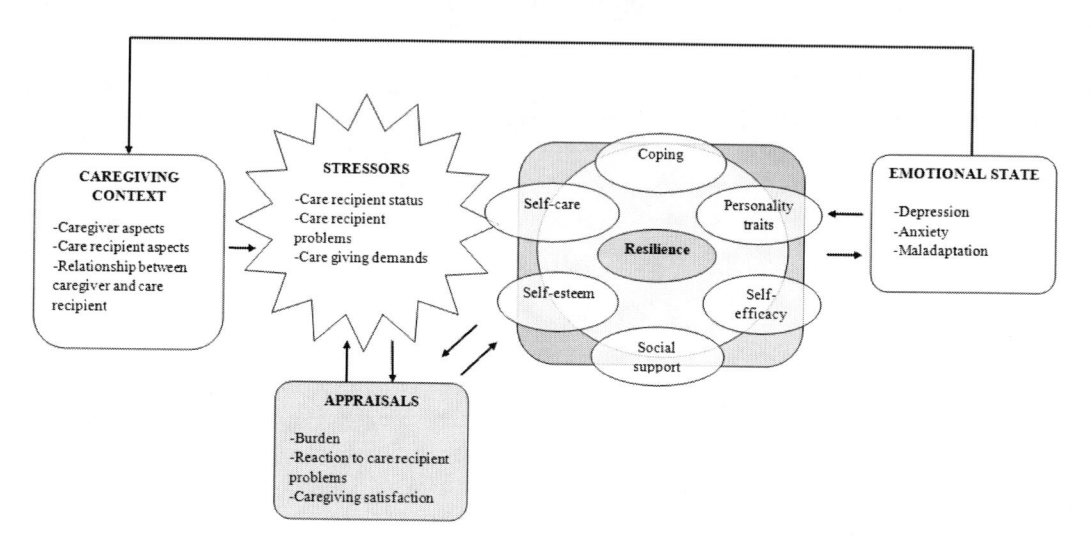

Figure 1. Caregiving stress and resilience model.

An integrative model of caregivers' resilience must contemplate reciprocal influences between different variables, and emphasizes the role of subjective aspects, rather than the one of objective aspects in the caregiving situation. Resilience could be understood as a protector factor that, in interaction with another mediator factors, would determine the emotional impact that stressors have on the caregiver. A hypothetical model of caregiver resilience can be outlined. As shown in Figure 1., resilience would be situated at the centre of the model. Primary and secondary stressors would be derived from the caregiving context. These stressors, related to the care recipient's state and number of demands of the situation, woul not have a direct effect in the caregiver's health. Appraisals will actually be determinant on results. People that evaluated stressors in a positive way (i.e. in terms of satisfaction, low burden and reaction) will see their resilience increased. Similarly, caregivers with high resilience will be more likely to assess stressors more positively. There would be a constellation of variables around the concept of resilience. These variables would comprise all resources that, as resilience (and thanks to their interaction with it), mediate the relationship between appraisal and consequences of caregiving. Hence, when an individual assesses stressors positively, and has high resilience, it can be predicted that he/she will develop less psychological symptoms, such as depression and anxiety, and will adapt better to the caregiver role.

The efforts of future research should focus on developing strategies to promote resilience in caregivers because fostering skills that integrate resilience should constitute an essential part of any psychological program for this population. The use of these strategies may be generalized to other populations that, as caregivers, suffer the devastating effects of chronic stress situations.

ACKNOWLEDGMENTS

Our thanks to all the caregivers involved in this study and their institutions: Alzheimer's State Reference Centre dependent on IMSERSO (Salamanca); Pamplona, Leñeros and Carmen Laforet Adult Day Services (Madrid City Council); Maria Wolff Adult Day Services (Madrid); Area 6 Teaching and Research Unit of Nursing (Madrid); Alzheimer Association of Zamora; and San Carlos Clinic Hospital (Madrid).

REFERENCES

Beck, A., Steer, R., & Brown, G. (1996). *Beck Depression Inventory Manual* (2nd. ed.). San Antonio, TX: Psychological Corporation.

Beckett, L.A., Brock, D.B., Lemke, J.H., Mendes de Leon, C.F., Guralnik, J.M., Fillenbaum, G.G., Branch, L.G., Wetle, T.T., & Evans, D.A. (1996). Analysis of change in self-reported physical function among older persons in four population studies. *American Journal of Epidemiology, 143*, 766-778. doi:10.1093/oxfordjournals.aje.a008814.

Bjelland, I., Dahl, A.A., Haug, T.T., & Neckelmann, D. (2002). The validity of the hospital anxiety and depression scale. An updated literature review. *Journal of Psychosomatic Research, 42*, 69-77.

Block, J., & Kremen, A. (1996). IQ and Ego-Resiliency. Conceptual and empirical connections and separateness. *Journal of Personality and Social Psychology, 70*, 349-361. doi:10.1037//0022-3514.70.2.349.

Bonanno, G. (2004). Loss, trauma, and human resilience: Have we underestimated the human capacity to thrive after extremely aversive events? *American Psychologist, 59*, 20-28. doi:10.1037/0003-066X.59.1.20.

Bonanno, G. A., Galea, S., Bucciarelli, A., & Vlahov, D. (2007). What Predicts Psychological Resilience After Disaster? The Role of demographics, resources, and life stress. *Journal of Consulting and Clinical Psychology, 75*, 671-682. doi:10.1037/0022-006X.75.5.671.

Bonanno, G. A., Moskowitz, T., Papa, A., & Folkman, S. (2005). Resilience to loss in bereaved spouses, bereaved parents, and bereaved gay men. *Journal of Personality and Social Psychology, 88*, 827-843. doi:10.1037/0022-3514.88.5.827.

Braithwaite, V. (2000). Contextual or general stress outcomes: Making choices through caregiving appraisals. *The Gerontologist, 40*, 706-717. doi:10.1093/geront/40.6.706.

Brody, E.M., Litvin, S.J., Hoffman, C., & Kleban, M.H. (1992). Differential effects of daughters' marital status on their parent care experiences. *Gerontologist, 32*, 58-67. doi:10.1093/geront/32.1.58.

Cacabelos, R. (1990). Neurobiología y genética molecular de la enfermedad de Alzheimer: marcadores diagnóticos y terapéutica [The neurobiology and molecular genetics of Alzheimer's disease: The diagnostic markers and therapy]. *Medicina Clínica, 95*, 502-516.

Caro, I., & Ibáñez, E. (1992). La escala hospitalaria de ansiedad y depresión [Hospital anxiety and depression scale]. *Boletín de Psicología, 36*, 43-69.

Carver, C. (1997). You want to measure coping but your protocol's too long: Consider the brief COPE. *International Journal of Behavioral Medicine, 4*, 92-100.

Cohen, C., Colantonio, A., & Vernich, L. (2002) Positive aspects of caregiving: rounding out the caregiver experience. *International Journal of Geriatric Psychiatry, 17*,184-188. doi:10.1002/gps.561.

Connor, K., & Davidson, J. (2003). Development of a new resilience scale: The Connor-Davidson Resilience Scale (CD-RISC). *Depression and Anxiety, 18*, 76-82. doi:10.1002/da.10113.

Costa, P., & McCrae, R. (1999). *Inventario de personalidad NEO revisado (NEO PI-R)*[Revised NEO Personality Inventory (NEO PI-R)]. Madrid:TEA Ediciones.

Crespo, M., & López, J. (2003). Cope Abreviado [Brief Cope]. In: M. Crespo, & F. Labrador (Eds.), *Estrés* [Stress] (pp. 98-99). Madrid: Síntesis.

Crespo, M., & López, J. (2007). *El apoyo a los cuidadores de familiares mayores dependientes en el hogar: desarrollo del programa «cómo mantener su bienestar»* [Support for caregivers of elderly relatives: development of program «How to mantein your well-being»]. Madrid: Imserso.

Cruz, A. (1991). El índice de Katz [The Katz Index]. *Revista Española de Geriatría y Gerontología, 26*, 338-348.

Echeburúa, E., & Corral, P (1998). *Manual de violencia* familiar [Manual of family violence]. Madrid: Siglo XXI.

Echeburúa, E., Corral, P., & Fernández-Montalvo, J. (2000). Escala de inadaptación (EI): propiedades psicométricas en contextos clínicos [Maladjustment Scale (MS): psychometric properties in clinical settings]. *Análisis y Modificación de Conducta, 26*, 325-340.

Fernández-Lansac, V., & Crespo, M. (2011). Resiliencia, personalidad resistente (hardiness) y crecimiento en cuidadores de personas con demencia en el entorno familiar: Una revisión [Resilience, hardiness and growth in dementia' patients family caregivers: A review]. *Clínica y Salud, 22*, 21-40. doi:10.5093/cl2011v22n1a2.

Fernández-Lansac, V.; Crespo, M.; Cáceres, R., & Rodríguez-Poyo, M. (2012). Resiliencia en cuidadores de personas con demencia: estudio preliminar [Resilience in caregivers of patients with dementia: A preliminary study]. *Revista Española de Geriatría y Gerontología, 47*,102-109. doi:10.1016/j.regg.2011.11.004.

Fleming, J.S., & Courtney, B.E. (1984). The dimensionality of self-esteem. II Hierarchical facet model for revised measurement scales. *Journal of Personality and Social Psychology, 6*, 404-421. doi:10.1037/0022-3514.46.2.404.

Garity, J. (1997). Stress, learning style, resilience factors, and ways of coping in Alzheimer family caregivers. *American Journal of Alzheimer's Disease,12*, 171-178. doi:10.1177/153331759701200405.

Gaugler, J., Kane, R., & Newcomer, R. (2007). Resilience and transitions from dementia caregiving. *The Journals of Gerontology: Psychological Sciences, 62 B*, 38-44. doi:10.1093/geronb/62.1.P38.

Hoge, E., Austin, E., & Pollack, M. (2007). Resilience: Research evidence and conceptual considerations for posttraumatic stress disorder. *Depression and Anxiety, 24*, 139-152. doi: 10.1002/da.20175.

Jew, C., Green, K., & Kroger, J. (1999). Development and validation of a measure of resiliency. *Measurement and Evaluation in Counseling and Development, 32*, 75-89.

Katz, S., Ford, A., Moskowitz, R., Jackson, B., & Jaffe, M. (1963). Studies of illness in the aged. The index of A.D.L., a standardized measure of biological and psychological function. *JAMA, 185*, 914-919.

Khoshouei, M.S. (2009). Psychometric evaluation of the Connor-Davidson Resilience Scale (CD-RISC) using Iranian students. *International Journal of Testing, 9*, 60-66. doi:10.1080/15305050902733471

Kinney, J., & Parris Stephens, M. (1989). Hassles and uplifts of giving care to a family member with dementia. *Psychology and Aging, 4*, 402-408. doi:10.1037//0882-7974.4.4.402.

Kobasa, S. C. (1979). Stressful life events, personality, and health: an inquiry into hardiness. *Journal of Personality and Social Psychology, 37*, 1-11. doi:10.1037//0022-3514.37.1.1.

Lawton, M., Moss, M., Kleban, M., Glicksman, A., & Rovine, M. (1991). A two-factor model of caregiving appraisal and psychological well-being. *Journals of Gerontology, 46*, 181-189.

Lawton, M., Kleban, M., Moss, M., Rovine, M., & Glicksman, A. (1989). Measuring caregiving appraisal. *Journal of Gerontology, 44*, 61-71.

López, J. & Crespo, M. (2003). *Salud física y mental en los cuidadores informales de enfermos con demencia. Análisis de la situación y factores asociados* [Physical and mental health in caregivers for dementia patients. Analysis of situation and associated factors]. Rafael Burgaleta award. Unpublished work: COP de Madrid.

López, J., Crespo, M., Arinero, M., Gómez, M., & Francisco, M. (2004). *Initial analysis of psychometric properties of the Brief-Cope in a sample of caregivers of older relatives.* Málaga: Poster presented at VII European Conference on Psychological Assesment.

López, J., López-Arrieta, J. & Crespo, M. (2005). Factors associated with the positive impact of caring for elderly and dependent relatives. *Archives of Gerontology and Geriatrics, 41*, 81-94. doi:10.1016/j.archger.2004.12.001.

Luthar, S., Cicchetti, D., & Becker, B. (2000). The construct of resilience. A critical evaluation and guidelines for future work. *Child Development, 71*, 543-562. doi:10.1111/1467-8624.00164.

Martín, M., Salvadó, I., Nadal, S., Mijí, L., Rico, J., Lanz, P., et al. (1996). Adaptación a nuestro medio de la Escala de Sobrecarga del Cuidador de Zarit [Spanish adaptation of Caregiver Burden Interview]. *Revista de Gerontología, 6*, 338-346.

Menezes de Lucena, V., Fernández, B., Hernández, L., Ramos, F., & Contador, I. (2006). Resiliencia y el modelo de Burnout-Engagement en cuidadores formales de ancianos [Resilience and the burnout-engagement model in formal caregivers of the elderly]. *Psicothema, 18*, 791-796.

Morano, C.L. (2003). Appraisal and coping: Moderators or mediators of stress in Alzheimer's stress disease caregivers? *Social Work Research, 27*, 116-128. doi:10.1093/swr/27.2.116

Ong, A., Bergeman, C., Bisconti, T., & Wallace, K. (2006). Psychological Resilience, Positive Emotions, and Successful Adaptation to Stress in Later Life. *Journal of Personality and Social Psychology, 91* , 730-749. doi:10.1037/0022-3514.91.4.730.

O'Rourke, N., Kupferschmidt, A.L., Claxton, A., Smith, J.Z., Chappell, N., & Beattie, B. L. (2010). Psychological resilience and depressive symptoms among spouses of persons with Alzheimer disease over time. *Aging and Mental Health, 14*, 984-993. doi:10.1080/13607863.2010.501063.

Pearlin, L., Mullan, J., Semple, S., & Skaff, M. (1990). Caregiving and the stress process: An overview of concepts and their measures. *The Gerontologist, 30*, 583-594. doi:10.1093/geront/30.5.583.

Pinquart, M., & Sörensen, S. (2003a). Differences between caregivers and noncaregivers in psychological health and physical health: A meta-analysis. *Psychology and Aging, 18*, 250-267. doi:10.1037/0882-7974.18.2.250.

Pinquart, M., & Sörensen, S. (2003b). Associations of stressors and uplifts of caregiving with caregiver burden and depressive mood: A meta-analysis. *The Journals of Gerontology: Series B: Psychological Sciences and Social Sciences, 58B*, 112-128. doi:10.1093/geronb/58.2.P112.

Reisberg, B., Ferris, S., De Leon, M., & Crook, T. (1982). The Global Deterioration Scale for assessment of primary degenerative dementia. *American Journal of Psychiatry, 139*, 1136-1139.

Rosenberg, M. (1965). *Society and the adolescent self-image*. Princeton: Princeton University Press.

Sanz, J., Navarro, M., & Vázquez, C. (2003) Adaptación española del Inventario para la Depresión de Beck-II (BDI-II): 1. Propiedades psicométricas en estudiantes universitarios [The spanish adaptation of Beck's Depression Inventory-II (BDI-II): 1. Psychometric properties with college students]. *Análisis y Modificación de Conducta, 29*,239-288.

Saranson, I. (1999). El papel de las relaciones íntimas en los resultados de salud [The role of close relationships on health]. In: J. Buendía (Eds.), *Familia y Psicología de Salud* [Family and Health Psychology] (pp. 113-131). Madrid: Pirámide.

Saranson, I., Saranson, B., Shearin, E., & Pierce, G. (1987) A brief measure of social support: practical and theoretical implications. *Journal of Social and Personal Relationships, 4*,497-510.

Steffen, A., McKIbbin, C., Zeiss, A., Gallagher-Thompson, D., & Bandura, A. (2002). The revised scale for Caregiving self-efficacy: reliability and validity studies *The Journals of Gerontology Series B: Psychological Sciences and Social Sciences, 57B*,74-86. doi:10.1093/geronb/57.1.P74.

Tedeschi, R., & Kilmer, R. P. (2005). Assessing strengths, resilience, and growth to guide clinical interventions. *Professional Psychology: Research and Practice, 36* , 230-237. doi:10.1037/0735-7028.36.3.230.

Teri, L., Truax, P., Logsdon, R., Uomoto, J., Zarit, S., & Vitaliano, P. (1992). Assesment of behavioral problems in dementia. The revised memory and behavior problems checklist. *Psychology and Aging, 7*, 622-631.

Vinaccia, S., Quiceno, J.M., & Remor, E. (2012). Resiliencia, percepción de enfermedad, creencias y afrontamiento espiritual-religioso en relación con la calidad de vida relacionada con la salud en enfermos crónicos colombianos [Resilience, illness perception of disease, beliefs and spiritual religious coping in relation to the health-related quality of life in chronic colombian patients]. *Anales de Psicología, 28,* 366-377.

Vitaliano, P., Young, H.M., & Russo, J. (1991). Burden: a review of measures used among caregivers of individuals with dementia. *Gerontologist, 31,* 67-75. doi:10.1093/geront/31.1.67.

Vitaliano, P., Zhang, J., & Scalan, J. (2003). Is caregiving hazardous to one's physical health? A meta-analysis. *Pychological Bulletin, 129,* 946-972. doi:10.1037/0033-2909.129.6.946.

Wagnild, G. M., & Young, H. M. (1993). Development and psychometric evaluation of the Resilience Scale. *Journal of Nursing Measurement, 1,* 165-178.

Werner, E., Smith, & R. (1982). *Vulnerable but invincible: A study of resilient children.* New York: McGraw-Hill.

White, B., Driver, S., & Warren, A. (2008). Considering resilience in the rehabilitation of people with traumatic disabilities. *Rehabilitation Psychology, 53,* 9-17. doi:10.1037/0090-5550.53.1.9.

Wilks, S., & Croom, B. (2008). Perceived stress and resilience in Alzheimer's disease caregivers: Testing moderation and mediation models of social support. *Aging & Mental Health, 12,* 357-365. doi:10.1080/13607860801933323.

Wilks, S., Little, K., Gough, H., & Spurlock, W. (2011). Alzheimer's aggression: Influences on caregiver coping and resilience. *Journal of Gerontological Social Work, 54,* 260-275. doi:10.1080/ 01634372.2010.544531.

Wilks, S., & Vonk, M. (2008). Private prayer among Alzheimer's caregivers: mediating burden and resiliency. *Journal of Gerontological Social Work, 50,* 113-131. doi:10.1300/J083v50n3_09.

Yu, X. & Zhang, J. (2007). Factor analysis and psychometric evaluation of the Connor-Davidson Resilience Scale (CD-RISC) with Chinese people. *Social Behavior and Personality, 35,* 19-30. doi:10.2224/ sbp.2007.35.1.19.

Zarit, S., Reever, K., & Bach-Peterson, J. (1980). Relatives of the impaired elderly: correlates of feelings of burden. *Gerontologist, 20,* 646-655. doi:10.1093/geront/20.6.649.

Zigmond, A., & Snaith, R. (1983). The Hospital Anxiety and Depression Scale. *Acta Psychiatrica Scandinavica, 67,* 361-370. doi:10.1111/j.1600-0447.1983.tb09716.x.

In: Caregivers: Challenges, Practices and Cultural Influences ISBN: 978-1-62618-030-7
Editors: Adrianna Thurgood and Kasha Schuldt © 2013 Nova Science Publishers, Inc.

Chapter 7

CAREGIVER BURDEN IN A HONG KONG CHINESE POPULATION: RISK FACTORS, CONSEQUENCES AND REMEDIES

P. H. Chau[1], T. Kwok[2] and J. Woo[2]*

[1]School of Nursing, Li Ka Shing Faculty of Medicine,
The University of Hong Kong, Hong Kong, China
[2]Department of Medicine & Therapeutics, Faculty of Medicine,
The Chinese University of Hong Kong, Hong Kong, China

ABSTRACT

To achieve the goal of ageing-in-place, informal family caregivers who look after older people at home are of crucial importance. In Hong Kong, over half of all elderly people who receive informal care are cared for by their children. Despite traditional Chinese beliefs concerned with filial piety, these caregivers, particularly if they have to deal with dementia or stroke patients, often face very heavy burdens, which may in turn lead to higher risk of institutionalization, and in some extreme cases abuse of the elderly. Deterioration in functional and cognitive status of the care recipient produces two of the main factors adding to the caregiver burden, while assistance from domestic helpers and a sense of self-efficacy may reduce it. Some initiatives, such as training programs for caregivers, which may ameliorate their situation have been established. In this chapter, existing and new evidence is presented on the risk factors and consequences of caregiver burden among the Hong Kong Chinese population, and strategies to tackle such burdens are discussed.

INTRODUCTION

Hong Kong, which is a Special Administrative Region of China, has a population of over 7 million, of whom 13.7% are aged 65 and above [1]. The proportion of the institutional

---

* Corresponding author. Email of corresponding author: phchau@graduate.hku.hk.

elderly population is much higher in Hong Kong than in New York or London [2]. In 2009, almost 7% of older people aged 65 and above were living in old age homes [3]. Nevertheless, over 90% of the older population still live in the community and, to achieve the goal of "ageing-in-place", informal family caregivers shoulder the bulk of the responsibility for looking after them [4-6].

Over 90% of the older Hong Kong population are Chinese [7], and as such they have certain traditional beliefs about informal care for family members. For example, women are expected to provide care for other family members, and elderly couples expect their adult children or children-in-law to do the same. There is a large imbalance between male and female caregivers, with women taking up most of the care-giving tasks [8,9]. The concept of filial piety also leads Chinese people to view caring for their older family members as an unavoidable obligation. However, both the increasing number of nuclear families and the rising proportion of women in the workforce pose challenges to such informal family caregiving. Although the influence of traditional Confucian filial piety tends to be diminishing, adult children still follow the practice in caring for their older parents and relatives [10]. However, the weakening of the filial piety concept may challenge the relationship between informal caregivers and older care recipients [11,12]. In a multi-centre study, there was no evidence that filial piety could reduce the occurrence of distress among those caring for dementia patients [13]. The younger generation frequently face a dilemma in caring for their parents, involving their own families and their work commitments, as well as difficult decisions about home versus institutional care [14,15].

According to a survey conducted by the Hong Kong Census and Statistics Department, about 37% and 27% of home-dwelling care recipients aged 60 and above were looked after, respectively, by their children or spouse as the major caregivers [16]. However, local research studies have found a higher percentage of caregivers being children or children-in-law of the recipients, with over half of elderly home-dwelling recipients being cared for in this way [17-21].

Care-giving is not an easy task, and the role could become a life-long commitment [22]. Sometimes, the relationship between family members deteriorates, and it is not uncommon to find caregiver stress. In this chapter, existing and new evidence is presented on the risk factors and consequences of caregiver burden among the Hong Kong Chinese population, and strategies to tackle the issue are discussed.

CAREGIVER BURDEN IN HONG KONG

Despite traditional Chinese beliefs concerned with filial piety, informal caregivers often face very heavy burdens. These primary caregivers face challenges of an emotional, social and physical nature [22]. Because there are now more chronic diseases and disabilities co-existing with longevity, fewer informal caregivers available, and more complexity in the caring regimes coupled with a lack of support services, health literacy and skills, stress among caregivers has become more acute than in the past [6].

Yip and colleagues found that women who needed to take care of or were worried about sick family members, relatives or friends had a higher risk of manifesting low back pain [23]. Another local study also showed consistent findings on adverse effects on health. Ho and colleagues conducted the first population-based cross-sectional study on informal caregivers to older people in Hong Kong [24]. The findings confirmed the fact that primary caregivers had poorer physical and psychological health than those not involved in care-giving. In terms of physical health, primary caregivers were more likely to report medical consultations, weight loss and worse health compared with the previous year. Illnesses such as osteoporosis, arthritis, digestive ulcers and bronchitis were more likely to exist. In terms of psychological health, primary caregivers were more likely to report poorer quality of life (as reflected by lower scores in SF-36 Health Survey), anxiety and depression; and symptoms such as headache, dizziness and loss of memory were more likely to occur. Furthermore, women were more affected than men by the burdens of care-giving. Stress among caregivers may also adversely affect their immune status. One study has shown that immune function, as measured by the lymphocyte (cell-mediated) and cytokine immune response to influenza vaccination, was lower among caregivers dealing with stroke, Parkinson's disease and/or dementia patients, compared with age- and gender-matched controls who were not caregivers but had a partner without a chronic illness [25].

Caregivers also face economic problems in caring for older people. A pilot study estimated the self-reported monthly expenses (excluding income loss) of care-giving to older people for one year [26], and found that about half of the caregivers spent more than HK$1,000 (US$128) on care-giving per month. In addition, 18% reported income reduction, 15% taking leave or absence from work, 14% working part-time, 11% routinely leaving work early and 9% early retirement. Wimo and colleagues estimated that informal care for home-dwelling people with dementia increased from US$602.6 million in 2005 to US$823.3 million in 2009, assuming an average 3.7 hours of caring per day [27,28]. Chau and colleagues also summarized estimates of the opportunity costs of informal caregivers to older people with chronic illness [29]. The opportunity cost (as compared with a full-time worker) of informal caregivers to elderly stroke patients aged 65 and above was projected to increase from HK$5.0 billion (US$0.6 billion) in 2010 to HK$13.3 billion (US$1.7 billion) in 2036, while in the case of elderly dementia patients aged 60 and above the increase would be from HK$10.4 billion (US$1.3 billion) in 2010 to HK$27.0 billion (US$3.5 billion) in 2036. These were conservative estimates which assumed the prevalence rate of the disease remained stable.

RISK FACTORS OF CAREGIVER BURDEN IN HONG KONG

Deterioration in functional and cognitive status produces two of the main factors contributing to the caregiver burden. Some diseases or conditions, such as stroke or dementia, are more demanding in terms of care-giving and require advice from specialized healthcare professionals, causing further hardship to the caregiver [6]. While there is a linear relationship between functional limitation levels and the caregiver burden, the relationship between cognitive impairment levels and the burden is more complex. Older care recipients with greater cognitive impairment are likely to have higher levels of functional limitation and more behavioral and psychological symptoms that affect caregivers indirectly. Fortunately, there exist some protective factors for the caregiver, domestic help and self-efficacy among them.

In 2007 to 2008, we conducted a survey on community-dwelling older people with limitations in functional and/or cognitive status and their caregivers in Hong Kong. The methodology is described in details elsewhere [19]. Older care recipients with a score of less than 6 on the Abbreviated Mental Test–Hong Kong version (AMT) (range: 0-10) or with a doctor's diagnosis of dementia were regarded in this study as having cognitive impairment [30]. The characteristics of both recipients and caregivers were collected. The caregiver burden was assessed by the Cost of Care Index (CCI)–Chinese version (range: 20-80), higher scores indicating heavier burdens [31]. Functional status was measured by the Multi-Dimensional Functional Assessment Questionnaire (MFAQ) (range: 14-42), with higher scores indicating better condition [32]. The behavioral and psychological symptoms of these cognitively impaired recipients were measured by the Chinese version of the Neuropsychiatric Inventory (NPI) (range: 0-144), higher scores indicating a worse condition [33]. In the survey, 705 caregivers were interviewed, with a response rate of 81.2%. In the following analysis, only main caregivers were included, 262 of older people with functional impairment only and 278 of older people with both functional and cognitive impairment. When comparing the two groups, we found that the caregiver burdens (as measured by the CCI) of the two groups were not statistically different, after controlling for their age and sex and for the age, sex and functional status of the recipients. This suggests functional status plays a more important role in adversely affecting caregivers than cognitive status.

The two groups of caregivers were then analyzed separately with multiple linear regressions to identify risk or protective factors. The factors examined included age, sex, income, education level, occupation and living arrangements (living together with care recipient or not) of the caregivers, relationship to the recipient, duration of the care-giving role, usage of community services, assistance from domestic helpers, as well as the age, sex and functional status of the recipients. In the case of caregivers to the cognitively impaired, behavioral and psychological symptoms were included as additional risk factors. We found that, for caregivers to functionally impaired recipients, a heavier burden was independently associated with poorer functional status among recipients (p-value<0.001) and shorter duration of care-giving role (p-value=0.014). For caregivers to both functionally and cognitively impaired patients, a heavier burden was independently associated with lower age in recipients (p-value=0.002), poorer functional status of recipients (p-value<0.001), more behavioral and psychological symptoms (p-value<0.001) among recipients, lack of support from domestic helpers (p-value=0.003), and higher education attainment among caregivers (p-value=0.012).

Our findings are consistent with the local literature in that, for caregivers to people with dementia, behavioral and psychological symptoms in the patient are predictive factors of an increasing caregiver burden [20]. In particular, caregivers to people with dementia face challenges concerned with confusion about their diagnosis, negative emotions, difficulties in coping with recipients' behavior, provision of their daily care needs, and conflicts among social roles [34]. Our results add two more findings to the literature. First, the assistance of a domestic helper was identified as a protective factor of the caregiver burden. This is an important observation since about 10% of households in Hong Kong employ domestic helpers [35]. Training these domestic helpers and supporting families to employ them could help to relieve the caregiver. Second, a shorter period of care-giving was identified as a risk factor for the caregiver. Shorter care-giving periods may imply that caregivers had less experience of the role, or that they had just taken it up and had not yet fully adapted. In this light, providing counseling and training in the early days of care-giving is clearly needed to stop the caregiver's burdens accumulating. Two further interesting findings were observed - lower age in recipients and higher educational attainment in caregivers were both associated with a heavier caregiver burden. The former finding may imply a perceived long period of care-giving, thus increasing the caregiver's worries. The latter may reflect busier lifestyles among caregivers, as those with higher education levels are more likely to be involved in the workforce, and the conflict between work commitments and care-giving may possibly increase the pressure.

Stroke is a major contributor to disability. A heavy burden on caregivers to stroke survivors is not uncommon [36]. In 2009-2012, we conducted a survey on older stroke survivors and their caregivers in Hong Kong, described in details elsewhere [21]. Here, we extract some data for an analysis of the burden on stroke survivor caregivers. Interviews were held with 125 caregivers to older stroke patients who had been discharged from public hospitals and continued rehabilitation at a public geriatric day hospital. About a quarter (25.8%) of these patients were discharged to old-age homes (nursing homes) and the remainder to their own homes. The patients had to travel to the geriatric hospital twice a week for rehabilitation treatment. The functional status of these people was measured by the Modified Barthel Index (MBI) (range 0-100), with higher scores indicating more independence in daily living activity [37,38]. The cognitive status of the care recipients was measured by the Mini-Mental Status Examination (MMSE) (range 0-30), with higher scores indicating better cognitive status [39]. The caregiver burden was measured by the Zarit Burden Interview (ZBI) (range 0-88), with higher scores indicating a greater caregiver burden [40,41].

Multiple linear regression was used to identify the risk or protective factors related to the caregiver burden. Potential factors to be examined included age, sex, income, education level and occupation of the caregivers, relationship with the recipient, payment of expenses, assistance from domestic helpers, and the age, sex, functional status, cognitive status and living arrangements (old age home or own home) of recipients. We found that poorer functional status (p-value=0.019) and the caregiver having to bear all the expenditure (p-value=0.005) were independently associated with a heavier burden on the caregiver.

Our findings, consistent with the existing local literature, suggest that the needs of caregivers to stroke patients may be different from those of people dealing with dementia patients. Mak and colleagues found that financial and psychological problems contributed to stress among stroke survivor caregivers in Hong Kong [42]. In our analysis, one risk factor was related to financial issues - a caregiver who had to bear all the expenditure had a greater burden than those who did not, or who did so only in part, highlighting the importance of providing financial support to this group of caregivers.

Louie and colleagues found that cognitive impairment and the functional impairment of the care recipients with stroke impacted caregivers in different ways - respectively related to higher levels of negative feeling and of personal distress (as measured by two subscales of Relatives' Stress Scale) [18]. We found that functional status was a better predictive factor than cognitive status to caregiver burden as a whole. The discrepancy between the two studies might be due to the method of analysis whereby Louie and colleagues did not control for other confounders when exploring the correlations between risk factors and caregiver stress. In fact, cognitive impairment could imply a higher level of dependency and lower level of physical activity. In addition, Louie and colleagues found that older caregivers sustained higher levels of stress, attributing these observations to a reduction in physical health and psychomotor function among caregivers and the sudden take up of the care-giving role without formal training.

It should be noted that residence in an old age home did not reduce the caregiver burden of the caregivers of the stroke patients (p-value=0.565), especially these caregivers continued to take an active role in caring for the patients. This suggests that caregiver burden not only occurred among those caregivers to home-dwelling older people, but it also applied to caregivers to institutionalized older people.

Besides the assistance of domestic helpers, the self-efficacy of caregivers (interpreted as a belief in their ability to master challenges in the care-giving role and tasks) is attracting more recognition for its role as a protective factor. Au and colleagues found that high self-efficacy might lead to well-being and reduce depressive symptoms among caregivers to people with dementia [17]. Cheng and colleagues reported that higher self-efficacy in controlling upsetting thoughts was associated with more positive gains and less caregiver burden among those caring for dementia patients when they were dealing with the behavioral problems of their care recipients [43]. Lui and colleagues had similar findings, that confidence in problem-solving among caregivers to stroke survivors was associated with their self-perceived social support and physical well-being [44]. These findings support the later development of interventions to reduce caregiver burden by increasing their self-efficacy.

CONSEQUENCES OF CAREGIVER BURDEN IN HONG KONG

These burdens not only affect the well-being of the caregivers themselves, but can in turn adversely affect the older people who are receiving care. If caregivers are physically exhausted, in poor health and suffering from depression, they may fail to deliver care for their relatives effectively [15]. When the caregiver burden is under control, the severity of the recipients' symptoms may well be reduced, as well as the frequency and duration of institutionalization in hospital or old age home [45,46]. In this way, symptoms and institutionalization could be seen as adverse outcomes of the caregiver burden. An overseas study has shown that caregiver training can reduce mortality and delay institutionalization of care recipients with dementia [47], implying on the other hand that less well-controlled caregiver burdens might lead to higher mortality and institutionalization rates.

The caregiver burden may lead to early institutionalization. In Hong Kong, Chau and colleagues conducted a survey on the preference for institutional care for the elderly [19]. It was found that caregivers with greater burdens (as measured by CCI) preferred to let their care recipients switch to an institution. The research team followed up the old people after a year to check whether they had been institutionalized or not [48]. By bivariate analysis, it was found that greater burdens on caregivers were associated with a higher risk of actual institutionalization of old people with both functional and cognitive impairments. However, when controlled for the functional status of the care recipients, caregiver burden was not a significant factor, suggesting higher caregiver burdens were probably related to greater functional impairment.

In some extreme cases, the conflicts between caregivers and recipients result in abuse of the elderly. In a local study, it was revealed that over a quarter (27.5%) of older people had experienced at least one instance of abusive behavior on the part of their caregivers: their adult children (88%), spouses (25%), grandchildren (9%) or domestic helpers (4%) [49]. It was found that over a quarter of the victims were abused by multiple abusers. While the study did not establish a relationship between caregiver burden and occurrence of abuse, it was shown that the more dependent the recipients, the more abuse.

REMEDIES FOR CAREGIVER BURDEN IN HONG KONG

There is a clear need to support caregivers in their roles, and to promote their effectiveness in caring for old people while coping with the caregiver burden [22]. However, only limited services such as caregiver support, day care and respite care are provided or subsidized by the Hong Kong Social Welfare Department. Researchers and service providers are still seeking the most cost-effective interventions to support caregivers and reduce their burdens. Nevertheless, it seems that, although much attention is paid to the caregivers of dementia patients, little is given to those who look after the elderly in general. In this section, some of the initiatives being pursued in Hong Kong will be discussed.

Some interventions focus on providing care for old people and hence relieving the caregiver burden. For example, dementia day care centers provide center-based care and support services during the day for those home-dwelling older people who are frail or suffer from dementia. Medical consultation, advice and referral for financial and social welfare support, training or talks about dementia care, and social and recreational activities are all provided for patients, together with support and assistance for caregivers. One self-financed day care center for people with dementia, the Jockey Club Centre for Positive Ageing, conducted a prospective study on newly admitted clients and found that the burdens (as measured by ZBI) on family caregivers were significantly reduced after a year's usage of the center [50].

Other interventions focus on providing trainings, support and assistance to caregivers directly. For example, mutual support groups, specially designed for family caregivers, serve as a platform for members to exchange personal experiences of care-giving challenges. Other components include education and training, sharing and discussion, psychological support, and problem-solving skills. Mutual support groups have been shown to be capable of achieving a greater reduction in distress levels among caregivers when managing their care recipients' problem behavior, and a greater increase in quality of life, both psychologically and socially, than conventional family services [46,51]. Fung and Chien also found that caregivers attending mutual support groups appreciated the opportunity to share their feelings and concerns, gained insights into problem-solving, and thus reduced the sense of guilt and distress involved in their care-giving [51]. Also, through sharing, they understood that they were not the only ones with problems. The team highlighted the importance of psycho-social support as a means of relieving the caregiver burden.

Another example is a psycho-educational program for caregivers to people with dementia. Au and colleagues developed and evaluated such a program via a cognitive-behavioral therapy approach [52]. The educational component was in line with the pragmatic characteristics of the Chinese caregivers, who were looking for practical problem-solving skills. Furthermore, flexibility in coping was also in line with the Chinese values of balance and integration, while they will adopt different strategies. The program proved to be effective in increasing caregivers' self-efficacy in controlling their own disturbing thoughts and handling problem behavior among their recipients. The caregivers also showed an increased use of problem-based and emotion-focused coping strategies, and the research team suggested future such programs should incorporate training in applying flexible coping skills according to specific situations, additional to practical problem-solving skills.

Many caregivers fail to join support services because of the costs in time and transport. To fill this service gap, a telephone-delivered psycho-educational program was developed by the Jockey Club Centre for Positive Ageing to enhance quality of life for caregivers of relatives with dementia. The intervention introduced ways to prevent or handle care-giving difficulties, with social workers cooperating with caregivers to improve the latter's relationship with care recipients. Communication skills, care planning, and tips for preventing or handling emotional distress were discussed over the phone. Findings from a pilot study showed that caregivers receiving the intervention experienced reduced levels of stress and improved efficacy in obtaining respite and responding to disruptive patient behavior, compared with those who had not received the intervention [53]. These positive results demonstrated the usefulness of telephone interventions in providing psycho-educational support for caregivers.

Apart from viewing interventions as directed solely towards problem-solving, some researchers promote an intervention for caregivers of elderly dementia patients that seeks to identify the benefits there might be [15]. Based on the belief that there are rewards, advances and gains in the caring process, the new intervention emphasizes the benefits rather than the losses and difficulties of the caring process. The trial is currently ongoing, but it is expected that through this new intervention caregivers will report a more positive side of caring, lower stress and depression, and less overload, as well as better subjective health and psychological well-being, than they experience with the usual routine treatment.

Some interventions target both care recipients and their caregivers. For example, a trial by Chung studied an empowering program for older people at an early stage of dementia and their caregivers that involved educational activities and other forms of support [54]. The educational component consisted of instruction on memory functions, practicing memory strategies, and participation in a task-oriented activity organized for recipients. Separate support groups were held for caregivers and care recipients. The caregivers learnt about caring strategies and community resources, shared their caring experiences and sought mutual support. It was clear that both caregivers and recipients shared pleasurable feelings and developed close relationships. In addition, caregivers came to see caring as a valuable and meaningful occupation. Chung suggested that educational and support programs for people at an early stage of dementia and their caregivers were important since the disorder was something new to both sides, and that the family should be used as the unit of participation to foster intra-family support and close bonding.

Chien and Lee [45], basing their work on Fung and Chien [51], developed a care management program for family caregivers of people with dementia. A case manager coordinated a tailored family care program according to the results of a family needs assessment. In parallel, routine dementia care was provided for the patients. It was shown that there were greater improvements in psychological distress levels and quality of life, and less use of family services, among the caregivers in the intervention group than in the standard care group. The care recipients in the intervention group also showed greater improvement in pathological behavior and shorter periods of institutionalization.

In the case of these interventions, the critical issue is how to motivate caregivers to seek help. Particularly in a Chinese population, caregivers tend to be reluctant to let professionals know about their problems and to seek formal help with them [42,55,56]. It was observed that the caregivers to people with dementia did not seek help until the problem behavior was already out of control [56]. In addition, the caregivers might be overwhelmed by tasks such that seeking help or receiving interventions became a challenge for them. Provision of a parallel comprehensive family service is therefore recommended, in order to release caregivers to attend mutual support groups or other psycho-social support programs; alternative ways of intervention, such as the telephone-delivered type, are also recommended [51,53].

CONCLUSION

Caregivers to older people face great challenges. The Chinese population in Hong Kong is no exception, although the concept of filial piety is recognized and practiced by the younger generation of caregivers. Consistent with the Western literature, the physical and psychological health problems and economic burdens are common to caregivers of the elderly in Hong Kong. Deterioration in functional and cognitive status produces two of the main factors contributing to the caregiver burden. Some diseases or conditions, such as stroke and dementia, are more demanding of care-giving, and require advices from specialized healthcare professionals, which lead to an increased burden on caregivers. Other risk factors include more behavioral and psychological symptoms among dementia patients, younger care recipients, higher educational attainment among caregivers, shorter experience of the care-giving role, and caregivers being solely responsible for all expenditure. Placing elderly people in homes does not seem to help reduce the caregiver burden, although the assistance of domestic helpers and self-efficacy are two positive factors.

The population is ageing rapidly, and family caregivers constitute a valuable resource for looking after the huge older population. However, ignoring the health impact of the caregiver burden will only contribute to the magnitude of those burdens as well as to a predisposition to institutionalize care recipients; or it may lead in extreme cases to abuse of the elderly. Some initiatives that may ameliorate the caregiver's lot have already been established, but the critical issue is still how to provide adequate community support in terms of services and accessibility, how to promote such services and motivate caregivers to seek help, and perhaps to put in place flexible work options to facilitate the care-giving task.

REFERENCES

[1] Hong Kong Census and Statistics Department. *Table 002: Population by Age Group and Sex*. Accessed on Nov 12, 2012. Available from: http://www.censtatd.gov.hk/showtableexcel2.jsp?tableID=002.

[2] Chau PH, Woo J, Gusmano MK, Weisz D, Rodwin VG. *Growing Older in Hong Kong, New York and London*. Hong Kong: The Hong Kong Jockey Club; 2012.

[3] Sau Po Center of Ageing and Department of Social Work and Social Administration, The University of Hong Kong. *Consultancy Study on Community Care Services for the Elderly - Final Report*. Accessed on Nov 12, 2012. Available from: http://www.elderlycommission.gov.hk/en/download/library/Community%20Care%20Services%20Report%202011_eng.pdf.

[4] Chow N. The changing responsibilities of the state and family toward elders in Hong Kong. *Journal of Aging & Social Policy*. 1993;5:111-126.

[5] Phillips DR. Ageing in the Asia-Pacific region: Issues, policies and contexts. In: Phillips DR, ed. *Ageing in the Asia-Pacific Region: Issues, Policies and Future Trends*. London: Routledge; 2000:1-34.

[6] Ngan R. Social care and older people. In: Stuart-Hamilton I, ed. *An Introduction to Gerontology*. Cambridge: Cambridge University Press; 2011:126-158.

[7] Hong Kong Census and Statistics Department. *Population by Ethnicity, 2001, 2006 and 2011 (A104)*. Accessed on Nov 12, 2012. Available from: http://www.census2011.gov.hk/en/main-table/A104.html.

[8] Ngan R, Wong W. Injustice in family care of the Chinese elderly in Hong Kong. *Journal of Aging and Social Policy*. 1996;7:77-94.

[9] Holroyd E. Hong Kong Chinese daughters' intergenerational caregiving obligations: a cultural model approach. *Social Science & Medicine*. 2001;53:1125-1134.

[10] Chow N. The practice of filial piety and its impact on long-term care policies for elderly people in Asian Chinese communities. *Asian Journal of Gerontology and Geriatrics*. 2006;1:31-35.

[11] Ng ACY, Phillips DR, Lee WKM. Persistence and challenges to filial piety and informal support of older persons in a modern Chinese society: A case study in Tuen Mun, Hong Kong. *Journal of Aging Studies*. 2002;16:135-153.

[12] Lee WKM, Kwok HK. Differences in expectations and patterns of informal support for older persons in Hong Kong: Modification to filial piety. *Ageing International*. 2005;30:188-206.

[13] Pang FC, Chow TW, Cummings JL, et al. Effect of neuropsychiatric symptoms of Alzheimer's disease on Chinese and American caregivers. *International Journal of Geriatric Psychiatry*. 2002;17:29-34.

[14] Ngan R, Cheng ICK. The caring dilemma, stress and needs of caregivers for the Chinese frail elderly. *Hong Kong Journal of Gerontology*. 1992;6:34-41.

[15] Cheng ST, Lau RWL, Mak EPM, et al. A benefit-finding intervention for family caregivers of persons with Alzheimer disease: study protocol of a randomized controlled trial. *Trials*. 2012;13:98.

[16] Hong Kong Census and Statistics Department . *Thematic Household Survey Report No. 21*. Hong Kong: Census and Statistics Department;2005.

[17] Au A, Lai MK, Lau KM, et al. Social support and well-being in dementia family caregivers: the mediating role of self-efficacy. *Aging & Mental Health*. 2009;13:761-768.

[18] Louie SWS, Liu PKK, Man DWK. Stress of caregivers in caring for people with stroke: Implications for rehabilitation. *Topics in Geriatric Rehabilitation*. 2009;25:191-197.

[19] Chau PH, Kwok T, Woo J, Chan F, Hui E, Chan KC. Disagreement in preference for residential care between family caregivers and elders is greater among cognitively impaired elders group than cognitively intact elders group. *International Journal of Geriatric Psychiatry.* 2010;25:46-54.

[20] Cheng ST, Lam LCW, Kwok T. Neuropsychiatric symptom clusters of Alzheimer's disease in Hong Kong Chinese: Correlates with caregiver burden and depression. *American Journal of Geriatric Psychiatry.* 2012;doi: 10.1097/JGP.0b013e318266b9e8

[21] Chau PH, Yeung F, Chan TW, Woo J. *Evaluation of a new service option for stroke patients in Hong Kong.* Poster presented at the 19th Annual Congress of Gerontology, Hong Kong; 2012.

[22] Mackenzie AE, Holroyd EE. An exploration of the carers' perceptions of caregiving and caring responsibilities in Chinese families. *International Journal of Nursing Studies.* 1996;33:1-12.

[23] Yip YB, Ho SC, Chan SG. Socio-psychological stressors as risk factors for low back pain in Chinese middle-aged women. *Journal of Advanced Nursing.* 2001;36:409-416.

[24] Ho SC, Chan A, Woo J, Chong P, Sham A. Impact of caregiving on health and quality of life: A comparative population-based study of caregivers for elderly persons and noncaregivers. *The Journals of Gerontology. Series A, Biological Sciences and Medical Sciences.* 2009;64A:873-879.

[25] Wong SYS, Wong CK, Chan FWK, et al. Chronic psychosocial stress: does it modulate immunity to the influenza vaccine in Hong Kong Chinese elderly caregivers? *Age.* 2012;doi: 10.1007/s11357-012-9449-z.

[26] You JHS, Ho SC, Sham A. Economic burden of informal caregivers for elderly Chinese in Hong Kong. *Journal of the American Geriatrics Society.* 2008;56:1577-1578.

[27] Wimo A, Winblad B, Jŏnsson L. An estimate of the total worldwide societal costs of dementia in 2005. *Alzheimer's and Dementia.* 2007;3:81-91.

[28] Wimo A, Winblad B, Jŏnsson L. The worldwide societal costs of dementia: Estimates for 2009. *Alzheimer's and Dementia.* 2010;6:98-103.

[29] Chau PH, McGhee SM, Woo J. Population ageing: Impact of common chronic diseases on health and social services. In: Woo J, ed. *Aging in Hong Kong:* A Comparative Perspective. New York: Springer; 2013:115-156.

[30] Chu LW, Pei CKW, Ho MH, Chan PT. Validation of the abbreviated mental test (Hong Kong version) in the elderly medical patient. *Hong Kong Medical Journal.* 1995;1:207-211.

[31] Tseh EOY. *Validation of Chinese version of the 'cost of care index'.* Unpublished M.Sc. Dissertation. Hong Kong: The Hong Kong Polytechnic University; 2003.

[32] Chiu HC, Chen YC, Mau LW, et al. An evaluation of the reliability and validity of the Chinese-version Oars multidimensional functional assessment questionnaire. *Chinese Journal of Public Health.* 1997;16:119-132.

[33] Leung VPY, Lam LCW, Chiu HFK, Cummings JL, Chen QL. Validation study of the Chinese version of the neuropsychiatric inventory (CNPI). *International Journal of Geriatric Psychiatry.* 2001;16:789-793.

[34] Chan WC, Ng C, Mok CC, Wong FLF, Pang SL, Chiu HFK. Lived experience of caregivers of persons with dementia in Hong Kong: A qualitative Study. *East Asian Archives of Psychiatry.* 2010;20:163-168.

[35] Hong Kong Census and Statistics Department. *Thematic Household Survey Report No. 5.* Hong Kong: Census and Statistics Department; 2001.
[36] Low JTS, Payne S, Roderick P. The impact of stroke on informal carers: a literature review. *Social Science and Medicine.* 1999;49:711-725.
[37] Shah S, Vanclay F, Cooper B. Improving the sensitivity of the Barthel Index for stroke rehabilitation. *Journal of Clinical Epidemiology.* 1989;42:703-709.
[38] Leung SOC, Chan CCH, Shah S. Development of a Chinese version of the Modified Barthel Index-- validity and reliability. *Clinical Rehabilitation.* 2007;21:912-922.
[39] Chiu HF, Lee HC, Chung WS, Kwong PK. Reliability and validity of the Cantonese version of the Mini-Mental State Examination: a preliminary study. *Journal of Hong Kong College of Psychiatrists.* 1994;4:25-28.
[40] Zarit SH, Reever KE, Bach-Peterson J. Relatives of the impaired elderly: correlates of feelings of burden. *The Gerontologist.* 1980;20:649-655.
[41] Chan TSF, Lam LCW, Chiu HFK. Validation of the Chinese version of the Zarit Burden Interview. *Hong Kong Journal of Psychiatry.* 2005;15:9-13.
[42] Mak AKM, Mackenzie A, Lui MHL. Changing needs of Chinese family caregivers of stroke survivors. *Journal of Clinical Nursing.* 2007;16:971-979.
[43] Cheng ST, Lam LCW, Kwok T, Ng NS, Fung AW. Self-efficacy is associated with less burden and more gains from behavioral problems of Alzheimer's disease in Hong Kong Chinese caregivers. *The Gerontologist.* 2012; doi: 10.1093/geront/gns062
[44] Lui MHL, Lee DTF, Greenwood N, Ross FM. Informal stroke caregivers' self-appraised problem-solving abilities as a predictor of well-being and perceived social support. *Journal of Clinical Nursing.* 2012;21:232-242.
[45] Chien WT, Lee YM. A disease management program for families of persons in Hong Kong with dementia. *Psychiatric Services.* 2008;59:433-436.
[46] Wang LQ, Chien WT. Randomised controlled trial of a family-led mutual support programme for people with dementia. *Journal of Clinical Nursing.* 2011;20:2362-2366.
[47] Mittelman MS, Ferris SH, Steinberg G, Shulman E, Mackell JA, Cohen J. An intervention that delays institutionalization of Alzheimer's disease patients: Treatment of spouse-caregivers. *The Gerontologist.* 1993;33:730-740.
[48] Chau PH, Woo J, Kwok T, Chan F, Hui E, Chan KC. Usage of community services and domestic helpers predicted institutionalization of the elders having functional or cognitive impairments: A 12-month longitudinal study in Hong Kong. *Journal of the American Medical Directors Association.* 2012;13:169-175.
[49] Yan ECW, Tang CSK. Elder abuse by caregivers: A study of prevalence and risk factors in Hong Kong Chinese families. *Journal of Family Violence.* 2004;19:269-277.
[50] Kwok T, Young D, Yip A, Ho F. Effectiveness of day care services for dementia patients and their caregivers. *Asian Journal of Gerontology & Geriatrics.* In press.
[51] Fung WY, Chien WT. The effectiveness of a mutual support group for family caregivers of a relative with dementia. *Archives of Psychiatric Nursing.* 2002;16:134-144.

[52] Au A, Li S, Lee K, et al. The Coping with Caregiving Group Program for Chinese caregivers of patients with Alzheimer's disease in Hong Kong. *Patient Education and Counseling*. 2010;78:256-260.

[53] Chui K, Yip A, Kwok T, Ho F. The effectiveness of telephone-delivered psycho-educational intervention to caregivers taking care of people with dementia. Poster presented at the 18th Annual Congress of Gerontology, Hong Kong; 2010.

[54] Chung JCC. Empowering individuals with early dementia and their carers: an exploratory study in the Chinese context. *American Journal of Alzheimer's Disease and Other Dementias*. 2001;16:85-88.

[55] Lui MHL, Mackenzie AE. Chinese elderly patients' perception of their rehabilitation needs following a stroke. *Journal of Advanced Nursing*. 1999;30:391-400.

[56] Chow TW, Liu CK, Fuh JL, et al. Neuropsychiatric symptoms of Alzheimer's disease differ in Chinese and American patients. *International Journal of Geriatric Psychiatry*. 2002;17:22-28.

In: Caregivers: Challenges, Practices and Cultural Influences
Editors: Adrianna Thurgood and Kasha Schuldt

ISBN: 978-1-62618-030-7
© 2013 Nova Science Publishers, Inc.

Chapter 8

MANAGING COMPASSION FATIGUE AMONG PROFESSIONAL CANCER CAREGIVERS: UNDERSTANDING THE PROBLEM AND POSSIBLE TREATMENT STRATEGIES

Amanda C. Kracen and Teresa L. Deshields
Siteman Cancer Center, Barnes-Jewish Hospital and Washington University,
St. Louis, Missouri, US

ABSTRACT

Professional cancer caregivers work with patients who are ill and vulnerable. Caregivers have opportunities to support and care for patients, and hopefully, to offer comfort and healing. However, as a result of the empathy and personal involvement they bring to their jobs, compassion fatigue (CF) is a common professional challenge. Recognizing that CF negatively affects many caregivers, as well as their colleagues and patients, this chapter provides an overview of recent research into CF in professional cancer caregivers. Specifically, the chapter defines CF and related constructs, reviews the prevalence and effects of CF, highlights why CF is a concern in oncology, and provides an overview of evidence-based interventions and personal coping strategies to ameliorate symptoms and enhance resiliency among caregivers.

INTRODUCTION

Professional caregivers are often drawn to their professions by a desire to care for others; however, a reality is that the work is accompanied by numerous demands on their limited resources of time, energy and empathy. This tends to be particularly true for professional caregivers – physicians, nurses, psychologists, social workers, chaplains and other allied staff – who work in oncology. In addition to the general stressors that affect staff working in medical settings, cancer caregivers cope with unique occupational tasks that, while rewarding, may further tax their personal and emotional resources (Grunfeld et al., 2005; Sherman et al.,

2006). For instance, they often partner with patients throughout their disease processes, thus serving as caregivers and witnesses to a great deal of pain and suffering (Najjar et al., 2009). As a result, compassion fatigue (CF) is a professional challenge for many cancer caregivers. CF has been defined as a combination of burnout and secondary traumatic stress (Stamm, 1995; Figley, 1995). Research demonstrates that it adversely affects caregivers, their colleagues, and the care they provide patients (Wolf et al., 1998; Vahey et al., 2004; Najjar et al., 2009). As CF is a challenge for many cancer caregivers, this chapter reviews current research regarding this important issue. Additionally, the chapter provides an overview of evidence-based interventions and supported recommendations to ameliorate symptoms and enhance resiliency among caregivers. Of note, as most of the research has been done in oncology with physicians and nurses, this chapter focuses on these professionals, while recognizing that allied staff members are also affected.

CONSTRUCTS

CF was first identified by Joinson (1992) in a study of burnout in nurses who worked in an emergency department. This researcher described behaviors characteristic of nurses who absorbed the traumatic stress of those they helped, including chronic fatigue, irritability, dread of going to work, aggravation of physical ailments, and diminished joy in life. In 1995, Charles Figley described CF as the combination of secondary traumatic stress and burnout, experienced by helping professionals and other care providers. Figley (2002) defined CF as a state of tension and of preoccupation with the individual or cumulative traumas of clients, described as the "cost of caring for others in emotional pain." CF has been described as the result of giving high levels of care and compassion over a prolonged period to those who are suffering the side effects of aggressive treatment or the end stages of cancer, particularly if there is little opportunity to experience the positive outcomes of seeing patients improve (McHolm, 2006).

In a concept analysis, Coetzee and Klopper (2010) defined CF as the final result of a progressive and cumulative process that is caused by prolonged, continuous and intense contact with patients, the "use of self" therapeutically, and exposure to stress. It is a condition that results in symptoms that are intrusive, cause agitation, and lead to avoidance (Gentry et al., 1997). The caregiver who is experiencing CF is often nervous, cynical, pessimistic, and angry toward coworkers; additionally he struggles with low self-esteem and dreads work. The stress of CF is not restricted to work. At home, the affected caregiver may be unable to sleep, has bad dreams, loses interest in social events or sexual activity, and experiences changes in appetite (e.g. weight loss or gain) and relations with others.

In contrast, burnout is cumulative stress from the demands of daily life – a state of physical, emotional, and mental exhaustion – caused by a depletion of the ability to cope with one's environment, particularly the work environment (Maslach, 1982). Burnout has been described as the chronic condition of *perceived* demands outweighing *perceived* resources (Gentry et al., 1997). Causative factors for burnout within a healthcare setting include insufficient resources (e.g. staff and supplies), poor design of work areas, poor inter-professional relationships, and management conflicts (Vahey et al., 2004). In the case of healthcare professionals, burnout has been shown to be associated with increased turnover, employee absenteeism, decreased performance, decreased patient satisfaction, and difficulty in recruiting and retaining staff (Garman et al., 2002; Medland and Howard-Ruben, 2004). In a study conducted by Leiter and colleagues (1998) a correlation was found between nurse burnout and patient evaluations of the quality of care. Patients cared for on units where nurses felt exhausted or frequently expressed a desire to quit were less satisfied with their care. In a study involving over 800 nurses and 600 patients, Vahey and colleagues (2004) also found that the overall level of nurse burnout affects patient satisfaction.

Secondary traumatic stress is the result of "bearing witness" by directly observing others being traumatized and/or hearing their stories of trauma (Gentry, Baranowsky, and Dunning, 1997). Secondary traumatic stress arises from repeated exposure to traumatic events, as is the case with the ongoing care of oncology patients. A caregiver's empathy is hypothesized to play a significant role in the transmission of traumatic stress from patient to nurse, with higher levels of empathy associated with greater vulnerability to secondary traumatic stress (Figley, 1995). Secondary traumatic stress has been shown to correlate highly with burnout (Vahey et al., 2004; Jones, 2004; Yoder, 2010).

The concepts of CF and burnout are closely related and sometimes confused. Definitions of burnout more often point to environmental stressors, while definitions of CF address the relational nature of the condition. Figley (2002) identifies CF as a form of burnout, while Szabo (2006) describes CF as the combination of burnout and secondary traumatization. The phenomena of burnout and CF are significant for health care organizations due to the demonstrated correlations to staff retention and turnover, patient satisfaction, and patient safety (Wolf et al., 1998; Garman et al., 2002; Halbesleben et al., 2008).

PREVALENCE AND EFFECTS

The prevalence of CF among registered nurses has been documented as ranging from 16% to 39%, with burnout ranging from 8% to 38% (Hooper et al., 2010; Potter et al., 2010; Yoder, 2010; Robins et al., 2009). The literature suggests that long-term effects of CF negatively impact the health and well-being of employees; these effects include potential mental and physical health issues, and increased use of alcohol or drugs (Stamm, 2002). Schwam (1998) reports that nurses who suffer from CF may experience changes in job performance, increased mistakes, noticeable personality changes, a decline in health, and the perceived need to leave the profession.

WORKING IN ONCOLOGY

Since CF has been identified and conceptualized, it has been recognized as a serious concern for professional caregivers working in oncology (Najjar et al., 2009). Oncology, as a career choice, can be fulfilling and satisfying for many physicians, nurses and allied healthcare professionals (Shanafelt, 2005). At the same time, it presents many challenges. Professional caregivers in oncology cope with occupational tasks that frequently drain personal and emotional resources (Grunfeld et al., 2005; Sherman et al., 2006). Lyckholm (2001, p. 750) argues that oncology is "inherently difficult and racked by emotional and psychological traumas." Shanafelt, Adjei and Meyskens (2003) suggest that healthcare professionals may be drawn to oncology because they are sensitive to the struggles of their patients. On the job, they may be at a higher risk of negative symptoms because of the specific nature of their work. They often develop close, long term relationships with patients, and many of these patients will die during care (Grunfeld et al., 2005; Shanafelt et al., 2003). Additionally, research has demonstrated that longer relationships between providers and patients are associated with stronger emotional reactions to patient death, particularly grief (Redinbaugh et al., 2003). Healthcare professionals working with cancer patients must continually negotiate closeness in their relationships with patients – not getting too attached but not becoming detached – for both can affect patient care and personal well-being (Wolpin et al., 2005). In addition to intense, relationship-based concerns, providers have identified other difficult aspects of their job. They struggle with relaying bad news, managing patients' pain, coping with angry and depressed patients, handling end of life care, and navigating family and cultural issues (Armstrong et al., 2004).

Early career healthcare professionals may be especially vulnerable to stressors on the job. For instance, in a study of 272 new oncology fellows, 50% of those surveyed reported moderate to significant concern regarding the stress of practice (Association of American Medical Colleges' Center for Workforce Studies [AAMC], 2006). The AAMC (2006) also found that higher job stress and lower job satisfaction are associated with early retirement or change in career among oncologists. This situation is particularly concerning as the AAMC already expects a major shortage of oncologists. Specifically, the AAMC (2006) reported that the demand for oncology services will increase 48% by 2020, while the supply of oncologists is forecasted to grow by only 20% in the same period. The AAMC considers the shortage to be an "acute" situation that will affect healthcare in the United States.

INTERVENTIONS

As research has documented the prevalence of CF in oncology staff (Hooper et al., 2010; Potter et al., 2010; Yoder, 2010; Robins et al., 2009), medical centers, teams and caregivers themselves have sought to learn how to enhance coping and resiliency. It is important to recognize that prevention, intervention and health promotion to combat CF will work best when multifaceted and directed at numerous levels (i.e., societal, organizational, familial, and individual level). For instance, healthcare organizations can help prevent the development of CF among its staff members by fostering a culture that supports self-care and wellbeing, as well as instituting corresponding policies and programs. While interventions at all levels most likely will have a beneficial cumulative effect, the focus in this chapter is on programs and strategies for the individual healthcare provider. Intervention at the individual level is critical as professional caregivers in oncology are likely to experience CF at some point during their career. Additionally, intervention is important as experts agree that that prevention and recovery from CF, like burnout, is possible (Boyle, 2011; Yoder 2010; Shanafelt et al., 2012).

Despite the magnitude of the problem, there are few structured interventions to help prevent and treat CF in healthcare workers (Potter et al., 2010). Additionally, of the programs that exist, it is unclear how much benefit they provide to participants, especially beyond the intervention period. A recent Cochrane Review evaluating the effectiveness of stress management training interventions to reduce job stress and prevent burnout among healthcare workers illustrated these concerns (van Wyk and Pillay-Van Wyk, 2010). They identified 10 studies involving 716 health workers (predominantly nurses) that sought to enhance stress management techniques in participants. While the authors conclude that four of these studies demonstrated reductions in job-related stress among participants, there were insufficient data to indicate if benefits are sustained over longer periods.

One of the more common interventions for CF is cultivating mindfulness, which is defined as "…paying attention in a particular way: on purpose, in the present moment, and nonjudgementally" (Kabat-Zinn, 1994, p.4). There is a growing recognition that mindfulness may be particularly useful for helping healthcare students and professional caregivers learn to manage stress. Epstein (1999, p. 833), a physician who is a major proponent of incorporating mindfulness in medical education and professional practice, defined a mindful clinician as one who "attends, in a nonjudgemental way, to his or her own physical and mental processes during ordinary everyday tasks to act with clarity and insight." He argued that mindful practitioners are more able to "listen attentively to patients' distress, recognize their own errors, refine their technical skills, make evidence-based decisions, and clarify their values so that they can act with compassion, technical competence, presence, and insight" (Epstein, 1999, p.833).

A number of clinical interventions involving mindfulness training have been developed with the express purpose of enhancing practitioners' health and well-being. One of the first interventions created was Mindfulness-Based Stress Reduction (MBSR), which was originally developed by Kabat-Zinn and colleagues (Kabat-Zinn, 1982; Kabat-Zinn et al., 1992) and is the model most frequently used to address CF. MBSR is a psycho-educational program that is taught over 8 weeks, including a day-long silent retreat; participants learn meditation practices and are requested to practice daily. Irving, Dobkin and Park (2009) provide a review of empirical studies of MBSR in healthcare professionals, including physicians, nurses, nurse aides, social workers, physical therapists, psychologists, and students across several disciplines. Findings from the 10 studies they review indicate that mindfulness training can help promote self-care and well-being among participants (Irving et al., 2009). MBSR is the most rigorously studied intervention that has been used to address symptoms of CF and stress among healthcare professionals.

Another program to target CF among professional caregivers is the Compassion Fatigue Prevention and Resiliency Program (Gentry, 2011). The program has been adapted from the Accelerated Recovery Program (ARP) developed by Gentry, Baranowsky, and Dunning (1997), which is an individual treatment model focused on mental health and trauma workers. Drawing on his earlier work, Gentry subsequently developed a systemic intervention to enhance resiliency among an entire staff population. Dubbed the Barnes-Jewish Model of Compassion Fatigue Prevention after its roll-out within the Barnes-Jewish Hospital in Missouri in 2011, the model has been designed specifically for healthcare workers and is currently taught in a 1-day course by peer trainers who were trained by Gentry. The focus of the training is to understand and recognize CF, learn coping skills to resolve symptoms, and develop self-care strategies to enhance personal resiliency (Gentry, 2011). Early research suggests it is effective at reducing CF symptoms in healthcare staff (Potter et al., in press).

Recognizing the costs of caregiving, the Canadian community cancer support organization, Wellspring, has developed a 1-day session called Care for the Professional Caregiver Program (CPCP). Although it was not developed specifically to combat CF, its design appears to address many of the associated concerns. According to its website, the program is designed to "...educate professional caregivers about burn-out, focusing on vicarious trauma and loss as a key contributor. The program also addresses how burnout can be recognized and prevented and teaches coping strategies specially designed for the workplace" (Wellspring, 2011). It has been delivered to more than 700 healthcare workers (Edmonds et al., 2012). A study evaluating its effectiveness among oncology nurses demonstrated a significant decrease in emotional exhaustion (Edmonds et al., 2012).

Similarly, offering healing for healers, VitalHearts: The Resiliency Training Initiative is a small charitable organization that provides training for professionals. The organization offers a 3-day training that "...helps normalize and attenuate secondary traumatic stress and reduce the shame often engendered by these stress reactions, while creating valuable mental health tools, increasing care-providers' ability to work from a place of compassion, enabling them to receive the full measure of self-esteem available from their work, and gaining resiliency regardless of the nature of their organization" (Vital Hearts: The Resiliency Training Institute, 2012). The training has been delivered more than 65 times since 1999 to over 1300 professionals (H. Tobey, personal communication, December 11, 2012).

Moreover, other interventions delivered to healthcare providers are discussed in the literature; however there is limited information about their success. Many of these interventions teach skills to professionals with the hope of decreasing stress and increasing resiliency. For instance, interventions have taught communication skills, coping skills, relaxation and guided imagery techniques, narrative writing, journaling strategies, and the development of an individualized wellness plan (Bragard et al., 2010; Kravits et al., 2010; Roth et al., 2011). Unfortunately, most of these interventional studies are small and often do not measure CF, but rather constructs of stress management and burnout.

Recognizing that prevention and early recognition of CF is ideal, there has been encouragement to include health promotion strategies within professional training programs. For instance, Dyrbye et al. (2012, p.1030) argue that "for the good of both society and individual students, medical schools should help students" develop skills to cope with the stresses of their work. Within professional cancer caregivers, the residency program for oncology nurses at the University of North Carolina is unique in that it has developed a four-hour presentation for nurses specifically on CF (Walton and Alvarez, 2010). The presentation combines didactic and experiential learning with personal reflection and fellowship to help raises awareness of the personal risks of caring for others. There is recognition by program developers that this single presentation is not exhaustive and that ongoing support would benefit oncology nurses (Walton and Alvarez, 2010).

PERSONAL COPING STRATEGIES

In addition to group interventions, educating individual caregivers about CF is key to ameliorating its impacts (Boyle, 2011; Yang and Kim, 2012). Caregivers benefit from learning about the symptoms and presentation of CF so that they may recognize it in themselves and colleagues. Education empowers them to intervene so that they may proactively reduce the effects of CF. Additionally, education about CF to individual professional caregivers helps normalize their experiences and clarify why they might be experiencing a constellation of CF symptoms. Therefore, when formal programs to treat CF are limited, developing personal strategies to cope with the demands of work as a professional cancer caregiver is critical.

Researchers have turned to professional caregivers to ask about strategies that protect their well-being and buffer them from job demands. In a recent study by Yoder (2010), 71 nurses in a community hospital were asked about strategies that they "...find helpful to deal with situations that trigger CF" (p.192). Their responses were categorized into work-related and personal strategies. In the former category, they reported altering how they engage with a patient (e.g. disengaging or engaging more), changing their workplace tasks to get some distance from stressors, debriefing with colleagues, taking a proactive role in addressing a stressor, and developing meaningful rituals. These nurses identified several prominent strategies to help them cope with stress at work. Strategies included maintaining activities and relationships outside of work, engaging in religious or spiritual practices, reviewing personal involvement in stressful situations, and modifying their attitudes if necessary. These strategies echo findings from earlier research, although other samples have reported several additional effective coping strategies including taking time off work, changing jobs, using humor, and taking part in self-care activities including hobbies, exercise and meditation (Maytum et al., 2004; Von Rueden et al., 2010).

Due to the paucity of studies assessing the construct of CF, it is helpful to turn to the much larger body of published literature about burnout, especially as there have been numerous studies asking healthcare workers how they cope with their stressful jobs. Their responses about self-care can benefit staff seeking to prevent or minimize CF symptoms. For instance, in a study of wellness promotion strategies used by primary care physicians, participants shared what buffered them from the stress they encountered (Weiner et al., 2001). The authors categorized physicians' responses into five main domains – relationships, religious beliefs/spiritual practices, work attitudes, life philosophy and self-care practices. These findings have been echoed in other studies and reviews of healthcare professionals (Lemaire et al., 2010; Lyckholm, 2001; Shanafelt et al., 2003; Shanafelt et al., 2012; Swetz et al., 2009). For instance, in a study of 241 oncologists (Shanafelt et al., 2005), respondents rated wellness promotion strategies. The top strategies identified by the physicians were, in decreasing order of popularity: developing a personal philosophy for end of life care, finding meaning in their work, protecting time with family, talking with family, taking time off work, maintaining a positive attitude, prioritizing recreational time for exercise and hobbies, striving for work-life balance, debriefing with colleagues, engaging in a religious/spiritual practice, looking forward to retirement, conducting research, working part-time, and meeting with a psychologist. Of course, self-care strategies vary by individual yet these studies highlight approaches adopted by colleagues in the field, and may be helpful for professional caregivers who are seeking to develop, enhance or augment the strategies that they currently use.

CONCLUSION

Professional cancer caregivers work in environments that provide interpersonal opportunities for both great rewards and enormous challenges. Unfortunately, due to the empathy that many caregivers bring to their jobs, a common challenge in oncology is managing compassion fatigue (CF). Despite the term 'compassion fatigue' being coined 20 years ago (Joinson, 1992), there is still limited information, conceptual clarity, research, and evidence-based interventions to support people who are affected by CF (Najjar et al., 2009). There has been little research about CF in professional cancer caregivers. However, as the United States' National Cancer Institute estimates that over 1.6 million American adults will be diagnosed with cancer and 577,000 will die of the disease in 2012 (Howlader et al., 2012), it is clear that thousands of professional cancer caregivers are involved in caring for these patients. Given the previously stated association between CF and the quality of patient care, further research into CF and possible prevention and treatment programs are needed. Currently, as the existing interventions are only available to a small proportion of cancer caregivers, individuals are encouraged to turn to their colleagues' recommendations that have been published in the literature. Developing personal coping strategies to avoid or ameliorate symptoms and enhance resiliency can benefit professional cancer caregivers, as well as their colleagues and patients.

REFERENCES

Armstrong, J., Lederberg, M. and Holland, J. (2004). Fellows' forum: A workshop on the stresses of being an oncologist. *Journal of Cancer Education, 19,* 88-90.

Association of American Medical Colleges' Center for Workforce Studies. (2006). *Forecasting the supply of and demand for oncologists.* Washington, DC: Author.

Aycock, N., and Boyle, D. (2009). Interventions to manage compassion fatigue in oncology nursing. *Clinical Journal of Oncology Nursing, 13*(2), 183-191.

Boyle, D., (Jan 31, 2011) "Countering compassion fatigue: A requisite nursing agenda." *OJIN: The Online Journal of Issues in Nursing, 16(1).* Retrieved from http://ana.nursingworld.org/MainMenuCategories/ANAMarketplace/ANAPeriodicals/OJIN/TableofContents/Vol-16-2011/No1-Jan-2011/Countering-Compassion-Fatigue.aspx

Bragard, I., Libert, Y., Etienne, A., Merckaert, I., Delvaux, N., Marchal, S., et al. (2010). Insight on variables leading to burnout in cancer physicians. *Journal of Cancer Education, 25,* 109-115.

Coetzee, S. K. and Klopper, H. C. (2010), Compassion fatigue within nursing practice concept analysis. *Nursing and Health Sciences, 12:* 235–243. doi: 10.1111 /j.14422018.2010.00526.x.

Cohen-Katz, J., Wiley, S., Capuano, T., Baker, D.M., and Shapiro, S. (2004). The effects of Mindfulness-based Stress Reduction on nurse stress and burnout. *Holistic Nursing Practice, 18(6),* 302-308.

Cohen-Katz, J., Wiley, S. D., Capuano, T., Baker, D. M., and Shapiro, S. (2005). The effects of mindfulness-based stress reduction on nurse stress and burnout, part II: A quantitative and qualitative study. *Holistic Nursing Practice, 19(2),* 78-76.

Dyrbye, L. N., Harper, W., Moutier, C., Durning, S. J., Power, D. V., Massie, F. S., Eacker, A., et al. (2012). A multi-institutional study exploring the impact of positive mental health on medical students' professionalism in an era of high burnout. *Academic Medicine, 87(8),* 1024-1031.

Edmonds, C., Lockwood, G. M., Bezjak, A., and Nyhof-Young, J. (2012). Alleviating emotional exhaustion in oncology nurses: an evaluation of Wellspring's "Care for the Professional Caregiver Program." *Journal of Cancer Education, 27(1),* 27-36.

Epstein, R. M. (1999). Mindful practice. *JAMA, 282,* 833-839.

Figley, C.R. (1995). *Compassion fatigue: Coping with secondary traumatic stress disorder in those who treat the traumatized.* New York, NY: Brunner Mazel.

Figley, C.R. (2002). *Treating compassion fatigue.* New York, NY: Brunner-Routledge.

Garman, A., Corrigan, P., and Morris, S. (2002). Staff burnout and patient satisfaction: Evidence of relationships at the care unit level. *Journal of Occupational Health Psychology, 7,* 235–241.

Gentry, J.E., Baranowsky, A., and Dunning, E. (1997). Accelerated Recovery Program for compassion fatigue. Presented at the 13th annual International Society for Traumatic Stress Studies Conference in Montreal, Quebec, Canada.

Gentry, J.E. (2011). *Compassion fatigue prevention and resiliency: Fitness for the frontline treatment manual.* Sarasota, FL: Compassion Unlimited.

Grunfeld, E., Zitzelsberger, L., Coristine, M., Whelan, T. J., Aspelund, F., and Evans, W. K. (2005). Job stress and job satisfaction of cancer care workers. *Psycho-Oncology, 14,* 61-69.

Halbesleben, J., Wakefield, B., Wakefield, D., and Cooper, L. (2008). Nurse burnout and patient safety perception versus reporting behavior. *Western Journal of Nursing Research, 30,* 560–577.

Hooper, C., Craig, J., Janvrin, D.R., Wetzel, M.A., and Reimels, E. (2010). Compassion satisfaction, burnout and compassion fatigue among emergency nurses compared with nurses in other selected inpatient specialties. *Journal of Emergency Nursing, 36*(5), 420-427.

Howlader N, Noone AM, Krapcho M, Neyman N, Aminou R, Altekruse SF, Kosary CL, Ruhl J, Tatalovich Z, Cho H, Mariotto A, Eisner MP, Lewis DR, Chen HS, Feuer EJ, Cronin KA (eds). SEER Cancer Statistics Review, 1975-2009 (Vintage 2009 Populations), National Cancer Institute. Bethesda, MD, http://seer.cancer.gov/csr/1975_2009_pops09/, based on November 2011 SEER data submission, posted to the SEER web site, April 2012. Accessed on July 11, 2012.Irving, J. A., Dobkin, P. L., and Park, J. (2009). Cultivating mindfulness in health care professionals: A review of empirical studies of mindfulness-based stress reduction (MBSR). *Complementary Therapies in Clinical Practice, 15*(2), 61-66.

Joinson, C. (1992). Coping with compassion fatigue. *Nursing, 22,* 116–120.

Jones, C. B. (2004). The costs of nurse turnover: Part 1: An economic perspective. *Journal of Nursing Administration, 34*(12), 562-570.

Kabat-Zinn, J. (1982). An outpatient program in behavioral medicine for chronic pain patients based on the practice of mindfulness meditation: theoretical considerations and preliminary results. *General Hospital Psychiatry, 4,* 33-47.

Kabat-Zinn, J. (1994). *Wherever you go there you are: Mindfulness meditation in everyday life.* New York: Hyperion.

Kabat-Zinn, J., Massion, A. O., Kristeller, J., Peterson, L. G., Fletcher, K. E., Pbert, L., et al. (1992). Effectiveness of a meditation-based stress reduction program in the treatment of anxiety disorders. *American Journal of Psychiatry, 149,* 936-943.

Kravits, K., McAllister-Black, R., Grant, M., and Kirk, C. (2010). Self-care strategies for nurses: A psycho-educational intervention for stress reduction and the prevention of burnout. *Applied Nursing Research, 23,* 130-138.

Leiter, M.P., Harvie, P., and Frizzell, C. (1998). The correspondence of patient satisfaction and nurse burnout. *Social Science and Medicine, 47,* 1611–1617.

Lemaire, J. B., and Wallace, J. E. (2010). Not all coping strategies are created equal: A mixed methods study exploring physicians' self reported coping strategies. *BMC Health Services Research, 10,* 208.

Lyckholm, L. (2001). Dealing with stress, burnout, and grief in the practice of oncology. *Lancet Oncology, 2,* 750-755.

Mackenzie, C. S., Poulin, P. A., and Seidman-Carlson, R. (2006). A brief mindfulness-based stress reduction intervention for nurses and nurse aides. Applied Nursing Research, 19, 105-109.

Maslach, C. (1982). *Burnout—The cost of caring.* Englewood Cliffs, NJ: Spectrum.

Maytum, J., Heiman, H., and Garwick, A. (2004). Compassion fatigue and burnout in nurses who work with chronic conditions and their families. *Journal of Pediatric Health Care, 18(4),* 172–179.

McHolm, F. (2006). Rx for compassion fatigue. *Journal of Christian Nursing, 23,* 12–19.

Medland, J., Howard-Ruben, J., and Whitaker, E. (2004). Fostering psychosocial wellness in oncology nurses: Addressing burnout and social support in the workplace. *Oncology Nursing Forum, 31,* 47–54.

Najjar, N., Davis, L.W., Beck-Coon, K., and Doebbeling, C.C. (2009). Compassion fatigue: A review of research to date and relevance to cancer-care providers. *Journal of Health Psychology, 14(2),* 267-277.

Potter, P., Berger, J., Clarke, M., Deshields, T., and Chen, L. (in press). Evaluation of a compassion fatigue resiliency program for oncology nurses. *Oncology Nursing Forum.*

Potter, P., Deshields, T., Divanbeigi, J., Berger, J., Cipriano, D., Norris, L., and Olsen, S. (2010). Compassion fatigue and burnout: Prevalence among oncology nurses. *Clinical Journal of Oncology Nursing, 14,* E56-E62.

Redinbaugh, E. M., Sullivan, A. M., Block, S. D., Gadmer, N. M., Lakoma, M., Mitchell, A. M., Seltzer, D., Wolford, J., and Arnold, R. M. (2003). Doctors' emotional reactions to recent death of a patient: Cross sectional study of hospital doctors. *British Medical Journal, 327,* 185-200.

Robins, P. M., Meltzer, L., and Zelikovsky, N. (2009). The experience of secondary traumatic stress upon care providers working within a children's hospital. *Journal of Pediatric Nursing, 24(4),* 270-279.

Roth M, Morrone K, Moody K, Kim M, Wang D, Moadel A, and Levy A. (2011). Career burnout among pediatric oncologists. *Pediatric Blood Cancer, 57(7),* 1168-1173.

Schwam, K. (1998). The phenomenon of compassion fatigue in perioperative nursing. *AORN Journal, 68,* 4, 642-648.

Shanafelt, T. D. (2005). Finding meaning, balance, and personal satisfaction in the practice of oncology. *Journal of Supportive Oncology, 3*, 157-162.

Shanafelt, T. D., Adjei, A., and Meyskens, F. L. (2003). When your favorite patient relapses: Physician grief and well-being in the practice of oncology. *Journal of Clinical Oncology, 21*, 2616-2619.

Shanafelt, T.D., Sloan, J.A., and Habermann, T.M. (2003). The well-being of physicians. *The American Journal of Medicine, 114*, 513-519.

Shanafelt, T. D., Novotny, P., Johnson M. E., Zhao, X., Steensma, D. P., Lacy, M. Q., Rubin, J., and Sloan, J. (2005). The well-being and personal wellness promotion strategies of medical oncologists in the North Central Cancer Treatment Group. *Oncology, 68(1)*, 23-32.

Shanafelt, T. D., Oreskovich, M. R., Dyrbye, L. N., Satele, D. V., Hanks, J. B., Sloan, J. A., and Balch, C. M. (2012). Avoiding burnout: The personal health habits and wellness practices of surgeons. *Annals of Surgery, 255(4)*, 625-633.

Sherman, A. C., Edwards, D., Simonton, S., and Hehta, P. (2006). Caregiver stress and burnout in an oncology unit. *Palliative and Supportive Care, 4*, 65-81.

Stamm, B.H., (1995). *Secondary traumatic stress: Self-care issues for clinicians, researchers, and educators*. Lutherville, MD: Sidran.

Stamm, B. H. (2002). Measuring compassion satisfaction as well as fatigue: Developmental history of the Compassion Satisfaction and Fatigue Test. Figley, C.R. (Ed.), *Treating compassion fatigue*, pp. 107-119. New York: Brunner-Routledge.

Swetz, K. M., Harrington, S. E., Matsuyama, R. K., Shanafelt, T. D., and Lyckholm, L. J. (2009). Strategies for avoiding burnout in hospice and palliative medicine: Peer advice for physicians on achieving longevity and fulfillment. *Journal of Palliative Medicine, 12(9)*, 773-777.

Szabo, B. (2006). Compassion fatigue and nursing work: Can we accurately capture the consequences of caring work? *International Journal of Nursing Practice:* 12: 136–142.

Vahey, D., Aiken, L., Sloane, D., Clarke, S., and Vargas, D. (2004). Nurse burnout and patient satisfaction. *Medical Care, 42*(2, Suppl.), II-57–II-66.

van Wyk, B. E., and Pillay-Van Wyk, V. *Preventive staff-support interventions for health workers*. Cochrane Database of Systematic Reviews 2010, Issue 3. Art. No.: CD003541. DOI: 10.1002/14651858.CD003541.pub2.

Vital Hearts: The Resiliency Training Institute. (2012). Retaining the expertise in healthcare institutions. Retrieved from http://www.vitalhearts.org/strtourtraining.html

Von Rueden, K. T., Hinderer, K. A., McQuillan, K. A., Murray, M., Logan, T., Kramer, B., Gilmore, R., et al. (2010). Secondary traumatic stress in trauma nurses: Prevalence and exposure, coping, and personal/environmental characteristics. *Journal of Trauma Nursing, 17(4)*, 191-200.

Walton, A. M. L., and Alvarez, M. (2010). Imagine: Compassion fatigue training for nurses. *Clinical Journal of Oncology Nursing, 14*, 399-400.

Weiner, E. L., Swain, G. R., Wolf, B., and Gottlieb, M. (2001). A qualitative study of physicians' own wellness-promotion practices. *Western Journal of Medicine, 174*, 19-23

Wellspring. (2011). Care for the professional caregiver. Retrieved from http://www.wellspring.ca/Centre-of-Innovation/Centre-of-Innovation-Programs/Care-for-Professional-Caregiver.aspx.

Wolf, Z., Colahan, M., and Costello, A. (1998). Relationship between nurse caring and patient satisfaction. *Medsurg Nursing: Official Journal of the Academy of Medical-Surgical Nurses, 7*(2), 99.

Wolpin, B. M., Chabner, B. A., Lynch, T. J., and Penson, R. T. (2005). Learning to cope: How far is too close? *Oncologist, 10,* 449-456.

Yang, Y. H., and Kim, J. K. (2012). A literature review of compassion fatigue in nursing. *Korean Journal of Adult Nursing, 24,* 38-51.

Yoder, E.A. (2010). Compassion fatigue in nurses. *Applied Nursing Research, 23*(4), 191-197.

In: Caregivers: Challenges, Practices and Cultural Influences ISBN: 978-1-62618-030-7
Editors: Adrianna Thurgood and Kasha Schuldt © 2013 Nova Science Publishers, Inc.

Chapter 9

CAREGIVING IN CLINICAL ONCOLOGY

Carola Locatelli,[1,*] *Marcella Cicerchia*[1] *and Lazzaro Repetto*[2,†]
[1]Research Department, INRCA-IRCCS, Rome, Italy
[2]Oncology Unit, ASL1 Sanremo Hospital, Sanremo, Italy

ABSTRACT

More often family play a central role in providing support to the complex needs of cancer patients: there are 4.6 million Americans who care for someone with cancer at home.

Informal caring may involve considerable physical, psychological and economic stresses. Several recent studies have examined the effect of caregiving on the health and well-being of cancer caregivers. These studies indicate that stress and demands associated with caregiving can cause problems and changes for caregivers in areas such as their psychological, physical, and financial well-being. This impairment has an important impact not only on the caregiver but also on the patient. We have to consider that caregivers who had high emotional distress in the course of illness had a significant negative effect on the adjustment of patients with cancer. Although many studies are set up to determine the link between the stressors in care-giving and the impact on the family caregiver and/or on the patient's outcomes, the results remained inconclusive. A range of supportive programmes for caregivers is being developed including psychological support and practical assistance. A recent (2011) and systematic review has detected an encouraging growth in the number of intervention studies that aim to improve outcomes for caregiver in cancer and palliative care and an improvement in the study designs used. However, this activity needs to continue to focus on mechanisms of intervention, powerful designs and a plurality of models and target populations/settings.

There is an urgent need for health care providers and policy makers to recognize the pivotal role of family caregivers in patients' care and a need to view them as care partners establishing tailored training programs. These intervention programs should give to caregivers the knowledge and skills to manage the patients' changing needs, also should grant tax credits or compensation for the care they provide and for the financial damages they make. A concerted effort is needed to train health professionals about the needs of

---

[*] Carola Locatelli: c.locatelli@inrca.it.
[†] Lazzaro Repetto: l.repetto@asl1.liguria.it.

caregivers and the importance of assessing them as part of routine cancer care. Training programs should ensure that clinicians are prepared to work with caregivers, to understand their needs, and to recognize the range of responsibilities being asked of them. For the caregivers training should incorporate strategies that would help caregivers to develop positive lifestyle behaviors, effective coping skills, and ways to access resources. Improved patient outcomes, including early detection or better management of adverse effects, increased adherence to oral medication, would result in reduced health care use and costs.

Respect to this topic we are performing a study aimed to demonstrate the mutuality of psychological distress in both cancer patients and their caregivers, by validation of a new assessment tool able to identify the risk factors to develop mental disorders in the caregivers' population.

We need to integrate a different point of view beginning to consider the patient-caregiver dyad as a unit of care. If the patient-caregiver dyad is treated as the unit of care, we can promote important synergies that can increase the well-being of both patients and caregivers.

1. INTRODUCTION

The world population is rapidly aging. The western developed countries of the world have been leading the process of population aging and, by 2050, the proportion of older people (60+years) in these countries is expected to be the double of the children population (under 15 years): 31.9% vs. 16.3% respectively. [1] Cancer increases with age, therefore we can expect more and more cancer patients over the age of 65.

The incidence of cancer worldwide among people over 65 is expected to grow from about 6 millions in 2008 to more than 11 millions during the coming decade. By 2030, individuals over 65 will account for 70% of all cancer patients in the western world. [2]

Literature review emphasizes that older cancer patients in active treatment and older cancer survivors suffer for more physical problems (comorbidities, complications of treatment) compared to younger cancer patients and for more physical and emotional problems compared to individuals without a history of cancer. [3]

The heterogeneity and severity of problems resulting from a diagnosis of cancer among senior patients give rise to increased demands from healthcare providers to achieve a continuative and constructive collaboration between geriatricians, family physicians and oncologists to improve the knowledges in the areas of geriatric oncology. [4]

An inevitable outcome of these demographic changes is a unavoidable increased financial pressure on public welfare and healthcare systems with a progressive restriction of formal care provided by governmental institutions. The natural consequence will lead to shift the assistance burden on the family members, such as partners and children.

In this context the role of caregiver is shaped: an unpaid person, frequently a family member, that provides assistance with daily activities, emotional support, managing complex care, navigating the health care system, and communicating with health care professionals.

There are 4.6 million Americans who care for someone with cancer at home. [5]

Family caregivers provide more than half the care needed by patients with cancer, without any training by health care system. [6]. Providing care with little or no preparation has a substantial impact on family caregivers' physical and mental well-being and can negatively influence patient and caregiver health outcomes. [7-9]

The burden of caregiving, combined with inadequate institutional support, places informal caregivers at high risk for psychological, social and physical difficulties [10].

Recent studies [11-13] found that caregivers' negative psychological status and/or physical impairment (including fatigue), not only may disrupt the informal caregiver's daily routine, and social and personal life [14] but also may compromise the effective management of patients' medications and have a negative effect on the adjustment of patients with cancer 1 year later.

2. EFFECT OF CAREGIVING ON THE HEALTH AND WELL-BEING OF FAMILY CAREGIVERS

Although such informal caregivers often undertake the role and derive personal rewards, being a caregiver may also involve considerable physical, psychological, economic and domestic challenges. Scarce evidence-based data exist concerning the quality of life and psychological distress among caregivers to older patients with cancer. Kim and Given report that there is clear evidence of the psychological impact of cancer upon family caregivers. Such stresses and demands associated with caregiving can affect not only aspects of caregivers' wellbeing, resulting in psychological impairment with a prevalence of mood disturbance, physical health changes like fatigue, sleeping problems, gastrointestinal disorders, loss of physical strength and appetite, weight loss, neuro-hormonal and inflammatory changes and an increased risk of death but also may affect their ability to care. [15-17] The results of a recent study of Goldzweig et al. [18], focused on the evaluation of levels of psychological distress among informal caregivers of older cancer patients conclude that the role of caring for older patients with cancer constitutes a considerable physical and psychological burden to caregivers, supporting other evidenced based studies. [19-20]

2.1. Psychological Impairment and Mood Disturbance

In a review of Stenberg et al. caregivers of older cancer patients were described as experiencing a wide range of emotional difficulties: as feelings of fear, uncertainty, hopelessness, powerlessness, and mood disturbances. [21] With an incidence of 39% and 40%, depression and anxiety are two of the most commonly reported problems related to the psychological consequences of caregiving. [22-23] In several studies [9, 24-25] the family caregiver's mental health burden was worst than the burden of the cancer patient. Caregivers' anxiety levels, depression, stress, and tension have all been shown to increase as the patient's functional status declines and at the end of life [26-27]. The analysis of the relationship between psychological distress of patients and their spouse caregivers found that each person affects the other's level of emotional well-being: i.e. emotional contagion. [28] Predictor variables for mental health problems among caregivers have been identified.

Caregiver depression seems to be correlated to several variables: caregiver age and gender, sleep deprivation, declines in their own health, perceived burden of caregiving and changes in caregivers' roles, responsibilities, social isolation, relationship to the patient, length of caregiving, patient's cancer type. All of which are risk factors. [29-36]

2.2. Symptoms Related to Sleep Disturbances

Sleep disturbance and fatigue among family caregivers of cancer patients is not well investigated. It's known that the intensity of the caregiver's schedule is associated with the severity of caregivers' fatigue while no correlation was found between caregiver's age, employment status, hours of daily care, or duration of care and severity of fatigue.

Carter et colleagues relieved that 95% of the caregivers experienced moderate to severe sleep disturbance [32; 37] underling a strong positive correlation between caregivers' sleep problems and their level of depression.

2.3. Physical Health Changes

Different studies found a positive association between caregivers' burden and an increased risk of morbidity, with a decline in personal health status. [38-39] A recent study of Rohleder et al. on the physiologic mechanisms related to caregiving [40] showed that a significant psychological distress marked changes in neurohormonal (salivary amylase and cortisol) and inflammatory (serum C-reactive protein and interleukin-6) parameters of caregivers. This study, although limited to a restricted sample of caregivers of patients with glioblastoma, opens a new perspective in the research of the physiological mechanisms implicated in the changes in caregivers' health status like outcomes of caregiving.

3. COPING STRATEGIES

Despite the paucity of data regarding coping strategies among caregivers of older cancer patients, it's known that coping strategies accounted for significant variances of patients' and caregivers' mental quality of life. Strategies that were found to be negatively correlated to caregivers' mental quality of life are avoidant strategies such as behavioral disengagement, denial and venting. On the other side, acceptance and utilization of social familial supports have been shown to be effective coping strategies to reduce psychological distress. Acceptance as a reality may provide caregivers with specific options to pursue different resources in an active way. Generally, female caregivers reported a broader spectrum of practical resources: planning, instrumental and emotional support, religious beliefs. [41-42]

3.1. High Risk Caregiver Situations

Caregivers at high risk for negative outcomes include: young female daughters, individuals with lower socioeconomic status, younger adult children with competing demands from career and individuals isolated with lack of social support.

Also the caregivers that provide more than 1,000 hours of care per year and caregivers who have a negative relationship with the care recipient, appear to be at risk. [43-44]

Caregivers with physical health care problems of their own are also at risk for negative outcomes on physical and mental health.

Crucial transitions points often threatening caregivers' emotional health, are especially observed at occurrence of disease progression, recurrence, or when moving through palliative or end of life care. The unavoidable adjustments in routines, decision making and skills at each of these points may cause a significant distress to the caregivers [45]

4. Cultural Influences

Cross-cultural differences may have an impact on cancer patients and their caregivers during the cancer care. [46-47]

There are ethnic differences in sociodemographic variables, stressors, family obligation beliefs, social support, coping strategies and caregivers outcomes. Usually ethnic minority caregivers reported more hours of caregiving, fewer financial resources and less educational attainment. However these caregivers reported also more informal support and more use of cognitive coping than white caregivers.

Singer and Wellish [48] have investigated ethnic differences of the breast cancer patients in their perceptions of the support received. The sample consisted of three ethnic groups: Euro-American (EA), Chinese-American (CA), and Japanese-American (JA) women. Results showed differences among the three groups. The qualitative evaluation pointed out that CA women were expected to be self-sacrificing and nurturing of husband and family, even in times of need, while EA women were able to be dependent. Indeed the traditional Japanese culture teaches women to sacrifice their emotional and physical needs for the family even when they are in need of care, so family members expect that their women continue to be self-sacrificers and nurturers even when their wives become affected of cancer. Otherwise, the EA women indicated that they expected that their husbands would support them, so they fell authorized to be dependent on them. [48]

Pinquart et coll. found that Africans Americans caregivers were more like to use cognitive strategies of coping than White, whereas Asian Americans were more like to use emotion-focused strategies of coping. In this meta-analysis they found worse physical health but better psychological health among ethnic minority caregivers than White caregivers, only Asian Americans caregivers were more depressed than White caregivers [49]. Lee et al. [50] have explained a similar result, assuming that higher levels of stress experienced by a consistent percentage of Asian-American caregivers may be explained by: (a) inconsistency between decisions based on cultural norms and their own beliefs (b) poor quality of their relationship with the care recipient and (c) the prevalent use of emotion-focused strategies of coping. This style of coping does not help to improve the management of the situation [51].

Compared with other ethnic groups African-American caregivers fared best psychologically, as indicated by lower levels of burden and depression and by higher levels of uplifts and subjective well-being. Several factors may contribute to this finding, such as high levels of intrinsic motivation to provide care, based on familism, the use of cognitive coping strategies that help caregivers to find personal and spiritual meaning in the caregiving experience, and greater availability of informal support.

Empirical studies show that not only sex and age, but also ethnicity, may affect the caregiver's risk to develop stress or mood disorders and to have physical and financial consequences. [52]

The goal in oncology practice is to develop individual and institutional sensitivity in order to be able to understand and appropriately respond to different health values and coping strategies of diverse cultural communities. For example, family- and community-centred cultures encourage a protective role of family assuming that a cancer patient has to be shielded from painful truths about his/her diagnosis and prognosis. In cultures centred on individuals' rights, on the other hand, full disclosure of medical information is deemed necessary to allow cancer patients to make autonomous decisions about their treatment and end-of-life choices [53-55].

Cross-cultural differences play an equally important role in communicating and planning psychosocial interventions for cancer patients. Formal teaching and training of patient-centred approach to cross-cultural care, based on assessing core cross-cultural issues, exploring meaning of illness to patient, determining patient's lived social context, and negotiating adherence to recommendations and treatments, is being implemented in many countries [56-58] To be effective, individual cultural competence must be accompanied by the establishment of culturally competent health care systems with the capacity to adapt their services to meet the culturally unique needs of their patients, also through the involvement of their different communities. [58-59].

5. Healthcare Programs to Support Informal Caregivers

Healthcare policies recognise that caregivers of cancer patients, especially caregivers of patients in the terminal phase may require a wide range of support, including clinical information about the disease process, social and psychological support, domestic help and financial support.

Whilst support for caregivers is a core of palliative care philosophy, and in some countries charitable organizations offer caregiver support. It is not uncommon that caregivers' psychosocial needs are more unmet than the patients' needs themselves [60-61]

Healthcare providers do not always know how or when to provide support to caregivers. Addressing caregivers' needs is not straightforward. Caregivers' needs are broad ranging and may change during the disease, especially in the bereavement phase. Caregivers may also not recognize or may be reluctant to seek support for their own needs, worried that health professionals might conclude that they are not able to care appropriately.

Current research suggests that, informal caregivers can benefit greatly from structured psychological interventions [62] but several systematic literature reviews have focused on interventions targeted at cancer caregivers [63]. To date, there is even more limited literature concerning caregiver interventions in older patients with cancer. [63-64]

A wide range of healthcare programs and strategies are being developed and implemented to support informal caregivers.

Three types of interventions were generally used:

1. Psycho-Educational Interventions, designed to provide information about management of patients' symptoms, physical aspects of patient care, and emotional aspects of care;

2 Skills Training, addressed to improve caregivers' coping, communication, and problem-solving skills;
3 Therapeutic Counseling, focused on strengthening patient-caregiver relationships, managing conflict, and dealing with loss.

The aims underpinning these intervention programs are:

- the contraction of the amount of care provided by a caregiver, by offering respite services;
- the improvement of coping skills;
- the improvement wellbeing, by providing psychological programs such as counselling, relaxation and psychotherapy.

There is some evidence on the impact of such interventions in related topics. In a narrative review of evaluations of interventions for caregivers of older patients with a chronic, severe and progressive disease, Sörensen and colleagues [65] noted that interventions which provided psychological support and/or aimed to enhance caregivers' coping skills appeared effective in the short term in ameliorating caregiver burden and depression as well as increasing caregiver satisfaction, ability and knowledge.

The evidence based on interventions designed to support family caregivers of patients in the terminal phase of disease has not been reviewed systematically, therefore remains unclear:

- which type(s) or combinations of interventions or services have been evaluated;
- which interventions provide greater potential benefit to caregivers and are more acceptable;
- which caregivers (such as those at higher risk) might benefit most.

5.1. Policy Implications and Conclusion

Health care providers and policy makers have to recognize the pivotal role of family caregivers in patients' care. Caregivers unmet needs not only compromise caregivers' QOL and distress, but also adversely impact on patients' distress.

Therefore, determining caregivers' unmet needs is the first step in the development of programs and services to enhance caregivers' and, indirectly, patients' illness adjustment. [12, 66-68]

We need programs to systematically assess caregivers' ability to give care and to provide them with resources, training and other forms of support.

In addition training caregivers to care for the cancer patients, health professionals must educate caregivers about self-care and personal health promotion practices. [69]

A concerted effort is needed to train health professionals about the needs of caregivers and the importance of assessing them as part of routine cancer care. Training programs should ensure that clinicians are prepared to work with caregivers, to understand their needs, and to recognize risk factors for psychological impairments.

To this aim we are implementing a new tool for the psychological assessment of caregivers of older cancer patients: The Multidimensional Caregiver Assessment.

The Multidimensional Caregiver Assessment, designed to evaluate different areas of caregivers' functioning (cognition, skills of communication-hearing-coping, mood and behavior disorders, social status, quality of life, health status), is developed with the specific aims to:

- plan tailored psycho-educational support groups to prevent mood disturbance, improve proximal outcomes (hopelessness and coping) and quality of life of both, patients and caregivers;
- improve the management of mood disorders, reducing the amount of requests for inappropriate health care (including inappropriate hospital admission and consultation and drug prescriptions).

A concerted effort is needed to integrate educational programs and support interventions for caregivers involved into the cancer patient's plan of care. Future research should include more comparison groups, larger samples, longitudinal studies, be more gender- and culture sensitive and exploit the caregivers experience along the trajectory of care.

REFERENCES

[1] World population prospects: the 2010 revision, highlights and advance tables. Working Paper No. ESA/P/WP.220. New York, NY: United Nations, Department of Economic and Social Affairs, Population Division; 2011).

[2] Ferlay, J., Shin, H. R., Bray, F., Forman, D., Mathers, C., Parkin, D. M. GLOBOCAN 2008, Cancer incidence and mortality worldwide: IARC cancer base No. 10 [Internet]. Lyon, France: International Agency for Research on Cancer; 2010. Available from: http:// globocan.iarc.fr.

[3] Avis, N. E., Deimling, G. T. Cancer survivorship and aging. *Cancer* 2008;113:3519–3529

[4] Puts, M. T., Girre, V., Monette, J.,Wolfson, C., Monette, M., Batist, G., et al. Clinical experience of cancer specialists and geriatricians involved in cancer care of older patients: a qualitative study. *Crit. Rev. Oncol. Hematol.* 2010;74:87–96

[5] National Alliance for Caregiving: Caregiving in the US, 2009. http://www.caregiving.org/data/)

[6] Blum, K., Sherman, D. W.: Understanding the experience of caregivers: A focus on transitions. *Semin. Oncol. Nurs.* 26:243-258, 2010

[7] Given, B., Wyatt, G., Given, C., et al.: Burden and depression among caregivers of patients with cancer at the end of life. *Oncol. Nurs. Forum.* 31:1105-1117, 2004

[8] Harding, R., Higginson, I. J.: What is the best way to help caregivers in cancer and palliative care? A systematic literature review of interventions and their effectiveness. *Palliat. Med.* 17:63-74, 2003

[9] McCorkle, R., Siefert, M. L., Dowd, M. F., et al.: Effects of advanced practice nursing on patient and spouse depressive symptoms, sexual function, and marital interaction after radical prostatectomy. *Urol. Nurs.* 27:65-77, 2007

[10] Haley, W. E. Family caregivers of elderly patients with cancer: understanding and minimizing the burden of care. *J. Support. Oncol.* 2003;1:25–29

[11] Lau, D. T., Berman, R., Halpern, L., et al.: Exploring factors that influence informal caregiving in medication management for home hospice patients. *J. Palliat. Med.* 13:1085-1090, 2010

[12] Park, S. M., Kim, Y. J., Kim, S., et al.: Impact of caregivers' unmet needs for supportive care on quality of terminal care delivered and caregiver's workforce performance. *Support Care Cancer* 18:699-706, 2010;

[13] Northouse, L., Templin, T., Mood, D.: Couples' adjustment to breast disease during the first year following diagnosis. *J. Behav. Med.* 24:115-136, 2001

[14] Haley, W. The costs of family caregiving: implications for geriatric oncology. *Crit. Rev. Oncol. Hematol.* 2003;48:151–158

[15] Kim, Y., Given, B. A. Quality of life of family caregivers of cancer survivors across the trajectory of the illness. *Cancer* 2008 Jun. 1;112 (11 Suppl.):2556-68.

[16] Kotkamp-Mothes, N., Slawinsky, D., Hindermann, S., Strauss, B.Coping and psychological well being in families of elderly cancer patients. *Crit. Rev. Oncol. Hematol.* 2005;55:213–229;

[17] Ho, A., Collins, S., Davis, K., Doty, M. A look at working-age caregivers roles, health concerns, and need for support (issue brief). New York, NY: The Commonwealth Fund; August 2005;(854):1-12

[18] Goldzweig, G., Merims, S., Ganon, R., Peretz, T., and Baider, L.: Coping and distress among spouse caregivers to older patients with cancer: An intricate path. *JGO* 3(2012)376–385

[19] Giacolone, A., Talamini, R., Fratino, L., Simonelli, C., Bearz, A., Spina, M., et al. Cancer in the elderly: the caregivers' perception of senior patients' informational needs. *Arch. Gerontol. Geriatr.* 2010;49:121–125.

[20] Locatelli, C., Piselli, P., Cicerchia, M., Raffaele, M., Abbatecola, A. M., Repetto, L. Telling bad news to the elderly cancer patients: The role of family caregivers in the choice of non-disclosure – The Gruppo Italiano di Oncologia Geriatrica (GIOGer) Study. *JGO* 2010; V(1), 2: 73–80

[21] Stenberg, U., Ruland, C. M., Miaskowski, C. Review of the literature on the effects of caring for a patient with cancer. *Psychooncology* 2010; 19: 1013–1025

[22] Braun, M., Mikulincer, M., Rydall, A., et al.: Hidden morbidity in cancer: Spouse caregivers. *J. Clin. Oncol.* 25:4829-4834, 2007

[23] Janda, M., Steginga, S., Langbecker, D., et al.: Quality of life among patients with a brain tumor and their carers. *J. Psychosom. Res.* 63:617-623, 2007

[24] Matthews, B. A.: Role and gender differences in cancer-related distress: A comparison of survivor and caregiver self-reports. *Oncol. Nurs. Forum* 30: 493-499, 2003

[25] Mellon, S., Northouse, L. L., Weiss, L. K.: A population-based study of the quality of life of cancer survivors and their family caregivers. *Cancer Nurs.* 29:120-131, 2006

[26] Ringdal, G. I., Ringdal, K., Jordhøy, M. S., et al.: Health-related quality of life (HRQOL) in family members of cancer victims: Results from a longitudinal intervention study in Norway and Sweden. *Palliat. Med.* 18:108-120, 2004

[27] Williams, A. L., McCorkle, R.: Cancer family caregivers during the palliative, hospice, and bereavement phases: A review of the descriptive psychosocial literature. *Palliat. Support Care* 9:315-325, 2011

[28] Hodges, L. J., Humphris, G. M., Macfarlane, G.: A meta-analytic investigation of the relationship between the psychological distress of cancer patients and their carers. *Soc. Sci. Med.* 60:1-12, 2005

[29] Kozachik, S. L., Given, C. W., Given, B. A., et al.: Improving depressive symptoms among caregivers of patients with cancer: Results of a randomized clinical trial. *Oncol. Nurs. Forum* 28:1149-1157, 2001;

[30] Carter, P. A.: Family caregivers' sleep loss and depression over time. *Cancer Nurs.* 26:253-259, 2003;

[31] Carter, P. A., Acton, G. J.: Personality and coping: Predictors of depression and sleep problems among caregivers of individuals who have cancer. *J. Gerontol. Nurs.* 32:45-53, 2006;

[32] Northouse, L. L., Mood, D., Kershaw, T., et al.: Quality of life of women with recurrent breast cancer and their family members. *J. Clin. Oncol.* 20:4050-4064, 2002;

[33] Kim, Y., Duberstein, P. R., So¨rensen, S., et al.: Levels of depressive symptoms in spouses of people with lung cancer: Effects of personality, social support, and caregiving burden. *Psychosomatics* 46:123-130, 2005;

[34] Rossi Ferrario, S., Zotti, A. M., Massara, G., et al.: A comparative assessment of psychological and psychosocial characteristics of cancer patients and their caregivers. *Psychooncology* 12:1-7, 2003;

[35] Cameron, J. I., Franche, R. L., Cheung, A. M., et al: Lifestyle interference and emotional distress in family caregivers of advanced cancer patients. *Cancer* 94:521-527, 2002;

[36] Goldstein, N. E., Concato, J., Fried, T. R., et al.: Factors associated with caregiver burden among caregivers of terminally ill patients with cancer. *J. Palliat. Care* 20:38-43, 2004

[37] Carter, P. A., Chang, B. L.: Sleep and depression in cancer caregivers. *Cancer Nurs.* 23:410-415, 2000;

[38] Kurtz, M. E., Kurtz, J. C., Given, C. W., et al.: Depression and physical health among family caregivers of geriatric patients with cancer: A longitudinal view. *Med. Sci. Monit.* 10:CR447-CR456, 2004;

[39] Lee, S., Colditz, G. A., Berkman, L. F., et al.: Caregiving and risk of coronary heart disease in US women: A prospective study. *Am. J. Prev. Med.* 24:113-119, 2003

[40] Rohleder, N., Marin, T. J., Ma, R., et al.: Biologic cost of caring for a cancer patient: Dysregulation of pro- and anti-inflammatory signaling pathways. *J. Clin. Oncol.* 27:2909-2915, 2009

[41] Holtslander, L., Duggleby, W. The psychological context for older women who were caregivers for a spouse with advanced cancer. *J. Women Aging* 2010;22:109–124;

[42] Hasson-Ohayon, I., Goldzweig, G., Braun, M., Galinsky, D., Baider, L. Religiosity and hope: path for women coping with a diagnosis of breast cancer. *Psychosomatics* 2009;50:525–533

[43] Yarbroff, K. R., Kim, Y. Time costs associated with informal caregiving for cancer survivors. *Cancer* 2009;115:4362-4373;

[44] Kim, Y., Spillers, R. L., Hall, D. L. Quality of life of family caregivers 5 years after a relative's cancer diagnosis: follow-up of the National Quality of Life Survey for Caregivers. *Psychooncology* 2012;21:273-281

[45] Given, B. A., Given, C. W., Sherwood, P. Family and caregiver needs over the course of the cancer trajectory. *J. Support. Oncol.* 2012;10:57-64

[46] Russell-Searight, H., Gafford, J. Cultural diversity at the end of life: issues and guidelines for family physicians. *Am. Fam. Phys.* 71:515–522; (2005)

[47] Surbone, A. Cultural aspects of communication in cancer care. *Supp. Care Cancer* (2008) 16:235–240

[48] Kagawa-Singer, M., Wellisch, D. K. Breast cancer patients' perceptions of their husbands' support in a cross-cultural context. *Psychooncology.* 2003 Jan-Feb.;12(1):24-37.

[49] Chilman, C. S., Hispanic families in the United States: Research perspectives. In: H. P. McAdoo (Ed.), *Family ethnicity: Strength in diversity* 1993 pp. 141–163. Newbury Park: Sage.

[50] Lee, Y. R. and Sung, K. T., Cultural influences on caregiver burden: Cases of Koreans and Americans. *International Journal of Aging and Human Development*, 1998 46, 125-141.

[51] Lazarus, R. S. and Folkman, S., *Stress, appraisal, and coping.* (1984). New York: Springer.

[52] Rhee, Y. S., Yun, Y. H., Park, S., et al. Depression in family caregivers of cancer patients: the feeling of burden as a predictor of depression. *J. Clin. Oncol.* (2008) 26:5890–5895

[53] Surbone, A. Persisting differences in truth-telling throughout the world. *Supp. Care Cancer* (2004) 12:143–146 82.

[54] Mystadikou, K., Parpa, E., Tsilika, E., et al. Cancer information disclosure in different cultural contexts. *Support Care Cancer* (2004) 12: 147–154.

[55] Surbone, A. Telling truth to patients with cancer: what is the truth? *Lancet Oncol.* (2006) 7:944–950

[56] Association of American Medical Colleges. Medical Education and Cultural Competence: A Strategy to Eliminate Racial and Ethnic Disparities in Health Care. Supported by The Commonwealth Fund. Division of Diversity Policy and Programs 2005. Accessible at www.AAMC.org.

[57] Kagawa-Singer, M., Kassim-Lakha, S. A strategy toreduce cross-cultural miscommunication and increase the likelihood of improving health outcomes. *Acad. Med.* (2003) 78:577– 587

[58] Betancourt, J. R., Green, A. R., Carrillo, J. E., Ananeh-Firempong, O. 2nd Defining cultural competence: a practical framework for addressing racial/ethnic disparities in health and health care. *Public Health Rep.* (2003) 118:293–302

[59] Nguyen, T. U., Kagawa-Singer, M. Overcoming barriers to cancer care through health navigation programs. *Semin. Oncol. Nurs.* (2008) 24: 270–278

[60] Osse, B. H., Vernooij-Dassen, M. J., Schadé, E., Grol, R. P. Problems experienced by the informal caregivers of cancer patients and their needs for support. *Cancer Nurs.* 2006;29(5):378-88;

[61] Soothill, K., Morris, S. M., Thomas, C., Harman, J. C., Francis, B., McIllmurray, M. B. The universal, situational, and personal needs of cancer patients and their main carers. *Eur. J. Oncol. Nurs.* 2003;7(1):5-13)

[62] Bessa, Y., Moore, A., Amey, F. Caring for a loved one with cancer: it is my job. *J. Psychosoc. Oncol.* 2012;30:212–238)

[63] Hudson, P., Remedios, C., Thomas, K. A systematic review of psychosocial interventions for family carers of palliative care patients. *BMC Palliat Care* 2010;9:1-5

[64] Baider, L., Balducci, L. Psychological interventions for elderly cancer patients. In: Watson, M., Kissane, D., editors. *Handbook of psychotherapy in cancer care*. West-Sussex, UK: J Wiley and Sons; 2011. p. 235–245

[65] Sörensen, S., Pinquart, M., Duberstein, P. How effective are interventions with caregivers? An updated meta-analysis. *Gerontologist* 2002;42:356-372

[66] Janda, M., Steginga, S., Dunn, J., Langbecker, D., Walker, D., Eakin, E. unmet supportive care needs and interest in services among patients with a brain tumour and their carers. *Patient Educ. Couns.* 2008;71(2):251–258,

[67] Kim, Y., Kashy, D. A., Spillers, R. L., Evans, T. V. Needs assessment of family caregivers of cancer survivors: three cohorts comparison. *Psycho-Oncology* 2010; 19 (6):573–582,

[68] Hodgkinson, K., Butow, P., Hunt, G., Wyse, R., Hobbs, K., Wain, G. Life after cancer: couples' and partners' psychological adjustment and supportive care needs. *Support Care Cancer* 2007;15(4):405–415

[69] Northouse, L., Williams, A. L., Given, B., and McCorkle, R. Psychosocial Care for Family Caregivers of Patients With Cancer. *JCO* 30:227-1234; 2011

In: Caregivers: Challenges, Practices and Cultural Influences
Editors: Adrianna Thurgood and Kasha Schuldt

ISBN: 978-1-62618-030-7
© 2013 Nova Science Publishers, Inc.

Chapter 10

CAREGIVER BURDEN OF OLDER ADULTS: A SOUTHEAST ASIAN ASPECT

Panita Limpawattana[*,1] *and Jarin Chindaprasirt*[2]

[1]Geriatric Medicine, Khon Kaen University, Thailand
[2]Oncology Department of Internal Medicine, Faculty of Medicine, Khon Kaen University, Thailand

ABSTRACT

Disability is common among the elderly; it worsens with age and erodes the well-being of the caregiver(s). Caregivers of the elderly with chronic illness (eg. dementia and stroke) will likely experience personal life strain, social isolation, financial burden, and lack of intrinsic reward. The perception of burden varies based on socioeconomic and cultural backgrounds. From a Southeast Asian perspective, a considerable burden for the care of older persons with disability is based on informal care by family members. It, however, varies considerably even within the region and data are limited. Developing a better understanding of the caregiving process—include all of the factors contributing to the caregiver's burden among these populations—would help allied-health workers provide support in dealing with the various stressors more effectively. Intervention(s) to lessen the caregivers' burden would include (a) assessment of the associated portions by focusing on acknowledged specific concerns (b) evaluating of caregivers' perspective regarding patients' illness and (c) management of a care plan with family members.

SOUTHEAST ASIAN COMMUNITY IN SOCIOECONOMIC DEVELOPMENT STATE

Southeast Asia is south of China, east of India, west of New Guinea, and north of Australia [1]. All of the countries in this area (excluding East Timor) are members of the Association of Southeast Asian Nations (ASEAN) established in 1967. The member states

---

[*] Corresponding author: Panita Limpawattana, email: lpanit@kku.ac.th.

include Brunei Darussalam, Cambodia, Indonesia, Lao PDR, Malaysia, Myanmar, Philippines, Singapore, Thailand and Viet Nam. Although the countries are close to each other, significant diversity exists vis-à-vis geography, language, religion, economics and politics [2].

Since the birth rate has declined and the life expectancy has increased in ASEAN, the proportion of elderly persons is rising. In 2007, those 60 years and over represented more than 5% in 5 ASEAN countries and more than 10% in 2, and these figures are expected to increase [3]. As life expectancy increases, communicable diseases account for a declining share of the gaps in longevity, while non-communicable diseases (NCDs) share grows. For example, the proportion of deaths due to NCDs in Indonesia increased dramatically from 42% in 1995, to 50% in 2001, to 60% in 2007 [4]. Among the NCDs, strokes, heart diseases, hypertension, diabetes and cancers account for the majority of deaths.

In the past, households predominantly comprised extended family in which there was reciprocal care giving: older physically capable, responsible person staking care of younger ones while the weak, infirm or extreme elderly were given supportive care [3]. Currently, ASEAN is urbanizing rapidly because of the migration of labor from agriculture to industry. According to United Nations data, the population in urban areas in Southeast Asia has increased from 32% of the total population in 1990 to 41% in 2005 and is estimated to reach 52.9% by 2025 [5]. As a result, the nuclear type family structure is becoming more common although overall the extended family persists. Females continue to be, therefore, the major informal caregivers and the majority of stroke patients live with family [3, 6].

Healthcare systems in ASEAN vary greatly. In 2003, the number of physicians (per 10,000 populations) ranged from 1 physician in Indonesia to 15 in Singapore [7]. Community healthcare service is insufficient and the number of hospices is very low, except in Singapore. Thus, family support plays an ongoing key role for informal care of older persons (65 years old or over). This could lead to a huge burden for family members in socioeconomic development state in ASEAN society.

CAREGIVER IMPACT OF OLDER ADULTS

Chronic illness clearly erodes the quality of the patient's life but it also impinges on the family and particularly the partner [8]. Compared to acute illness, the caregiver must bear a longer duration of care with possibly increasing responsibilities and negative consequences beyond caregiving; as the natural history of chronic illness is usually progressive [8]. Caregivers often experience reduced physical and psychological health, worsened quality of life and compromised immunity and mortality [9].

Perceived caregiver burden and stressors can be divided into 4 domains (1) personal life strain (2) social isolations (3) financial burden and (4) intrinsic rewards [8]. Caregivers of patients with cancer, musculoskeletal and digestive disorders are risk for perceiving greater impact on the consequences of chronic illness. Depending on the disease characteristics, those inflicting physical disabilities are associated with a greater personal life strain and financial burden on the caregiver while those resulting in social impairment can affect on all 4 domains. The impact on caregivers of patients afflicted with fatigue experience erosion of their personal life, social isolation and intrinsic rewards; whereas caregivers of patients experiencing mostly a burden of pain mainly experience a diminishment of their social relations [8]. Currently, there are fewer studies about caregiver burden in the Southeast Asian context than in other regions. Evidence from a nationwide, cross-sectional household survey—the Singapore Mental Health Study (SMHS) investigating the prevalence of psychiatric disorders in Singapore—revealed that caregivers of patients with any chronic physical illness perceived a greater physical burden in terms of time spent in caring and associated costs whereas caregivers of patients with any mental illness perceived a greater burden in terms of eroded psychological, social and emotional (embarrassment and worry) health [10].

In Thailand, the prevalence of negative impact variables on caregivers of older persons/with chronic illness was studied at the community level. The Zarit Burden Interview (ZBI) was used to assess the subjective psychological, social and emotional burden. 'Guilt' (35.6±15.5%) was the most frequently cited factor, followed by the 'strain on personal life' (22.8±18.3%).

The 'consequences for their privacy conflict' (17.4±12.5%) and 'uncertain attitude' (13.6±14.5%) were reported least frequently [6]. This might be due to the legacy of the extended family values and/or possibly a religious merit; that is, family members see the responsibility of caring for elderly parents as an unavoidable duty [11, 12].

HOW TO MEASURE CAREGIVER BURDEN?

Since a high degree of the caregiver burden can in turn have an impact on patient care—including adverse physical, psychological, psychosocial, social, and economical aspects—careful evaluation of the ramifications of caregiving on the informal caregiver's health would help allied-healthcare workers to better understand patients and their informal caregivers vis-à-vis their diverse circumstances; thus suggesting more appropriate interventions in order to alleviate the burden as well as to assess their effectiveness [13, 14].

Table 1. Main dimensions of assessment regarding the impacts of caregiving

Positive impact	Negative impact	Neutral impact
Appraisal	Burden	Coping
Quality of life	Strain	Help
Competence	Stress	Impact
Well-being	Depression	Hassles and uplifts
Satisfaction	Grief	Management assessment
Self-efficacy	Risk	Preparedness
Social support	Role overload	Reaction
Reward	Guilt	
Mastery	Loss of self	
Meaning	Task difficulty	
Effectiveness	Role captivity	
Gain		

Note: modified from [14].

Several tools for assessing the caregiver burden of older adults are available; most of which focus on older adults with dementia, cancer, chronic illness and stroke [14].

These instruments impact on the caregiver including (a) burden (b) needs and (c) quality of life. Such can then be categorized into 3 main dimensions: (1) positive (e.g., appraisal of caregiving scale, caregiver competence scale); (2) negative (e.g., caregiver burden scale, Zarit burden interview); and, (3) neutral (e.g., caregiver reaction assessment, perceived health index) [13, 14].

The components of each dimension are presented in Table 1. According to the literature review, ~100 validated scales are in clinical use and vary considerably in their internal consistency (range, 0.48-0.99). These scales and tools are predominantly from Europe and America but a few have been developed for the Asian context (viz., Japan, Taiwan and South Korea) [14].

The Zarit Burden Interview-22 (ZBI) which comprises 22 items is one of the most commonly used scales for research and clinical use because it is user-friendly and has had widespread international validation, including a Thai version. It mainly assesses the negative dimension vis-à-vis the aspect of burden. The internal consistency (Cronbach's alpha) is 0.85 (0.92 and 0.93 for Thai and Singaporean version, respectively). It mainly assesses in the caregiver burden dimension [14-18]. The short version of ZBI (ZBI-12, ZBI-8, ZBI-7, ZBI-6, ZBI-4, and ZBI-1) has also been broadly validated among caregivers of older adults but not for Thai people until now [19, 20]. The ZBI-12 is accepted as the best short-form version and the ZBI-1 is recommended for screening: it is, however, less sensitive for caregivers of patients with cancer [19].

WHAT ARE FACTORS ASSOCIATED WITH CAREGIVER BURDEN OF OLDER PERSONS WITH CHRONIC ILLNESS

Generally, existing studies document several variables influencing caregivers' quality of life. These factors can be classified into two areas; patient characteristics and caregiver characteristics. Caregiver characteristics are stronger factors with respect to burden on caregiving.

Caring for a person who requires more assistance with daily tasks—like a patient-to-child relationship—and the need for more communication with a patient's doctor are associated with a high burden.

Some factors, however, do not reach statistical significance in some studies including female sex, income, educational level, relationship quality, health status, experience of adverse life events, neuroticism, caregiver confidence, self-efficacy, coping strategies, family functioning and social support.

Thus, a high burden to the caregiver is related to their performance status or the severity of illness (i.e., shortness of breath and physical discomfort). Possible related factors include: depression, age, male sex, and type of illness [6, 8, 9, 21]. Focusing the caregiver burden on the specific illness is summarized in Table 2: the influencing factors are dissimilar for different conditions.

Table 2. Factors influencing the burden to the caregiver for specific illnesses

Domain	Cancer	Heart disease	Stroke	Alzheimer's disease	Chronic mental illness
Patient characteristics					
Illness severity	✓	✓	✓	✓	✓
Prior hospitalization		✓			✓
Length of recovery period		✓			✓
Degree of impairment/illness stage	✓		✓	✓	✓
Prognosis	✓				
Caregiving demands	✓				
Time since diagnosis	✓ (some)				✓ (some)
Amount of patient change/distress	✓	✓	✓	✓	✓
Suddenness of onset	✓	✓	✓		
Caregiver characteristics					
Demographic variables					
Sex	✓	✓	✓	✓	✓
Relationship to patient		✓ (non-spouse)	✓ (spouse)	✓ (spouse)	✓ (parent)
Caregiver health	✓		✓		✓
Household size					✓
Age of caregiver	✓ (younger)	✓ (younger)	✓ (younger)		
Socioeconomic status		✓ (higher)	✓ (higher)		✓ (higher)
Work status of caregiver	✓				
Life status variables					
Other life stressors	✓			✓ (financial concerns)	
Prior psychological problems		✓			
Relationship quality	✓	✓		✓	
Family life stage	✓				
Social support	✓	✓	✓	✓	

Note: modified from [22].

FACTORS ASSOCIATED WITH CAREGIVER BURDEN FROM A SOUTHEAST ASIAN PERSPECTIVE

Since both (a) cultural and society diversity influences the perceptions of the caregiver burden and (b) long-term institutional care is generally limited in Southeast Asia, informal care from family members (particularly children and spouses) is a core component of care for the elderly, including those with chronic illness. A substantial burden is, therefore, placed on families [6]. Moreover, compared to other areas of the world, there has been relatively little research focusing on the caregiver burden from a psychosocial perspective. Most studies have been conducted in Singapore and Thailand. In general, existing studies—regarding the factors influencing the informal caregiver burden for community-dwelling older persons—agree with prior reports that show caregiver characteristics are related to the high burden more than the patient characteristics [6, 10].

In Thailand, a cross-sectional study reported that informal care was performed predominately by female family members followed by sons/daughters. Based on the Zarit Burden Interview (ZBI), the majority of caregivers perceived that they had no burden (52%), followed by mild burden (44%). The mean ZBI scores were 20.8±11.3, 95%CI 19.0-22.7. Caregivers of older adults with cerebrovascular disease, dementia, cancer, renal failure and psychiatric conditions accounted for the 'mild caregiver burden' whereas other chronic illnesses including diabetes mellitus, hypertension, chronic insomnia, musculoskeletal disease were reported as 'no caregiver burden'. The prevalence of the impact variables on the caregivers—including personal strain, privacy conflict, guilt, and uncertain attitudes—showed that guilt was the most frequently reported factor (35.6±15.5%), followed by the strain on personal life (22.8±18.3%), privacy conflict (17.4±12.5%) and uncertain attitudes (13.6±14.5%).

In sum, a high burden for caregivers was associated with 4 factors: (1) older age of caregiver (2) perceived poor health status (3) perceived financial problems and (3) longer duration of care. Poor perceived health status was the highest factor impact on caregiver burden, followed by poor perceived financial problems, older age, and longer duration of care [6]. Other caregiver characteristics—including, sex, educational level, types of illness, kinship, employment status, caregiver income, number and types of assistance in daily tasks—did not have any significant association. Based on this report, caregiver burden in Thailand appears modest; however, it should be interpreted carefully because the majority of the study areas had few chronic illnesses including few high burden conditions such as dementia, cerebrovascular disease, or advanced cancer [6].

A large cross-sectional survey in Singapore mainly on Chinese (77.3%) and some Malays (11.5%) (~50% female) reported that a perceived high burden was associated with having at least 1 close family member with a chronic illness for whom the trouble was mainly a memory problem (86.9%), followed by physical disability (74.8%), heart ailment (74.1%), and cancer (62.2%). Based on a bivariate analysis, age, sex, ethnicity, marital status, education, income, "being able to open up", having dysthymia, major depressive, bipolar, generalized anxiety and obsessive compulsive disorder were related to perceived burden. A multivariate analyses, however, revealed that there were only 4 predictors associated with high burden; viz., ethnicity (Chinese; OR 1.0) vs. Malay; OR 0.68), female (OR 1.58), caregivers who could speak about (ventilate) their concerns/burden (OR 1.65) and dysthymia (OR 4.91) [10].

In the social support domain, the results from Vaingankar et al. (2012) study were not in agreement with previous studies as caregivers who were able to express their feelings to others were less likely to perceive burden than others. Since social interaction is different in each culture, further research into this area may lead to a better understanding of this element.

The factors influencing caregiver burden in Southeast Asia vary from country to country so direct comparison might be difficult. The variation might be the result of (a) cultural and/or religious perceptions (b) study design and/or (c) the different tools used to measure the impact of informal caregiving. The results may even be underestimated since, in traditional Southeast Asian societies, caregivers are bound by duty to care their ageing parents or spouses. As such, they may be reluctant to express their feelings openly as it might imply failure of filial duty [6, 23].

CAREGIVER BURDEN VIS-A-VIS DEMENTIA IN SOUTHEAST ASIA

Dementia is a progressive, degenerative brain syndrome that affects memory, thinking, behavior and emotion. It is one of the common geriatric syndromes in which its prevalence has been rising in relation to the increasing age [24]. The number of new cases of dementia in Southeast Asia is projected to rise as with that of other regions [25]. Based on existing data for Indonesia, Malaysia, Singapore and Thailand, the prevalence of dementia per 1,000 populations is estimated to increase from 2005 to 2050 by: 606.1 to 3,042 for Indonesia; 63 to 453.9 for Malaysia; 22 to 186.9 for Singapore; and, 229.1 to 377 for Thailand [25]. The impact of dementia is not only upon persons with dementia but also on informal caregivers [24].

In Singapore, there is evidence that about one-half of caregivers experience burden in caring for patients with mild to moderate dementia, indicating a significant burden even in the early phase of the disease. The main concerns among caregivers were both physical and psychological issues that led them to consider institutionalization for the patients [26]. Most of the caregivers were female (68%) and the majority of them the offspring or spouse of the elderly person being cared for.

Using bivariate analyses, patient characteristics (viz., patient behavioral problems and functional dependence and caregiver with clinical depression) had more impact on their perceived burden than their own caregiver characteristics. The predictive factors—based on multiple logistic regressions—revealed 4 factors: urinary incontinence, repetition, agitated behavior and caregiver depression. The highest factor predicting caregiver burden of mild to moderate dementia patients was urinary incontinence (OR 7.69), followed by caregiver depression (OR 5.74), agitation (OR 4.31), and repetition (OR 3.4) [26].

From the Thai perspective, the perceived burden in caregiving of patients with dementia using Caregiver Burden Inventory as a multidimensional tool for assessment revealed that: (a) the majority of caregivers were female (86%) (b) serving elderly parents needing continuous care (57%)(c) had a Bachelor degree or higher and (d) worked outside the home (69%) [12]. As with the Singaporean study, after adjusting for sex and kinship only caring for demented patients with dependency significantly increased the odds ratio (to 7.48; 95%CI 1.42, 39.53).

The most troubling behaviors for caregivers were memory problems, repetitions, insomnia, impaired activities of daily living, and irritability. The study by Muangpaisan et al. was conducted in Bangkok—the highly urban, capital city—so the results might not be generalized to the whole country.

FACTORS ASSOCIATED WITH CONSIDERING INSTITUTIONALIZATION FOR PATIENTS FROM A SOUTHEAST ASIAN PERSPECTIVE

Although institutionalization for the aged is limited in Southeast Asia as most families prefer to look after their elderly at home, the number of institutionalized elderly is increasing [23]. The factors associated with caregivers' preference for institutionalization were studied in the Singapore Dementia Caregiver Profile Study. Three factors were identified (1) working outside home (OR 6.32) (2) absence of domestic maid (OR 3.27) and (c) caring for a dementia patient with behavioral problems (OR 1.01). These results, however, were limited to families of Chinese ethnicity educated in Singapore.

CHALLENGES OF CAREGIVING FOR ALLIED-HEALTHCARE WORKERS: POLICY AND SERVICE RECOMMENDATIONS

The perceived burden of caring for the elderly with chronic illness(es) in Southeast Asia is different from other regions of the world. Such a perception is subjective and individuals and different cultures interpret it in different ways. Acquiring a better understanding of family burdens, however, is a key when strategizing how best to care for both the elderly person and their family who deliver much of the care at home. Always incorporating a care plan which includes an assessment of the caregiver burden along with the comprehensive geriatric assessment (CGA) would be invaluable.

Strategies for dealing with the burden of caregivers of elderly persons can be categorized as: (1) coping strategies; (2) improving patients' functional status; (3) family and social support; (4) caregiver health checkup program; and, (5) support of further research in Southeast Asia.

COPING STRATEGIES

Allied-healthcare workers should acknowledge the specific issues arising for caregivers of persons with chronic natural disease and in particular dementia. There is limited technical awareness of dementia in Southeast Asia as it is considered an ordinary part of ageing. More consideration needs to be given the role change (offspring taking care of parents) and the related uncertainty and perceptions of autonomy loss. Focusing on caregiver strain is not as fruitful as providing time for caregivers to share their perspective and contribute to the care plan. In addition, caregivers need to feel: (a) that all family members are expected and empowered to join in problem-solving; (b) acknowledged for previously effective strategies; (c) welcome to contribute potential approaches; (d) that plans are practicable; and, (e) that desired outcomes are open for discussion. These strategies could help caregivers to recover or to feel more at ease with the illness(es); particularly chronic illness with high disability, including stroke and dementia with neuropsychiatric symptoms [6, 21, 25]. In addition, using religious teachings to deal with their daily burden and solve complicated circumstances can bring consolation [6, 27, 28].

Improving Patients' Functional Status

Patients' functional status is one of the patient-dependent factors influencing the caregiver burden [26]. Reducing total dependency helps to mitigate the caregiving burden. For example, older persons with urinary incontinence, can schedule toileting, undergo bladder training and be educated on appropriate individualized approaches. For mobility, providing a suitable gait aid and elderly-friendly environment can be useful. In elderly persons, major neuropsychiatric problems (principally dementia) lead to functional dependency. Non-pharmacologic interventions employed at first followed by pharmacologic treatment(s), which are associated with significant adverse effects and only moderate efficacy [25].

Family and Social Support

Family and social support should: (1) establish and encourage the standard needs assessments for caregivers be given in their own homes;(2) develop multidisciplinary community-based care teams—including support from family members and neighbors; (3) encourage caregivers to persevere in giving care; (4) schedule caregiver training; and, (5) set up daycare and short-term respite for the elderly with chronic illness to give caregivers a break. For example, in Singapore, domestic help is arranged in order to delay institutionalization [23].

Caregiver Health Checkup Program

Caregiver depression or anxiety, and poor self-reported health status are associated with burden among caregivers. Health check-ups and caregiver burden should be evaluated periodically in order to determine what interventions would best suit each caregiving situation.

Support Further Research in Southeast Asia

The cultural context also has a bearing on caregiver burden so needs to be characterized regionally (in Southeast Asia) and country by country and probably region by region. For enhanced understanding, further studies need to be done in primary healthcare settings on: (a) prevalence; (b) associated factors; (c) outcomes;(d) impact of each chronic illness in the community; and,(e) cost-effectiveness of introducing interventions alongside disease prevention [25].

CONCLUSION

Each society and culture influences the perception of the burden of caregiving. Although many countries in Southeast Asia are currently in the course of rapid economic development and urbanization, the traditional, extended family remains the basic unit of society. Informal care from family members therefore remains the heart of care for the elderly at home.

The burden of caring can have serious, long-term adverse physical, psychological, psychosocial, social and economical consequences on the caregiver. The Zarit Burden Interview (ZBI) is one of the most extensively used tools for research and general practice. The perception of burden evidently varies according the socio-economic and cultural background of the caregiver.

Studies on the caregiver burden from the Southeast Asian perspective are limited. Existing evidence, however, indicates that caregiver characteristics have more influence on the perception of burden than the symptoms of chronic illness of the elderly person cared for. The opposite is trended when the patient has cognitive and functional disabilities as with dementia.

By taking all these aspects into consideration AND by assessing the actual burden on caregivers during visits, healthcare providers can more accurately target interventions that lessen the caregiving burden. The five recommended strategies to better manage burdens are: (1) to provide coping strategies; (2) to improve the patient's functional status; (3) to support the family and community; (4) to schedule caregiver health check-ups; and, (5) to support further research in Southeast Asia.

CONFLICT OF INTEREST

None to our knowledge.

ACKNOWLEDGMENTS

The authors thank the Department of Medicine at the Faculty of Medicine, Khon Kaen University for its support and Mr. Bryan Roderick Hamman and Mrs. Janice Loewen-Hamman for assistance with the English-language presentation.

REFERENCES

[1] WHO. History of the WHO South-east Asia region. 2012 [updated April 26th, 2006; cited 2012 September 30th]; Available from: http://www.searo.who.int/ EN/Section898 /Section1443.htm

[2] The Association of Southeast Asian Nations (ASEAN). Evolving Towards ASEAN 2015: ASEAN annual report 2011-2012. Jakarta: The Association of Southeast Asian Nations (ASEAN); 2012. Available from: http://www.aseansec.org/documents/annual% 20report%202011-2012.pdf

[3] Podhisita C. Thai family and household changes: What we don't know? In: Punpuing S, Sunpuwan S, editors. Thailand's population in transition: a turning point for Thai society. 1st ed. Bangkok: October press; 2011. p. 23-41.

[4] WHO: regional office for the South-east Asia region. Health and Development Challenges of Non-communicable Diseases in the South-East Asia Region. *Report of the Regional Meeting*; March 1-4, 2011; Jakarta, Indonesia: India; 2011.

[5] United Nations. World Urbanization Prospects, the 2011 Revision. New York: September 14th; 2011. Available from: http://esa.un.org/unup/pdf/ FINAL-FINAL _REPORT%20WUP2011_Annextables_01Aug2012_ Final.pdf

[6] Limpawattana P, Theeranut A, Chindaprasirt J, Sawanyawisuth K, Pimporm J. Caregivers Burden of Older Adults with Chronic Illnesses in the Community: A Cross-Sectional Study. *J. Community Health* 2012 Jun 12 [Epub ahead of print].

[7] WHO data. Physicians density (per 10 000 population). 2010 [updated November 19th, 2010; cited 2012 September 20th]; Available from: http://data.un.org/ Data.aspx?d=WHOandf=MEASURE_CODE%3aWHS6_125

[8] Baanders AN, Heijmans MJ. The impact of chronic diseases: the partner's perspective. *Fam. Community Health* 2007 Oct-Dec;30(4):305-17.

[9] Garlo K, O'Leary JR, Van Ness PH, Fried TR. Burden in caregivers of older adults with advanced illness. *J. Am. Geriatr Soc.* 2010 Dec;58(12):2315-22.

[10] Vaingankar JA, Subramaniam M, Abdin E, He VY, Chong SA. "How much can I take?": predictors of perceived burden for relatives of people with chronic illness. *Ann. Acad. Med. Singapore* 2012 May;41(5):212-20.

[11] Limpanichkul Y, Magilvy K. Managing caregiving at home: Thai caregivers living in the United States. *J. Cult. Divers* 2004 Spring;11(1):18-24.

[12] Muangpaisan W, Praditsuwan R, Assanasen J, Srinonprasert V, Assantachai P, Intalapaporn S, et al. Caregiver burden and needs of dementia caregivers in Thailand: a cross-sectional study. *J. Med. Assoc. Thai.* 2010 May;93(5):601-7.

[13] Deeken JF, Taylor KL, Mangan P, Yabroff KR, Ingham JM. Care for the caregivers: a review of self-report instruments developed to measure the burden, needs, and quality of life of informal caregivers. *J. Pain Symptom Manage* 2003 Oct;26(4):922-53.

[14] Van Durme T, Macq J, Jeanmart C, Gobert M. Tools for measuring the impact of informal caregiving of the elderly: A literature review. *Int. J. Nurs Stud.* 2011 Nov 10.

[15] Toonsiri C, Sunsern R, Lawang W. Development of the Burden Interview for Caregivers of Patients with Chronic Illness. *Journal of nursing and education* 2011;4(1):62-75.

[16] Arai Y, Kudo K, Hosokawa T, Washio M, Miura H, Hisamichi S. Reliability and validity of the Japanese version of the Zarit Caregiver Burden interview. *Psychiatry Clin Neurosci* 1997 Oct;51(5):281-7.

[17] Zarit SH, Reever KE, Bach-Peterson J. Relatives of the impaired elderly: correlates of feelings of burden. *Gerontologist* 1980 Dec;20(6):649-55.

[18] Seng BK, Luo N, Ng WY, Lim J, Chionh HL, Goh J, et al. Validity and reliability of the Zarit Burden Interview in assessing caregiving burden. *Ann. Acad. Med. Singapore* 2010 Oct;39(10):758-63.

[19] Higginson IJ, Gao W, Jackson D, Murray J, Harding R. Short-form Zarit Caregiver Burden Interviews were valid in advanced conditions. *J. Clin. Epidemiol.* 2010 May;63(5):535-42.

[20] Bedard M, Molloy DW, Squire L, Dubois S, Lever JA, O'Donnell M. The Zarit Burden Interview: a new short version and screening version. *Gerontologist* 2001 Oct;41(5):652-7.

[21] Lim JW, Zebrack B. Caring for family members with chronic physical illness: a critical review of caregiver literature. *Health Qual Life Outcomes* 2004;2:50.

[22] Sales E. Family burden and quality of life. *Qual Life Res.* 2003;12 Suppl 1:33-41.

[23] Tew CW, Tan LF, Luo N, Ng WY, Yap P. Why family caregivers choose to institutionalize a loved one with dementia: a Singapore perspective. *Dement Geriatr Cogn Disord* 2011;30(6):509-16.

[24] Limpawattana P, Tiamkao S, Sawanyawisuth K. The performance of the Rowland universal dementia assessment scale (RUDAS) for cognitive screening in a geriatric outpatient setting. *Aging Clin. Exp. Res.* 2012 Feb. [Epub ahead of print].

[25] Asia Pacific Members of Alzheimer's Disease International: Dementia in the Asia Pacific region: the epidemic is here2006 [cited 2012 August 14]: Available from: http://www.alz.co.uk/research/files/ apreportexecsum.pdf

[26] Lim PP, Sahadevan S, Choo GK, Anthony P. Burden of caregiving in mild to moderate dementia: an Asian experience. *Int. Psychogeriatr 1999* Dec;11(4):411-20.

[27] Limpawattana P, Theeranut A, Chindaprasirt J, Sawanyawisuth K, Pimporm J. Caregivers Burden of Older Adults with Chronic Illnesses in the Community: A Cross-Sectional Study. *J. Community Health2012* Jun 12 [Epub ahead of print].

[28] Greenwood N, Mackenzie A. Informal caring for stroke survivors: meta-ethnographic review of qualitative literature. *Maturitas* 2010 Jul;66(3):268-76.

Chapter 11

COMMUNITY-BASED EDUCATION CONCERNING PALLIATIVE CARE FOR THE ELDERLY IN JAPAN

Yoshihisa Hirakawa and Kazumasa Uemura
Nagoya University Hospital Center for Postgraduate Clinical Training and Career Development, Nagoya, Japan

ABSTRACT

Japan is confronted with shifting preferences of elderly patients and their families regarding their care. Namely, an increasing number of elderly people are now opting to spend their last few years of life in community settings such as long-term care facilities or in their own home. The community is therefore expected to assume a growing responsibility in caring for the dying elderly. Improving the quality and quantity of palliative care provision at home or at long-term care facilities has become an urgent priority in Japan. We believe that community-based palliative care education is one of the most important aspects of palliative care for the elderly.

Although a number of palliative care educational intervention programs have reportedly been implemented, many of these programs were formulated for university education rather than for community-based education.

In this paper, we described the current situation of community-based education concerning palliative care for the elderly in Japan. We also explained the details of community-based education programs concerning palliative care for the elderly, with special focus on community staff education.

BACKGROUND

Japan is currently one of the most quickly aging countries in the industrialized world. In 1970, only 7% of the Japanese population was aged 65 years or older, but by 1990 this rate had climbed to 12%. By 2006, 20.8% of the Japanese population was aged 65 or older - the highest rate in the world at the time [1,2]. Further complicating the situation, the number of elderly deaths has climbed very rapidly in Japan in recent years. The number of overall

Japanese deaths is expected to continue rising from 1.1 million in 2007 to 1.7 million in 2040, a surge associated with the steady growth in elderly deaths [1,2].

Aside from the rapid aging of the population, Japan is confronted with shifting preferences of elderly patients and their families regarding their care. Namely, an increasing number of elderly people are now opting to spend their last few years of life in community settings such as long-term care facilities or in their own home [2,3]. The community is therefore expected to assume a growing responsibility in caring for the dying elderly. Improving the quality and quantity of palliative care provision at home or at long-term care facilities has become an urgent priority in Japan [2-7]. We believe that community-based palliative care education is one of the most important aspects of palliative care for the elderly.

Community-based education refers to instructional and social development work with individuals and groups in their communities using a wide range of formal and informal methods [8,9]. In response to findings that community-based education was effective in fostering health personnel who are responsive to community needs, community-based education has been started in many medical schools around the globe as an innovative approach to medical education [9]. Although a number of palliative care educational intervention programs have reportedly been implemented [10-15], many of these focused mainly on palliative care for cancer patients and did not target non-cancer elderly patients; furthermore, these programs were formulated for university education rather than for community-based education. As highlighted by the position statement of the Japan Geriatric Society [5,6], there has been insufficient support for research or education contributing to the improvement of palliative care for the elderly in Japan.

In 2011, a project for the development of a comprehensive educational program for long-term care staff delivering palliative care for the elderly was launched in Japan with the financial support of the Ministry of Education, Culture, Sports, Science and Technology. Aside from this initiative, we have continuously performed community-based palliative care education focusing on multidisciplinary care since 2001 [16,17].

In this paper, we would like to describe the current situation of community-based education concerning palliative care for the elderly in Japan. We also wish to explain the details of community-based education programs concerning palliative care for the elderly, with special focus on the above-mentioned educational program launched in 2011.

1. COMMUNITY STAFF EDUCATION

a) Long-Term Care Facility Staff Education

Caring staff education is central to providing quality end-of-life care at long-term care facilities, where a growing number of elderly people are opting to spend their last years of life [1,18]. In Japan, many caring staff start working without having been sufficiently educated and trained on end-of-life care at university or college. Additionally, due to the growing number of nuclear families in Japan and well as the rising number of hospital deaths, caring staff have for the most part never personally witnessed the death of a family member and therefore have little practical experience. As a result, many caring staff are ill-prepared to provide elderly residents with quality end-of-life care.

A number of important studies on end-of-life care education for caring staff at long-term care facilities have so far been carried out worldwide. Henderson et al. developed a training manual for nursing home staff to improve nursing home end-of-life care [19]. Kortes-Miller et al. developed a 15-hour end-of-life care education program for long-term care facility staff [20]. Arcand et al. conducted a pilot study of long-term care facility staff education programs concerning dementia palliative care, and reported that the programs improved residents' family satisfaction [21]. Also, Parks et al reported that a pilot end-of-life care educational program improved caring staff attitudes [22]. However, there is currently no standardized caring staff educational program concerning end-of-life care for the elderly in Japan.

As detailed in the position statement of the Japan Geriatric Society, Japan has a distinct cultural background which differs from that of western countries [5,6]. It is characterized by a high degree of obedience from elderly people toward their physicians and a fatalistic attitude toward death (Japanese people generally resign themselves to their fate if they face an unfortunate situation). Therefore, we have devised a Japanese-style end-of-life care educational program for caring staff. In 2003, we conducted a questionnaire survey targeting 2876 chief nurses at long-term care facilities which highlighted a number of important concerns concerning end-of-life care staff education: residents' living will, communication skills, progressive clinical course of advanced diseases and accompanying symptoms, physical care, and psychological support to patients and families [23]. In 2006, Hirakawa et al conducted an opinion survey of caring staff at long-term care facilities about end-of-life care staff education, which revealed that dementia care, physical care, communication with residents and families, psychological aspects of dying, and pain/symptom control were top educational priorities for caring staff [18].

Based on the above-mentioned educational needs, we developed a number of pilot educational programs. From 2007 to 2008, we gave seven consecutive lectures concerning end-of-life care for the elderly to the caring staff of a long-term care facility [24]. The lectures centered on elderly first-aid, presentation skills in emergency situations, dementia care, terminology and definitions about end-of-life care, background of end-of-life care for the elderly at long-term care facilities, residents' living will, communication skills with residents and families, (bereaved) family care, among others. Lecture participants thought the initiative was rewarding, but felt that it did not have much of an impact on their attitude toward death. Therefore, we decided to introduce picture books concerning death or dying as an educational tool to engage participants on a deeper level [25]. Participants read a few picture books to each other and discussed the illustrations in detail. This proved to be a positive step in bringing about a change in attitudes among caring staff toward death.

Because caring staff lack the time to follow a lengthy program, what is needed is a short but effective and comprehensive educational strategy for them to acquire key knowledge and a wide range of skills concerning end-of-life care. In Canada, Gagliese ea al. et al developed a brief educational intervention about pain and ageing for older members of the community and health care workers and revealed that the intervention could potentially improve pain management for older people [26]. However, the intervention was not comprehensive. In addition, because end-of-life issues involve complicated decisions and feelings, caring staff should be educated about the attitudes and skills that would best allow them to confidently provide quality end-of-life care for the elderly. We thus opted for workshops as an educational method. In Japan, a project to develop an educational program for long-term care staff delivering palliative care for the elderly was launched in 2011 under the scheme of a research project funded by the Ministry of Education, Culture, Sports, Science and Technology. The program was developed based on a pilot trial [28], and consisted of a 6-hour basic course and a 5-hour advanced course. The basic course covered the following topics: signs and symptoms of death or dying, definition of end-of-life, do-not-resuscitate (DNR) order, families of end-of-life elderly residents, percutaneous endoscopic gastrostomy (PEG), and caring for bed-ridden elderly residents. During the session focusing on "signs and symptoms of death or dying", the participants were divided into groups of 7 to 8 people. We used the brainstorming method whereby participants took turns stating at least one sign, symptom or premonition of death or dying. During the session "definition of end-of-life of the elderly", the participants engaged in a group discussion and made a presentation. At the conclusion of the session, the workshop facilitator explained that it is difficult to define the "end-of-life process of the elderly" because not only is the end-of-life clinical course of non-cancer elderly patients complex [27], it is also more difficult to predict than that of cancer patients.

During the "DNR" session, the participants took part in a group discussion revolving around a case where caring staff provided cardiopulmonary resuscitation (CPR) to an end-of-life elderly resident with a DNR order who suffered from a sudden cardiopulmonary arrest during a meal.

During the session "families of end-of-life elderly residents", each participant shared a story about a family that had impacted them profoundly; each group then chose the most impressive case and presented it through role playing. During the PEG session, the facilitator explained the following excerpt of the position statement of the Japan Geriatric Society 2012 [29]: "indication for tube feeding including PEG, tracheotomy, or mechanical ventilation should be carefully considered."

Namely, if these therapies were found to impair the dignity of the patient or to worsen the patient's pain, the possibility of withholding or stopping such interventions should be considered. Finally, the participants engaged in a micro debate concerning the suitability of PEG for end-of-life elderly. During the session "care for bedridden elderly residents", the facilitator showed the participants a trigger video of a caring staff dealing with his bedridden elderly patient in a mechanical fashion. Through small group discussions, the participants were encouraged to share their thoughts about what constitutes a positive attitude in caring for bed-ridden elderly.

The Advanced Course was developed under the concept of "teaching is learning". Namely, the course aimed at allowing participants to gain greater confidence in their own skills by educating a newcomer caring staff on end-of-life care for the elderly. During the course, the participants made videos showing how to care for end-of-life elderly and how to nurture positive feelings with patients at long-term care facilities. Next, because caring staff generally lack confidence in making presentations about emergency patients to medical professionals, the participants were taught how to make a presentation about a first-aid case through role playing. Finally, the participants discussed a number of complicated issues concerning institutional end-of-life care for elderly using the KJ pulse discussion method [30].

The pulse discussion method is widely used as a brainstorming method in Japan, and constitutes a really useful method to hold an inspirational discussion without a recording clerk. In a general meeting, recording clerks document the participants' statements, but in a pulse discussion the participants can discuss any other issue that was not brought up during in the discussion.

b) Sputum Suction Training System for Caring Staff Cosponsored by University Hospital and Community

In Japan, providing caring staff with medical care training has become an urgent necessity due to the fast-growing number of end-of-life elderly residing in community settings. Sputum suction is one of the top priority medical care skills in end-of-life care settings [31,32]. Until recently, only medical professionals could perform certain procedures such as sputum suction; now, caring staff may also carry out sputum suction (under certain conditions) provided they undergo an authorized sputum suction training. However, many caring staff feel that they lack the confidence to provide sputum suction safely. Nagoya University and Nagoya University Hospital were the first to implement a sputum suction simulation training system for caring staff working in Nagoya and surroundings; caring staff were thus provided with the opportunity to receive regular sputum suction training throughout the year [32].

The lecturers for this program are recruited from long-term care facilities and the Nagoya University Hospital. This recruiting system contributes to the promotion of cultural exchange between university and community and to the expansion of the educational skills of experienced caring staff.

2. COOPERATION BETWEEN UNIVERSITY HOSPITAL AND LOCAL GOVERNMENT

The Nagoya University Hospital and Aichi prefecture established a community care support system in 2010. In collaboration with Aichi prefecture, Nagoya University set up an information desk to provide support on a wide variety of elderly care questions for care/welfare professionals [33]. For example, one care manager placed the following e-mail query: *"we have an elderly client who cannot communicate with us due to advanced dementia. His family wishes for him to use our short-stay service for lengthy periods of time, but the client seems to be against it. I am afraid that we are not serving the client's needs but those of his family.*" Nagoya University responded as follows: *"Elderly people are sometimes erratic in their choices, and they might suddenly begin to enjoy a service that they previously disliked. In addition, short stay or day service fall under the category of respite care services. The main purpose of respite care services is to lessen the caregiver's burden. The client's wishes are important, but the family's desires should also be given careful consideration to provide quality care for elderly. Quality care that is focused on the family enhances the quality of life of elderly clients"*.

As part of this cooperative effort, Nagoya University and the Nagoya University Hospital also send lecturers to rural areas and organize workshops or seminars for medical professionals and caring staff on end-of-life care or dementia care. These activities contribute to upgrading end-of-life skills and knowledge of medical, caring, and welfare staff in community settings.

3. Improving Motivation of Caring and Welfare Staff Working in End-of-Life Care Settings

Career development is a great incentive toward high quality end-of-life care for the elderly, promoting greater job motivation among caregivers [34]. However, in Japan, most career education programs focus primarily on the development of proper caring skills, and very little on motivation maintenance or life career development [34]. Therefore, we organized a series of workshops and lectures for caring or welfare staff in Aichi prefecture which covered the following topics: self-analysis, self-care, leadership, education, etc. We reported elsewhere on the effectiveness of this initiative in enhancing caring or welfare staff's awareness of their professional responsibilities [34].

4. End-of-Life Care Education Program for Community Residents

Death education by participatory learning is needed in the community. Although community death education helps enhance the quality of home end-of-life care, only a few of community death education programs have been reported [35,36]. Therefore, in April 2010, we carried out a 75-minute pilot program targeting middle-aged and elderly residents. The program consists of picture book reading sessions lead by a facilitator, lectures on the dying process and living wills, and group discussions on death or dying. The program was helpful in reducing the participants' fear of death. Our results were published elsewhere [37]. Additionally, we used a leaflet we had previously published (details published elsewhere [38]) concerning living wills as a teaching tool. We developed this leaflet to help physicians provide a standardized explanation of the concept of living wills, as we felt that the wishes of elderly patients and their family were often influenced by the personal views of their own physicians or by the limited information they provided [39]. From 2008 to 2010, the Outreach Palliative care Trial of Integrated regional Model (OPTIM) [40] was set up to educate community residents about palliative care through lecture meetings and role-playing workshops. This education program was instrumental in reducing negative attitudes and feelings toward home palliative care. Thus, the development of educational tools and the implementation of community-based learning opportunities appear helpful in changing the attitude of residents toward death and end-of-life care.

5. Community-Based Inter-Professional Education (IPE)

As stated in the position statement of the Japan Geriatric Society [29], a multidisciplinary approach to the care of dying patients is preferable. In Japan, the public long-term care insurance system promotes the use of multidisciplinary care conferences [41]. Comprehensive geriatric assessment (CGA) is a useful tool for health care providers who offer long-term and palliative care for elderly [42]. In Japan, this assessment tool is widely used in geriatric care settings including hospitals, long-term care facilities, and the community. CGA is a multidimensional, interdisciplinary diagnostic process to determine the medical, psychological and functional capabilities of a frail elderly person leading to the development of a coordinated and integrated plan for treatment and long-term follow up [42]. However, due to a lack of guidelines for the use of CGA as an inter-professional educational tool, education in this area has so far been experience-based. Subsequently, under the scheme of a comprehensive research project on longevity sciences funded by the Ministry of Health, Labor and Welfare, a research team has developed a CGA-based tool for discharge support [43].

Many important issues need to be addressed before a multi-professional network can be successfully launched. One report suggests that subject extraction, IPE, information transmission, and network management are central to the promotion of a multi-professional network [44]. Also, according to the OPTIM report [40], inter-professional networks are strongly based on face-to-face relations. OPTIM held community-based inter-professional conferences to foster face-to-face relations, and reported that most of the participants regarded the initiative as an effective means of strengthening inter-professional networks.

Another source of concern is moral harassment in the workplace, which refers to hostile treatment, verbal or otherwise, from peers or superiors. Moral harassment is an especially important educational topic concerning end-of-life care for the elderly because it hampers the establishment of a solid inter-professional network which is necessary to provide comprehensive, quality care. In an effort to curb this problem, we launched a series of community-based IPE conferences on gerontology from 2001 [16,17]. According to a report issued following a small inter-professional seminar on moral harassment, the best approach for community physicians to adopt is to pay close attention to the opinions and concerns of caring and welfare staff as well as patients. Thus, the findings deriving from IPE seminars or workshops are very useful for the improvement of moral education for medical professions.

CONCLUSION

In this paper, we described the current situation of community-based education concerning palliative care for the elderly in Japan. We also explained the details of community-based education programs concerning palliative care for the elderly, with special focus on community staff education.

REFERENCES

[1] National Institute of Population and Social Security Research. Population Statistics 2011, 01.08.2011, Available from http://www.ipss.go.jp/syoushika/tohkei/Popular/Popular2011.asp?chap=0.

[2] Hirakawa, Y (2012). Palliative Care for the Elderly:A Japanese Perspective, Contemporary and Innovative Practice in Palliative Care, Esther Chang and Amanda Johnson (Ed.), InTech, Available from: http://www.intechopen.com/articles/show/title/palliative-care-for-the-elderly-a-japanese-perspective.

[3] Hirakawa, Y.; Kuzuya, M.and Uemura, K. (2009) Opinion survey of nursing or caring staff at long-term care facilities about end-of-life care provision and staff education. *Archives of Gerontology and Geriatrics, Vol.49*, pp.43-48.

[4] Hirakawa, Y.(2009) End-of-life care at long-term care facilities for the elderly in Japan. *Hallym International Journal of Aging (HIJA)* 11: 1-12.

[5] Iguchi, A. (2001) How the terminal care in the elderly: a position statement from the Japan Geriatric Society started. *Nippon Ronen Igakkai Zasshi, Vol.38*, pp.584-586,(In Japanese).

[6] Japan Geriatric Society(2001). Announcement from The Japan Geriatrics Society Ethics Committee: The Terminal Care of the Elderly-position statement from the Japan Geriatrics Society,01.28.2012 (in Japanese) Available from http://www.jpngeriat-soc.or.jp.

[7] Iijima, S.(2009). The terminal care in the elderly: a position statement from the Japan Geriatric Society and how it will develop. *Geriatric Medicine, Vol.47*.

[8] Ladhani, Z.; Scherpbier, AJ.; and Stevens, FC. (2012) Competencies for undergraduate community-based education for the health professions - A systematic review. *Med. Teach.* 34:733-43.

[9] Okayama, M. and Kajii, E. (2011) Does community-based education increase students' motivation to practice community health care? - a cross sectional study. *BMC Medical Education* 11:19.

[10] Lloyd-Williams, M. and MacLeod, RD. (2004) A systematic review of teaching and learning in palliative care within the medical undergraduate curriculum. *Med. Teach* 26:683-690.

[11] Irwin, SA.; Montross, LP.; Bhat, RG.; Nelesen, RA. and von Gunten, CF. (2011) Psychiatry resident education in palliative care: opportunities, desired training, and outcomes of a targeted educational intervention. *Psychosomatics*, 52:530-536.

[12] Ahmed, NN.and Farnie, M. and Dyer CB. (2011) The effect of geriatric and palliative medicine education on the knowledge and attitudes of internal medicine residents. *J. Am. Geriatr. Soc.*, 59:143-147.

[13] Yacht, AC.; Suglia, SF. and Orlander, JD. (2006) Evaluating an end-of-life curriculum in a medical residency program. *Am. J. Hosp. Palliat. Care*, 23:439-446.

[14] Hirakawa, Y.; Masuda, Y.; Uemura, K.; Kuzuya, M.; Noguchi, M.; Kimiata, T. and Iguchi A.(2005) National survey on the current status of programs to teach end-of-life care to undergraduates of medical and nursing schools in Japan. *Nippon Ronen Igakkai Zasshi, Vol.42*, pp.540-545, (In Japanese).

[15] Sullivan, AM.; Warren, AG.; Lakoma, MD.; Liaw, KR.; Hwang, D. and Block, SD. (2004) End-of-life care in the curriculum: a national study of medical education deans. *Acad. Med.*, 79:760-768.

[16] Hirakawa, Y. and Yasui, H. (2011) Scheme for inter-professional network development in the community. *Nippon Ronen Igakkai Zasshi*,48:713.

[17] Hirakawa, Y.; Kuzuya, M.; Masuda, Y.; Asahi, T. and Iguchi, A. (2007) Seminar "introduction to Gerontology"-Future directions. *Hospice and Home care*,15:201-207.(In Japanese).

[18] Hirakawa, Y.; Kuzuya, M. and Uemura, K. (2009) Opinion survey of nursing or caring staff at long-term care facilities about end-of-life care provision and staff education. *Archives of Gerontology and Geriatrics, Vol.49*, pp.43-48.

[19] Henderson, ML. ; Hanson, LC. and Reynolds, KS. (2003) Improving nursing home care of the dying: a training manual for nursing home staff. *NY: Springer Publishing Company.*

[20] Kortes-Miller, K. ; Habjan, S. ; Kelley, ML. and Fortier, M. (2007) Development of a palliative care education program in rural long-term care facilities. *Journal of palliative care. Vol.23*, pp.154-162.

[21] Arcand, M.; Monette, J.; Monette, M.; Sourial, N.; Fournier, L.; Gore, B. and Bergman, H. (2009) Educating nursing home staff about the progression of dementia and the comfort care option: impact on family satisfaction with end-of-life care. *J. Am. Med. Dir. Assoc.*, 10:50-55.

[22] Parks, SM.; Haines, C. ; Foreman, D.; McKinstry, E. and Maxwell, TL.(2005) Evaluation of an educational program for long-term care nursing assistants. *J. Am. Med. Dir. Assoc.*, 6:61-65.

[23] Hirakawa, Y.; Masuda, Y.; Kuzuya, M.; Iguchi, A. and Uemura, K. (2007) Non-medical palliative care and education to improve end-of-life care at geriatric health services facilities: a nationwide questionnaire survey of chief nurses. *Geriatrics and Gerontology International, Vol7*, pp.266-270.

[24] Hirakawa, Y.; Kuzuya, M. and Uemura, K. (2009) Evaluation of an educational program on end-of-life care for the staff of geriatric health service facilities. *Medical Education Japan*, 40::197-200.

[25] Hirakawa, Y.; Kuzuya, M. ; Kato, T. and Uemura, K. (2009) The effect of death education using picture books on elderly care workers. *Hospice and Home Care*, 17:14-16.

[26] Gagliese, L. and et al. (2012) A brief educational intervention about pain and ageing for older members of the community and health care workers. *The Jounal of Pain*, 13:849-856.

[27] Lunney, JR.; Lynn, J.; Foley, DJ. and Lipson, S. (2003) Guralnik JM. Patterns of functional decline at the end of life. *JAMA*,289:2387-2392.

[28] Hirakawa, Y.; Yasui, H.; Aomatsu, M. and Uemura, K. (2011) Effect of an end-of-life care workshop program for upper-class care staff. *Hospice and Home Care*, (in press), (In Japanese).

[29] Japan Geriatric Society (2012). The Terminal Care of the Elderly- position statement from the Japan Geriatrics Society, 01.28.2012, (in Japanese) Available from http://www.jpngeriat-soc.or.jp.

[30] Kawakita, J. (1967). Idea creation-for creativity development. *Chuokouronsha*. (in Japanese).

[31] Hirakawa, Y. and Uemura, K. (2012) Care staffs perceptions in providing sputum suction, *Nippon Ronen Iggakai Zasshi*, 49:253.

[32] Hirakawa, Y. and Uemura, K. (2012) Construct of sputum suction training system for long-term care facility staff and home helper. *Medical Education Japan,* 43:322.

[33] Nagoya University graduate school of medicine community medicine support center, Available from http://www.med.nagoya-u.ac.jp/edu/msc/about/index.html.
[34] Hirakawa, Y. ; Yasui, H. ; Aomastu, T. ; Yoshida, M. and Uemura,K.(2011) Development of career awareness workshop program for caring staff. *Hospice and Home Care,* 19:33-37.
[35] Matsui, M. (2010) Effectiveness of end-of-life education among community-dwelling older adults. *Nursing Ethics, Vol.17*, pp.363-372.
[36] Hirakawa, Y. ; Masuda,Y. ; Kuzuya, M. ; Iguchi,A. and Uemura, K. (2006b) [Attitude of middleaged healthy elderly toward location of end-of-life care and living will. *Hospice and Home Care, Vol.14*, pp.201-205, (In Japanese).
[37] Hirakawa, Y. and Uemura, K. (2012) Educational program about end of life for older people of the community and caring staff. *Hospice and Home care*,20:63-66.(In Japanese).
[38] Hirakawa, Y. ; Uemura, K. ; Kato, T. and Kuzuya, M. (2008) Development of living will leaflet for patient and family- trial at University hospital department of geriatrics. *Hospice and Home care*,16:209-212.
[39] Hirakawa, Y. ; Masuda, Y. ; Kuzuya, M. ; Iguchi, A. and Uemura, K. (2007) [Decision-making factors regarding resuscitate and hospitalize orders by families of elderly persons on admission to a Japanese long-term care hospital]. *Nippon Ronen Igakkai Zasshi, Vol.44*, pp.497-502, (In Japanese).
[40] Morita, T. ; Miyashita, M. ; Yamagishi, A. ; Akizuki, N. ; Kizawa, Y. ; Shirahige, Y. ; Akiyama, M. ; Hirai, K. ; Matoba, M. ; Yamada, M. ; Matsumoto, T. ; Yamaguchi, T. and Eguchi, K.(2012) A region-based palliative care intervention trial using the mixed-method approach: Japan OPTIM study. *BMC Palliat Care*, 11;11:2.
[41] Hara, K. (2011) [Multidisciplinary approaches for the elderly at the end-of-life stage]. *Nippon Ronen Igakkai Zasshi, Vol.48*, pp.257-259, (in Japanese).
[42] Ellis, G. ; Whitehead, MA. ; O'Neill, D. ; Langhorne, P. and Robinson, D. (2011) Comprehensive geriatric assessment for older adults admitted to hospital. *Cochrane Database of Systematic Reviews*, 6;7:CD006211.
[43] Hirakawa, Y.; Uemura, K. and Kuzuya, M. (2010) Comprehensive geriatric assessment (CGA)-based tool for discharge support. *Nippon Ronen Igakkai Zasshi, Vol.47*,pp.162, (In Japanese).
[44] Hirakawa, Y. and Yasui, H. (2011) Scheme for inter-professional network development in the community. [Article in Japanese]. *Nippon Ronen Igakkai Zasshi*, 48:713.
[45] Hirakawa, Y. ; Kuzuya, M. and Uemura, K. (2012) Skills and aptitude required for physician who specializes in the care of older adults, *Nippon Ronen Iggakai Zasshi*,49:375.
[46] Hirakawa, Y. (2011) Required ability and morality physicians working at rural hospitals, *Medical Education Japan*,42:158.

In: Caregivers: Challenges, Practices and Cultural Influences
Editors: Adrianna Thurgood and Kasha Schuldt

ISBN: 978-1-62618-030-7
© 2013 Nova Science Publishers, Inc.

Chapter 12

DOES CAREGIVER PERCEPTION REFLECT ORAL HEALTH IN CEREBRAL PALSY CHILDREN?

Renata Oliveira Guaré[*],
Daniel Cividanis Gomes Nogueira Fernandes
and Maria Teresa Botti Rodrigues Santos
[1]The Discipline of Dentistry, Persons with Disabilities Division,
Universidade Cruzeiro do Sul, Brazil

ABSTRACT

Purpose: This study aimed to evaluate the quality of life of children with CP concerning oral health/dental caries and their caregivers' perception. *Methods:* Forty-three children with CP, aged 1-15 years-old (8.7 ±3.7) were evaluated regarding dental caries experience (DMF Index; WHO 1997) and grouped as Group I (GI, n=20; carie-free; DMFT=0), and Group II (GII, n=23; with caries, DMFT≥1). Caregivers completed the questionnaire Early Childhood Oral Health Impact Scale (B_ECOHIS) composed of 13 questions with frequency scores ranging from 0 to 4, such that the higher the score, the greater the impact on the child, the family and the overall value. Comparison between the groups was performed by the Fisher Exact and Mann-Whitney tests, with the significance level set at 5%. *Results:* Significant differences were observed between the group impact scores for child (GI 0.95 ±1.67 and GII 3.00 ±3.93, p=0.044), family (GI 0.05 ±0.22 and GII 1.13 ± 1.84, p=0.007) and overall (GI 1.00 ±1.78 and GII 4.14 ±4.82, p=0.004), with higher values for Group II. *Conclusion:* Caregiver perception does not reflect the real condition of the child's oral health and caries increase the impact and diminish the quality of life in children with CP.

Keywords: Cerebral palsy, quality of life, oral health

---

[*] Adress for correspondence: Renata de Oliveira Guaré. Rua Jorge Tibiriçá, no74, apto 113. CEP:04126-000 São Paulo (SP), Brazil. e-mail:renataguare@uol.com.br.

INTRODUCTION

Cerebral palsy (CP) describes a group of movement and posture development disorders, which are attributed to nonprogressive disturbances that occur in the developing fetal or infant brain that cause activity limitation and may be accompanied by disturbances of sensation, cognition, communication and seizure disorders [1]. CP is the most common cause of severe physical disability in childhood [2], with an estimated prevalence of 2.4 per 1000 children [3]. The severity of CP motor impairment and presence of associated conditions lead to reduced self-cleaning function of the oral cavity identified as a negative factor for oral health [4]. The consumption of a soft diet, rich in carbohydrates, mastication by pressure at the back of the tongue and palate, incoordination of the muscles of mastication, food remaining in the oral cavity and decreased salivary flow, are some of the factors responsible for the increased prevalence of dental caries in individuals with CP. [5,6,7,8] Moreover, the fact that an expressive part of caregivers show difficulties in performing proper oral hygiene on CP individuals and that most of these individuals are fed on a semi-solid diet, means the dental biofilm tends to accumulate and becomes a caries risk factor for these individuals [9]. Maintaining the oral health of these individuals requires systematic hygiene practices, demanding supervision or even the realization of their oral hygiene by the caregivers. The child's development demands the participation, involvement and support of the family, which, when well structured, will positively contribute to the child's quality of life. [10] However, when CP individuals are considered, this process of participation, involvement and support is not restricted to the development period. The task of taking care of a child with complex disabilities at home might be somewhat daunting for caregivers [11, 12] and may sometimes reflect in the way these individuals are cared for.[13] Since dental caries are still widespread in CP children, it is important to recognize the caregiver perception regarding the real condition of the oral health of children with CP. Thus, the aim of this study was to evaluate the quality of life of children with CP in relation to oral health/dental caries and their caregivers' perception.

METHODS

This study was approved by the Ethics Committee on Human Research of the Cruzeiro do Sul University under protocol number 136/2009. After being informed of the aim of the investigation, written informed consent for participation and publication was obtained from the adult responsible for each child who agreed to participate in this study.

Participants

Ninety-six noninstitutionalized individuals with a medical diagnosis of CP attending the Rehabilitation Center Lar Escola São Francisco, São Paulo, Brazil, were invited to participate in this study; 43 of these responded to the invitation. The inclusion criteria were individuals with a clinical medical diagnosis of cerebral palsy, aged 1-15 years-old, of either sex, whose parents/caregivers provided informed consent. Patient medical records were reviewed for demographic and clinical data, including sex, age and type of movement disorder (spasticity, dyskinesia or ataxia), clinical patterns of involvement among the spastic individuals (quadriplegia, diplegia, hemiplegia) and Gross Motor Function Classification System: GMFCS level I indicates walking without restrictions with limitations in more advanced gross motor skills; II indicates walking without assistive devices with limitations walking outdoors and in the community; III indicates walking with assistive mobility devices with limitations walking outdoors and in the community; IV indicates self-mobility with limitations, the patient is transported or uses a power mobility outdoors and in the community; level V indicates that self-mobility is severely limited even with assistive technology.

Questionnaire

Caregivers responded to the Brazilian version of the Early Childhood Oral Health Impact Scale (B_ECOHIS) [14] which is reliable and valid for assessing the impact of oral disorders on the quality of life of preschool children. [15] It consists of 13 issues with frequency scores ranging from 0 to 4, such that the higher the score, the greater the impact on the child, the family and the overall value. To our knowledge, no published studies have used a questionnaire specific to oral health-related quality of life in a study involving children with CP. Thus a validated questionnaire for preschool children was used requiring the caregiver to answer, since not all the CP children were able to answer the questions. Du and Yiu [16] also used the ECOHIS questionnaire to evaluate CP individuals.

Dental Examination

For dental evaluation, the teeth were dried with compresses air and examined by a single calibrated examiner (Kappa = 0.87) under artificial light. Dental caries experience was recorded as decayed, missing and filled teeth using the DMF-T index. [17] The CP children were divided into two groups: Group I, caries-free (DMFT = 0), and Group II, with caries (DMFT ≥ 1).

Statistical Analyses

All data were presented as mean and standard deviation (±SD). Comparison between the groups was performed by the Fisher Exact and Mann-Whitney tests, with the significance level set at 5%.

RESULTS

In this study, 43 children aged between 1 and 15 years-old (8.7 ± 3.7) were evaluated, 24 (55.8%) males and 19 (44.2%) females. The CP children were divided into two groups:

Group I (n=20), and Group II (n=23). The descriptive characteristics of the individuals with CP are presented in Table 1.

Table 1. Distribution of CP individuals according to movement disorder, clinical pattern and GMFCS (I-V)

Movement Disorder	Clinical Pattern	I	II	GMFCS III	IV	V
Spastic	Quadri-plegia	0 (0%)	0 (0%)	0 (0%)	0 (0%)	14 (32.7%)
	Diplegia	0 (0%)	0 (0%)	2 (4.6%)	17 (39.7%)	3 (6.9%)
Dyskinetic		0 (0%)	0 (0%)	0 (0%)	2 (4.6%)	2 (4.6%)
Ataxic		0 (0%)	1 (2.3%)	1 (2.3%)	1 (2.3%)	0 (0%)
Total		0 (0%)	1 (2.3%)	3 (6.9%)	20 (46.6%)	19 (44.2%)

The B-ECOHIS responses of children's caregivers showed that that caregiver perception concerning the CP child's oral health is compromised (Table 2). The three impact section values of the B-ECOHIS differed significantly between the groups in relation to dental caries, with Group II (with caries) presenting the highest scores, suggesting that that caries affects the quality of life of children with CP. (Table 3).

In order to elucidate caregiver perception concerning the oral health of children with CP, this study was conducted to obtain relevant information regarding the quality of life related to oral health in children with CP.

The distribution of children with CP among the GMFCS classifications revealed that 72.4% of our sample were nonambulant (GMFCS IV and V), characterizing a sample from a high complexity rehabilitation center. These patients require greater personal care and are totally dependent on their caregivers. [18]

The Brazilian version of B_ECOHIS [14] evaluates the impact of oral disease on quality of life of preschool children. [15] Since there is no specific questionnaire to assess caregiver perception in relation to the oral health of children with CP, in this study, the B_ECOHIS was answered by the caregivers.

It should be noted that for these caregivers, the high degree of severity of the children and greater demand for care represent a negative impact on the way these children are cared for [19].

Analysis of the results of this study indicate that caregiver perception does not represent the real oral health status of the CP child, since in all 13 questions of the B_ECOHIS, the answer "never" predominated, ranging from 67.5% to 97.7%, even for CP children with caries. Assessment of the caregivers' perception concerning the quality of life of children with CP showed that the severity of the child's disability required other rehabilitation approaches, resulting in diminished perception of the importance of the health of the oral cavity.

Oral problems reported in individuals with CP that have been described in the literature include: reduced intraoral self-cleaning due to the presence of abnormal pathological reflexes, such as biting [20]; lack of understanding concerning the importance of oral hygiene, possibly due to mental deficit; and greater difficulty in opening and maintaining the mouth open for cleaning. [21,22]

Table 2. B-ECOHIS responses of children's caregivers (n=43)

Impacts	Never	Hardly ever	Occasionally	Often	Very Often
Child impacts, n (%)					
How often has your child had pain in the teeth, mouth or jaws	29 (67.5%)	4 (9.3%)	9 (20.9%)	-	1 (2.3%)
How often has your child. because of dental problems or dental treatment? had difficult drinking hot or cold beverages	33 (76.8%)	3 (7.0%)	5 (11.6%)	1 (2.3%)	1 (2.3%)
had difficult eating some foods	36 (83.7%)	2 (4.7%)	5 (11.6%)	-	-
had difficult pronouncing any words	40 (93.0%)	-	2 (4.7%)	-	1 (2.3%)
missed preschool, daycare or school	42 (97.7%)	1 (2.3%)	-	-	-
had trouble sleeping	40 (93.0%)	1 (2.3%)	2 (4.7%)	-	-
been irritable or frustrated	37 (86.0%)	2 (4.7%)	4 (9.3%)	-	-
avoided smiling or laughing	42 (97.7%)	-	1 (2.3%)	-	-
avoided talking	41 (95.3%)	-	2 (4.7%)	-	-
Family impacts, n (%)					
How often have you or another family member because of your child's dental problems or dental treatment? been upset	36 (83.7%)	1 (2.3%)	4 (9.3%)	-	2 (4.7%)
felt guilty	41 (95.4%)	1 (2.3%)	-	1 (2.3%)	-
taken time off from work	42 (97.7%)	1 (2.3%)	-	-	-
How often has your child had dental problems or dental treatment that had a financial impact on your family?	41 (95.4%)	-	1 (2.3%)	1 (2.3%)	-

Table 3. Comparison of the three impact sections of the B-ECOHIS for children from Group I (DMFT = 0) and Group II (DMFT ≥ 1)

Impact section	Group I (n=20)	Group II (n=23)	P value
Child	0.95 ± 1.67	3.00 ± 3.93	0.044*
Family	0.05 ± 0.22	1.13 ± 1.84	0.007*
Overall	1.00 ± 1.78	4.13 ± 4.82	0.004*

DMFT: Decay, Missing, Filled Tooth Index; (*) Statistical significance, $P < 0.05$ by the *Mann-Whitney* test.

In some cases, the involvement of upper limbs that hinder the movement of brushing facilitates the accumulation of biofilm [6], while the presence of spasticity in masticatory muscles is an aggravating factor for the onset of oral abnormalities, leading to the increased risk of dental caries observed in this study.

In this study, more than half of the sample presented dental caries. Worse dental health was described in CP children compared with normal children of the corresponding age group for primary permanent dentitions. [8] Although the caregivers denied oral problems, important expression of impact was observed for all three impact sections of the B-ECOHIS for children with and without dental caries. This finding clearly suggests that the caregivers do not correlate oral health with general health.

CP individuals represent a high-risk group for caries, our goal as health professionals should be to motivate caregivers to modify this high caries experience; however, this is a difficult task, since caregivers themselves exhibit a low quality of life, which is reflected in the care dispensed to CP individuals. Healthcare professionals should be aware of the important relationship between the individual with disability, the caregiver and the professional team.

The caregiver's role in the medical treatment of the CP individual is of great importance and their participation in establishing early preventive measures and adequate maintenance for this population is essential. [9].

Children with special needs require continuous care of a complex nature, constituting a challenge for caregivers. Enhancing the quality of life of mothers, fathers and other caregivers, the rehabilitation team can set up strategies, not only for the purpose of improving well-being, but can directly influence the life of children with CP.

Conclusion

Caregiver perception does not represent the real condition of the child's oral health and dental caries increase the impact and diminish the quality of life of children with CP.

Acknowledgments

This study was supported by AUX-PE-PROSUP-CAPE grants 2198/2010.

References

[1] Bax, M, Goldstein, M, Rosenbaum, P, Leviton, A, Paneth, N, Dan, B, Jacobsson, B and Damiano D (2005). Executive Committee for the Definition of Cerebral Palsy. Proposed definition and classification of cerebral palsy. *Developmental Medicine and Child Neurology*, 47, 571-576.

[2] Kuban, KC and Leviton, A. Cerebral palsy (1994). The New England *Journal of Medicine*, 330, 188-195.

[3]   Hirtz, D, Thurman, DJ, Gwinn-Hardy, K, Mohamed, M, Chaudhuri, AR and Zalutsky R (2007). How common are the "common" neurologic disorders? *Neurology*, 68, 326-337.

[4]   Dos Santos, MT and Nogueira, ML (2005). Infantile reflexes and their effects on dental caries and oral hygiene in cerebral palsy individuals. *Journal of Oral Rehabilitation*, 32, 880-885.

[5]   Dos Santos, MT, Masiero, D and Simionato, MR (2002). Risk factors for dental caries in children with cerebral palsy. *Spec Care Dentist*, 22, 103-107.

[6]   Rodrigues dos Santos, MT, Masiero, D, Novo, NF and Simionato, MR (2003). Oral conditions in children with cerebral palsy. *Journal of Dentistry for Children Chicago*, 70, 40-46.

[7]   Guaré, RO and Ciamponi, A (2003). Dental caries prevalence in the primary dentition of cerebral palsied children. *The Journal of Clinical Pediatric Dentistry*, 27, 287-292.

[8]   De Camargo, MA and Antunes, JL (2007). Untreated dental caries in children with cerebral palsy in the Brazilian context. *Int. J. Paediatr. Dent*, 18, 131-138.

[9]   Rodrigues dos Santos, MTB, Bianccardi, M, Celiberti, P and Guaré, RO (2009). Dental caries in cerebral palsied individuals and their caregivers' quality of life. *Child: Care, Health and Development*, 35, 475–481.

[10] Pal, DK (1996). Quality of life assessment in children: a review of conceptual and methodological issues in multidimensional health status measures. *Journal of Epidemiology Community Health*, 50, 391–396.

[11] Manuel, J, Naughton, MJ, Balkrishnan, R, Smith, BP and Koman, A (2003). Stress and adaptation in mothers of children with cerebral palsy. *Journal of Pediatric Psychology*, 28, 297–301.

[12] Raina, P, O'Donnell, M, Rosenbaum, P, Brehaut, J, Walter, SD, Russel, D, Swinton, M, Zhu, B and Wood, E (2005). The health and well-being of caregivers of children with cerebral palsy. *Pediatrics*, 115, 626–636.

[13] Benedict, MI, Wulff, LM and White, RB (1992). Current parental stress in maltreating and nonmaltreating families of children with multiple disabilities. *Child Abuse and Neglect*, 16, 155–163.

[14] Tesch, FC, Oliveira, BH and Leão, A (2008). Semantic equivalence of the Brazilian version of the Early Childhood Oral Health Impact Scale. Cad Saude Publica, 24, 1897-1909.

[15] Scarpelli, AC, Oliveira, BH, Tesch, FC, Leão, AT, Pordeus, IA and Paiva, SM (2011). Psychometric properties of the Brazilian version of the Early Childhood Oral Health Impact Scale (B-ECOHIS). *BMC Oral Health,* 11,19.

[16] Du, RY, McGrath, C, Yiu, CK and King, NM (2010). Health- and oral health-related quality of life among preschool children with cerebral palsy. *Qual Life Res*, 19, 1367-1371.

[17] World Health Organization (1997). WHOQOL – measuring quality of life. The World Health Organization quality of life instruments. Geneva: World Health Organization.

[18] Palisano, RJ, Kang, LJ, Chiarello, LA, Orlin, M, Oeffinger, D and Maggs, J (2009). Social and community participation of children and youth with cerebral palsy is associated with age and gross motor function classification. *Phys. Ther*, 89, 1304-1314.

[19] Santos, MT, Biancardi, M, Guaré, RO and Jardim, MD (2010). Caries prevalence in patients with cerebral palsy and the burden of caring for them. *Spec. Care Dentist*, 30, 206-210.

[20] Santos, MT, Manzano, FS, Ferreira, MC and Masiero, D (2005). Development of a Novel Oral-Facial Motor Function Assessment Scale for Children with Cerebral Palsy. *J. Dent. Child* (Chic), 72, 113-118.
[21] Dos Santos, MT and De Oliveira, LM (2004). Use of cryotherapy to enhance mouth opening in patients with cerebral palsy. *Spec. Care Dentist*, 24, 232-234.
[22] Manzano, FS, Granero, LM, Masiero, D and Dos Santos, MT (2004). Treatment of muscle spasticity in patients with cerebral palsy using BTX-A: a pilot study. *Spec. Care Dentist*, 24, 235-239.

In: Caregivers: Challenges, Practices and Cultural Influences ISBN: 978-1-62618-030-7
Editors: Adrianna Thurgood and Kasha Schuldt   © 2013 Nova Science Publishers, Inc.

Chapter 13

ROLE OF ASSISTIVE TECHNOLOGIES FOR PERSON-CENTERED DEMENTIA CARE: AN EXPLORATORY CASE STUDY IN JAPAN

Taro Sugihara* and Tsutomu Fujinami
School of Knowledge Science,
Japan Advanced Institute of Science and Technology, Japan

Abstract

This article discusses potential role of assistive technologies for dementia care. Despite urgent needs for person-centered care, it is difficult for care houses in Japan to achieve it because of a lack of resources and fatigue caused by the shortage of funds and caregivers. Assistive technologies for dementia care are fruitful in helping care work. However, little attention has been focused on the influence of these technologies on person-centered care. To investigate effects of assistive technologies on the care house, we installed a video monitoring system for caregivers in three homes and observed the effects of applying the system to caregiving by interviews and video observations. As results, the video monitoring system enabled caregivers to optimize their work and helped them concentrate on their tasks at hand, reducing both mental and physical stresses. Finally, we established the concept of a triage support environment, which can augment dementia care.

Keywords: person-centered dementia care, assistive technologies, system development and deployment

AMS Subject Classification: 53D, 37C, 65P

1. Introduction

According to a United Nations report [1], many countries are expected to become gsuper-agedh societies by 2050, when more than 20% of the world population will be 65 years or older. As the probability of becoming cognitively impaired increases with age, the number

---
*E-mail address: sugihara@jaist.ac.jp

of people developing dementia will also increase. A report by the WHO [2] indicates that 35.6 million people worldwide currently suffer from dementia, and this number will double by 2030 and more than triple by 2050.

Elderly persons with dementia (PWD) require special attention because they are vulnerable to unexpected events and changes in their environment and become uncomfortable when they do not recognize their surroundings. Thus, caregivers need to create a peaceful environment. They need to be well trained and experienced and need to pay particular attention to the needs of PWD. Person-centered care [3, 4] is an approach to dementia care whereby the person cared for is central; through observation and communication, the caregiver becomes keenly aware of the needs of the patients and the reasons for their actions. Then, the caregiver can assist that person in accomplishing his or her goal. PWD exhibit unpredictable behavior, such as aimless wandering and agitation. The physical security of a person with dementia is a top priority for caregivers.

Most caregiver tasks are predictable. The daily activities of PWD do not vary significantly. Routinely, caregivers assist residents in a care facility with their meals and personal hygiene. However, some tasks are hard to anticipate and need to be performed unpredictably and urgently. For example, caregivers may have to deal with a resident who insists on going to his/her previous home in the evening and persists in that desire no matter how strongly caregivers try to persuade them to stay. This sort of task places an extra burden on caregivers because of its unpredictability. It may also become a cause of stress because they cannot estimate the duration of residents' unexpected behaviors. Caregivers need to coordinate with each other to deal with these types of incidents. For example, more than one caregiver may have to attend to a resident when he or she insists on leaving the care home.

A normal house is the best place for those with dementia to live their lives peacefully. However, converting a normal house into a care home inevitably increases the risk of some residents being involved in accidents, which may result in injuries, when they are unattended by caregivers. We place the highest value on residents' privacy, and our approach involves a balance between privacy and safety. To ensure safety, we install a video-monitoring system to solve the problem of blind spots, which are locations that are difficult to observe.

The use of video-monitoring systems in care homes for PWD is not particularly innovative. Several monitoring systems have been developed [5, 6, 7, 8, 9, 10, 11, 12]. In this study, we emphasize the system's usage and effects on caregivers to clarifying the utility of such monitoring systems and to explore the design of a better system. Thus far, little attention has been focused on the augmentation of caregivers' ability to administer care by information and communication technologies; most efforts have focused solely on the systems. In this study, we focus on caregivers rather than particular technologies or systems.

Monitoring systems not only help caregivers care for PWD but also reduce the physical and mental stress associated with caregiving. If we respect the concept of personhood, as advocated by Kitwood and Bredin in their pioneering studies [3, 4], we must equally consider both the patient and caregiver. The basic human rights of both caregivers and PWD must be observed.

This study aims to increase the utility of monitoring systems for caregivers. In our field study, we installed video-monitoring systems into three care homes and qualitatively analyzed the systems' effects on caregivers [13, 14]. In addition to a video observation of their caregiving, we conducted a series of interviews with 16 caregivers and 3 managers. Hereafter, we refer to care homes as group homes according to the custom in Japan.

2. Challenges and Difficulties for Person-Centered Dementia Care in Japan

2.1. Dementia and Person-Centered Care

Dementia is a broad term referring to a decline in cognitive ability that interferes with daily life and activities [15]. The majority of people with dementia have Alzheimer's disease (60–80% of PWD) and vascular dementia [16]. Therefore, this study mainly focuses on these types of dementia.

The cognitive ability of PWD is predominantly impaired in two ways: memory and higher brain function. If a person's memory is impaired, he or she has difficulty remembering recent events, not uncommon ones, but recent as a few hours past. Such a person also has difficulty in recognizing a consequence of his or her situation. In other words, such a person can recognize what he or she is seeing, but cannot understand what it means. For example, such persons know that they have to wash their hands after going to the lavatory, but do not understand the relationship between opening the tap and running water.

The ill-formed behavior described above results from difficulty with memory and inference. This sort of behavior directly stems from the disability and can be solely explained by referring to it. Such collective behaviors are known as the core symptoms of dementia.

The complex behavior of PWD is attributed to the influence of their environments and personal histories. Wandering around the residence is a typical symptom; to caregivers and family members, this may appear to be aimless wandering. Such behavior may not be persistent; that is, PWD may not constantly wander. Such types of ill-formed behavior are called behavioral and psychological symptoms of dementia (BPSD).

Person-centered care [3, 4] is an approach to dementia care whereby the person cared for is central; the caregiver keenly observes and communicates with the patient to determine the type of tasks and the reasons for which he or she wants to perform them. The caregiver can then help them accomplish their goal. The core idea of person-centered care is to respect gpersonhood,h i.e., to understand the individual needs, considering his or her motivation and background. Person-centered care is most prevalent and is regarded by many caregivers as the most important approach to dementia care because it treats PWD in relation to others, especially to caregivers.

2.2. Shortage of Funds and Caregivers

In this study, we discuss the issues associated with financial difficulties in the field of caregiving in the context of Japan, which is one of the most advanced countries in terms of services for the aging.

Increased demand for care housing has resulted in greater demands on caregivers. However, financial constraints make it difficult to employ more caregivers. Figure 1 shows that between 2004 and 2009, the budget for elderly benefits has been constant–6,000-7,000 billion yen per year. The ratio of benefits for the elderly relative to social insurance has also remained constant at approximately 70%. The budget for other benefits, including medical care and pensions, is continuously rising, with a one trillion yen increase between 2004 and 2009. The graph indicates that there is no room for the government to spend more money to increase the number of caregivers.

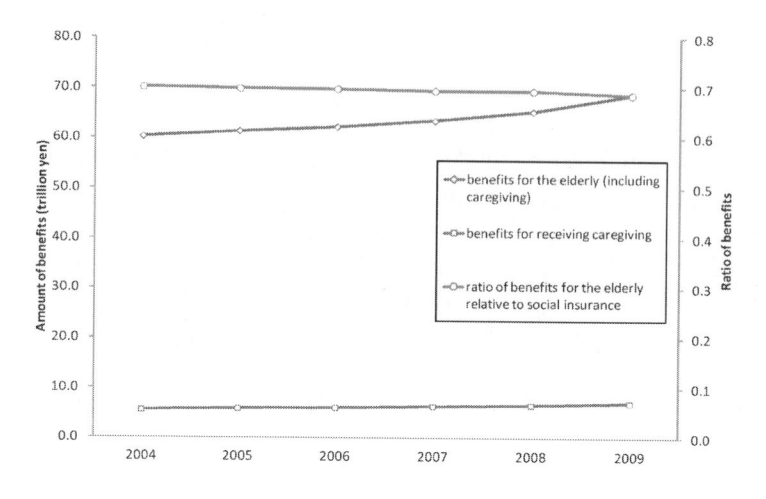

Figure 1. Expenses for care [17].

Since the number of care institutions increases and the budget to employ caregivers does not, the demand for caregivers naturally increases. Figure 2 shows that 20% of care workers leave their jobs every year and almost three quarters of them do so within three years of commencing work at a care institution [18, 19, 20, 21, 22, 23]. This trend shows the difficulty in recruiting new workers for these jobs. It is also difficult for care institutions to consistently provide high-quality caregiving services because many workers quit soon after they have acquired a certain amount of experience, and inexperienced newcomers make up a significant percentage of the workforce.

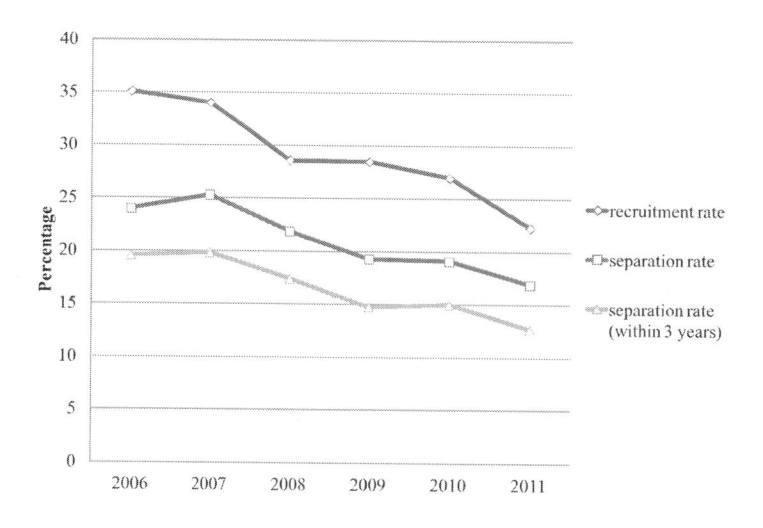

Figure 2. Trends in caregivers' employment [18, 19, 20, 21, 22, 23].

To solve these problems, we need to make caregiving more efficient and to provide caregivers with systematic ways to acquire and improve their skills. Therefore, we believe it is preferable for organizations, rather than families or individuals, to provide caregiving services. Systematic care provided by professionals in organizations should benefit the elderly with dementia. Organizations can provide more efficient caregiving, counterbalancing the shortage of caregivers and funds.

2.3. What are the Challenges and the Difficulties?

To adequately achieve person-centered care, a group home needs to employ a sufficient number of caregivers, especially skilled ones. However, it is difficult to hire caregivers in Japan because of the shortage of funds, as described in the previous section. According to the latest report on labor condition [23], of 53.1% ($n = 4,675$) of informants who answered a question about staffing levels indicated that there were no sufficient caregivers in their institutions. When questioned about the availability of quality caregivers, 50.4% informants ($n = 7,070$) answered that it is difficult to employ quality caregivers, and 49.8% informants ($n = 7,070$) pointed out that managers cannot pay employees a salary that is sufficient to retain them in the workforce because of inadequate government subsidies.

Caregiving is high-level knowledge work; it heavily depends on contexts, such as the individual person with dementia, the type of care work, the equipment used, and the relationships among PWD and their caregivers. Person-centered care is extremely demanding. To effectively implement person-centered care, caregivers must focus on everything that occurs in the facility. To fulfill the responsibilities associated with respecting personhood, caregivers must carefully observe their patients, and based on training and experience, they must try to discern the patients' needs and react appropriately. Caregivers accommodate various BPSDs to realize person-centered care.

In addition, often caregivers also encounter ethical dilemmas in various situations. Typically, these situations involve having to prioritize competing demands for their assistance. For instance, a caregiver who is helping a patient go to the lavatory will hear a sensor-detected alarm, which is installed in a room occupied by a person with severe dementia, and has to decide whether to respond to the alarm. These types of dilemmas frequently occur throughout the day and are extremely stressful. As described by Kahn et al., this type of work stress is known as role stress [24]. Role stress, especially role ambiguity and role conflict, is a well-known predictor of burnout [25].In healthcare settings, several studies show that role ambiguity and role conflict are causally related to emotional exhaustion (*e.g.* [26, 27, 28]).

If caregivers have adequate knowledge and skill, they can learn to cope with the role stress that results from the various dilemmas they face. However, novices cannot cope with them. While managers may recognize this problem, because of limited budgets, they are unable to provide sufficient caregivers to alleviate the situation. In addition, individual group homes are continually obliged to train new employees because of the high separation rate, as shown in Figure 2.

3. Assistive Technologies for Dementia Care

In this section, we focus on the various technologies that are currently available for developing assistive technologies for dementia care.

Technologies for assisting PWD and their caregivers are classified into five groups: screening, memory aid, monitoring health or safety, information sharing and tele-care, and communication support and therapy.

Screening technology enables the elderly to become aware of symptoms that may indicate the onset of cognitive impairment. It is intended for the elderly in general, not specifically for PWD. Typically, a person's cognitive ability is evaluated by various cognitive impairment-screening techniques or a simple exercise [29, 30, 31].

Memory aid includes a number of systems that help PWD in remembering things they experience daily. The intended user is one whose condition is mild and relatively stable. This technology can be employed in a wide range of places, including at home and in institutions. Usually, it includes aids for decision making and planning. This technology targets both fixed dementia [32] and the initial phase of progressive dementia, such as mild cognitive impairment [33, 34].

Health and safety monitoring technologies aim to keep the elderly healthy and to identify when their safety is at risk. They are most effective for monitoring people who tend to leave a group home without being noticed. The devices consist of various sensors, such as GPS-enabled mobile phones. Several monitoring systems have been developed to ensure the safety of PWD. Such systems focus on preventing residents from performing risky actions, such as wandering [6, 8, 9, 10]. A smart home with a sensor network enables caregivers to monitor the position of residents. It can also help them to identify the risks associated with residents' unusual behaviors, such as wandering and agitation [5, 7, 11, 12].

Information-sharing technologies include websites from which caregivers can obtain specialized knowledge about dementia and required care. Other types of websites specialize in providing caregivers with information on services available from various organizations. Research on information-sharing technologies includes investigation methods for seeking social support, such as studies that focus on accessibility [35, 36].

Services related to telecare involve persons who intervene on behalf of PWD or caregivers to improve the quality of care. Unlike information sharing, telecare services require professionals from the fields of caregiving and medicine. An integrated computer-telephone system is implemented to fortify social support for caregivers [37, 38, 39].

Some researchers employ audio-visual systems to stimulate PWD to help them recall past events or friends. This can include reminiscence sessions during which a facilitator encourages the elderly to recall past events and to understand and accept their behavior's consequences [40, 41, 42].

Although such assistive technologies are fruitful in helping care work, little attention has been focused on the influence of these technologies on person-centered care. When a system is implemented, it is highly probable that the impact on person-centered care will be significant.

4. Case Study

4.1. Overview

Table 1. Overview of this study

		GH-A	GH-B	GH-C
Configuration		renovated		purpose-designed and newly established
Number of residents		9	6	9
Total caregivers		9	5	8
Number of informants		6	5	5
Caregivers in daytime		2 or 3	2	2 or 3
Caregivers in nighttime		1	1	1
Residential areas		first and second floor	first floor	first floor
Start of operation		December 2006	January 2005	March 2008
Time of interview	before	—	—	November and December 2007
	after		June 2007	May 2008
Time of video observation	before	—	—	March 2008
	after	—	—	December 2008

The installed monitoring systems were slightly different in each of the three group homes (Table 1). Hereafter, the three homes will be referred to as GH-A, -B, and -C. The system installed in GH-A permitted video recording, and its devices were wired. The systems installed in GH-B and GH-C used wireless devices and did not permit video recording. In this section, we focus on the system deployed in GH-C.

4.2. Case Study of a Video Monitoring System

4.2.1. Research Design

Group Home. The notion of a group home has been imported to Japan from northern Europe, from countries such as Sweden. A typical group home in Japan accommodates 9 residents who are cared for by 2-3 caregivers. The primary characteristic of a group home is its small size, making residents feel as though they are residing in a household similar to their previous home.

From an architectural standpoint, group homes in Japan are categorized into two types. One type is converted from an old house that was built for a family, not originally intended to be used as a care home. This type of home tends to have many blind spots. The other type is a purpose-built home to accommodate the elderly with dementia. This type of home is built to eliminate as many blind spots as possible, thereby reducing safety concerns.

Video Monitoring System and Its Deployment. We designed the system to be as simple as possible because the caregivers in GH-C were not familiar with computers. The system consisted of four wireless cameras, a portable monitor, and a laptop PC functioning as server. Visual data from the cameras were collected on the server and were displayed on a Web browser. A down-scan converter was employed to transfer the information displayed on the Web browser to a portable monitor. Possible malfunctions due to mishandling by the

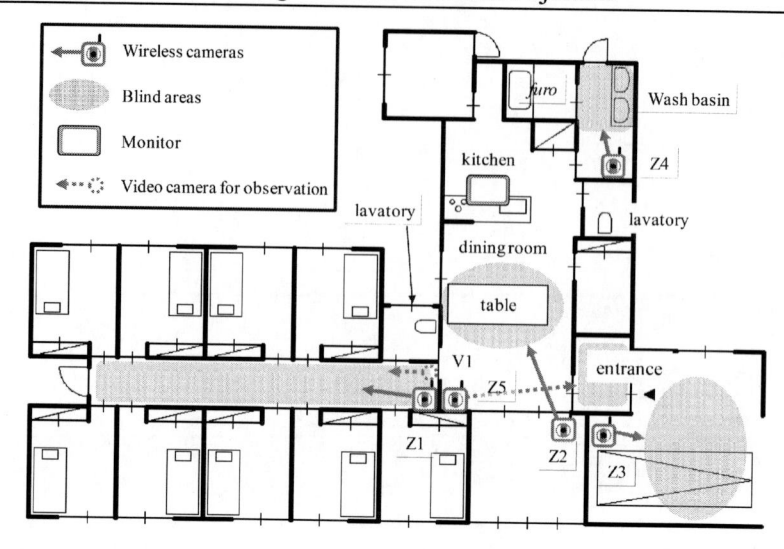

Figure 3. The plan of GH-C and arrangement for cameras and a monitor.

caregivers or residents were minimized because it was impossible for them to operate the system through the monitor. The cameras and monitor were placed as shown in Figure 3.

Before the installation, a preliminary investigation was carried out to identify both blind spots in the group home and system's requirements. The manager and caregivers were concerned about the invasion of privacy and were especially concerned about avoiding any unwanted effects that might be caused by video recording. Consequently, we gave preserving residents' privacy the highest priority, and as a result, we decided to set the cameras in common spaces only, such as the entrance hall, entrance hall corridor, and living room. These locations are denoted as Z1 to Z5 in Figure 3. Furthermore, we decided not to include any video-recording functionality in the system. Through our discussion with the manager of GH-C, we determined that Z1-Z5 locations were often difficult to observe.

Interview. A series of semi-structured interviews was carried out before and after the system had been installed in GH-C. Five caregivers and two managers were interviewed; they were questioned about their opinions of the system and the aspects that they regarded as the most valuable in terms of dementia care. Specifically, they were asked the following questions: Q1: What is the burden of dementia care? (before)
Q2: What is/are the most demanding task(s) in dementia care? (before)
Q3: How do you use the video-monitoring system? (after)
Q4: What do you think of the system? (after)
Q5: How has the system affected your work stress? (after)

Questions Q3-Q5 were focused on the change from the conventional situation and were compared with the responses to Q1 and Q2.

At full capacity, each group home accommodates 9 residents, and as required by law, the number of caregivers is usually two or three. All the interviews were recorded with an digital voice recorder and were fully transcribed for ease of reference. A continual comparison process was used to analyze the transcriptions. The transcriptions were repeatedly read to identify commonalities and differences among the interview data. Similar data were classified into a category. In this process, when similar categories were recognized, they were integrated. This process was repeated until no new categories emerged.

Video Observation and Its Analysis. We recorded and observed the behavior of caregivers and residents. The caregivers and managers allowed us to record their activities with two additional video cameras that were not part of the video-monitoring system. We collected data two days before installation and another two days after installation. We analyzed behaviors in the corridor (V1 in Figure 3) and in the living room to focus our investigation on the events that were closely related to daily activities, such as assistance in the lavatory.

Every 90 min, from four o'clock in the afternoon to half past five in the early morning (16:00 to 5:30), we calculated the frequency of the performance of an action by each resident and the response of the caregiver. We studied the behaviors observed in the evening and at night because we assumed that the effects of the system could be best evaluated during that period. The number of caregivers was limited to one at night, and the video-monitoring system was expected to be most effective then. Previous studies also suggest that caregivers receive the most benefit from monitoring systems at night [13, 14].

Ethical Considerations. In this study, we strictly observed informed consent guidelines in asking individual caregivers and managers of the group homes for data collection. Likewise, a letter of consent was obtained from the residents' families. Video cameras were never set in private residential areas such as inside a resident's room, the lavatory, *furo* (Japanese-styled bathroom), etc., to maintain privacy. The ethics committee of the Japan Advanced Institute of Science and Technology approved the data collection method used in this study.

4.2.2. Results of Case Study

Results of Interview: Release from Restrictions. During both day and night shifts, caregivers reported that the video-monitoring system helped them make decisions and refrain them from interaction with residents excessively. Before the intallment of the monitoring system, residents' activities were limited to secure their physical safety. For instance, when a resident leaves their room and walk toward the lavatory (depicted in the center of Figure 3) at night, caregivers in the kitchen may not be aware of the event. If they notice that a resident is heading toward the lavatory, they leave their work and take any necessary action.

Even if two or three caregivers are working during the day, blind spots are unavoidable in group homes. Although the caregivers have limitations regarding resources for observing residents, caregivers are obligated to ensure residents' safety. Before the system was installed, caregivers often disturbed residents' activities to ensure their physical safety. A veteran caregiver (a3) noted that she always asked residents about where they wanted to go when they stood up or showed signs of heading in a direction that did not have an identified and safe objective. She felt apologetic for this behavior and felt that it became a source of stress for her and for the residents. Another caregiver (a6) described that she used the system to take preemptive actions. When she noticed a resident going out to take a walk, she rushed to the back door and was able to approach the resident from the front and greet them. In the case of GH-C, two caregivers (c4 and c5) and a manager said that it was easy for them to observe residents entering or exiting the lavatory during both the day and night.

Both the PWD and caregivers were under fewer restrictions when the system was installed.

Results of Interview: Alleviating Stresses. The interviews revealed that the system reduced caregivers' physical and mental stress, as previously reported [13, 14]. Caregivers reported that some areas became blind spots at night because fewer caregivers were available. The video-monitoring system was most effective at night, particularly from midnight to early morning. Caregivers who worked at night were very anxious about blind spots. They were afraid that some residents might be seriously injured. For example, they were concerned that a resident could suffer a bone fracture if they fell down.

Such accidents are always a possibility, but they must be avoided because being injured and confined to a bed may cause further cognitive impairment. Caregivers were so worried about accidents that they would experience anxiety in the evenings.

Two caregivers and a manager said that it was easy for them to observe residents entering or exiting the lavatory both during the day and at night. A veteran caregiver (c3) reported that the elderly residents' peace of mind improved in response to the increased level of caregiver attention. This alleviated stress for both the residents and the caregivers.

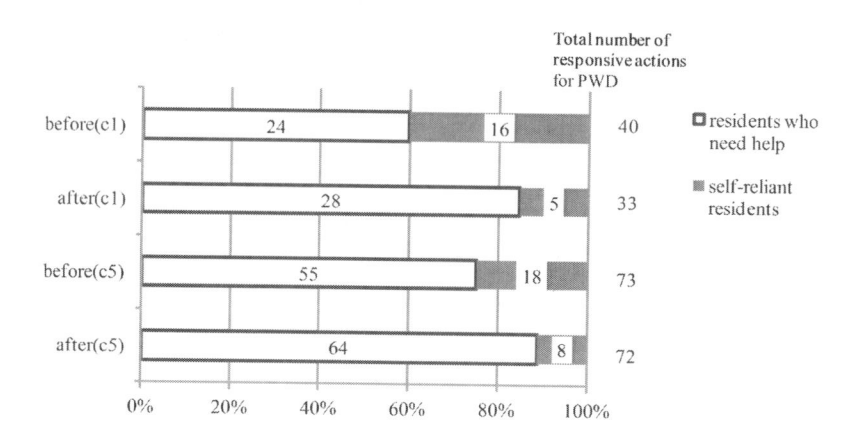

Figure 4. Change in responsive action for people with dementia.

Results of Video Observation: Changing Work Style. Figure 4 shows the behaviors of two caregivers. This figure indicates that the caregivers' responses to the residents' behaviors were optimized. Although the total number of responsive actions is slightly different, the proportion of actions changed: caregivers could adequately judge whether they needed to take action and assist residents. In fact, the system helped the caregivers in adjusting their efforts to the residents' demands and allowed caregivers to wait until residents truly needed help.

The monitoring system clarified caregivers' roles. A caregiver working in the kitchen, where one of the video monitors was placed, played the role of a watcher, while other caregivers were involved in household chores. Those caregivers were helped by the caregiver who was watching because they could concentrate on their work even if there were several areas they could not see. Caregivers felt that the system had significantly improved their work styles because it enabled them to focus on the tasks at hand, such as helping another resident to use the lavatory.

Having an employee monitor residents from the kitchen indicates that caregivers and managements could specify tasks more clearly than before the system was installed. Previously, if the staff suspected that something unusual had happened, they had to investigate by physically moving to the location. The staff who reacts to an incident caused by a resident receives information on the spot through the monitor. The video-monitoring system enabled caregivers to observe blind spots and remotely monitor incidents. Note that there were no cases in which a caregiver watches an incident with being there before the installment of the system.

One of the difficulties in dealing with PWD is that they may unexpectedly perform unusual activities. Consequently, caregivers have to focus on the residents at all times. However, they cannot always watch them directly. For example, when they take a resident to the lavatory, they are not able to observe other residents. The video-monitoring system provides a wider view of activities in the group home by decreasing the times when no caregiver is able to directly observe residents. This increases the likelihood of caregivers responding to residents' sudden unusual behaviors.

5. Discussion

Figure 5 presents a summary of the results and illustrates the proposed concept of a *triage support environment*. Triage refers to the prioritization of allocation of resources for medical treatment according to the severity of a patient's condition. The term is used in computer science to categorize vast amounts of information [43], documents [44], and e-mail [45, 46]. The term can also be applied to research into assistive technologies for person-centered dementia care.

The group homes we investigated were strained because of a lack of resources and fatigue caused by the shortage of funds and caregivers, respectively, as described in Section 2. Caregivers had to constantly observe residents to maintain their safety. Whenever they detected certain behaviors, especially when residents attempted to go outside, caregivers had to ask the residents to confirm where they wanted to go and what they wanted to do. In order to attend to this situation, the caregiver had to suspend their task at hand, such as cooking, cleaning, or assisting with personal hygiene. As there were always demands on caregivers' time and attention, often they could not take the time to carefully and thoroughly evaluate an individual resident's actions. If caregivers did not become aware of a resident's unusual and potentially risky behavior in a timely manner, they were forced to immediately suspend their current task and attend to the resident who may be at risk. It is quite difficult to make appropriate decisions under stressful conditions. The lack of redundancy in the workforce, which would allow caregivers to effectively respond to residents' unanticipated and erratic behavior, was ascribed as a cause of stress.

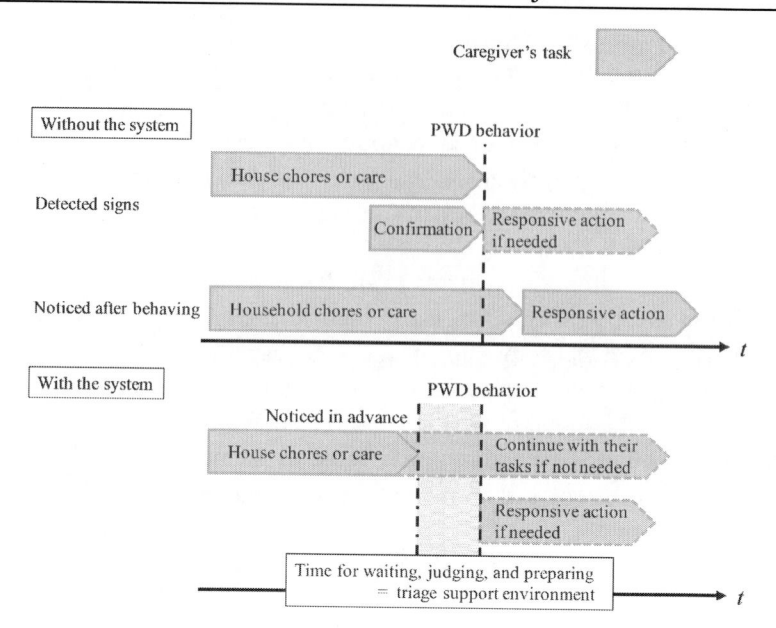

Figure 5. Emerging triage support environment.

However, caregivers were more at peace and were able to effectively respond to residents' needs while the system was in use. These benefits were the result of increased time for waiting, judging, and preparing that came from the system. The time that caregivers need to determine who needs help and to prioritize their actions is an important factor in their job performance.

Caregivers were less stressed and more comfortable and were able to effectively respond to residents' needs while the system was in use. These benefits were the result of increased time for waiting, judging, and preparing. The time that caregivers need to determine who needs help and to prioritize their actions is an important factor in their job performance.

When using the video-monitoring system, caregivers could observe residents and take action ac- cording to the urgency of their need. In other words, the video-monitoring system helped in creating a triage support environment. However, note that, as opposed to the original meaning of triage, which is to aggressively treat on the basis of severity, the most important aspect of the triage support environment herein is the time it allows caregivers to wait until action is necessary, which enhances the independence of PWDs. In brief, the triage support environment can improve the quality of person-centered dementia care.

The triage support environment also has the potential to meet the needs of PWD. User needs identified for person-centered care are (a) attachment, (b) comfort, (c) identity, (d) occupation, and (e) inclusion [3]. These points stem from the approach to dementia inherent in person-centered care; that is, appreciating the uniqueness of each person; this approach is in contrast with conventional approaches in which individuality was often disregarded in the face of tasks that needed to be immediately performed. One of the significant effects of assistive technologies is to meet the needs of comfort, identity, and inclusion because these technologies create the time required to wait and observe PWD.

6. Conclusion

We analyzed the influence of the video-monitoring system on caregivers in terms of the contribution of the system to the field of caregiving. The results of interviews showed that the stress felt by the caregivers was decreased. This decrease was probably caused by increased control they had over observing the residents' behaviors with the video-monitoring system. Ironically, the video-monitoring system liberated both PWD and caregivers from oppressive surveillance. The video observation allowed caregivers to efficiently respond to residents' activities. Finally, we established the concept of a *triage support environment*, which can augment dementia care.

Because all of our data was derived from a limited set of interviews and observations, further data collection is required to verify our findings. We also need to improve the video-monitoring system by investigating caregivers' needs with additional field studies.

This study has two noteworthy limitations: data collection and external validity. Our data were collected through semi-structured interviews and video observation; an observational study would have added to the validity of the findings.

Acknowledgments

Our research was partly supported by the Grant-in-Aid for Scientific Research (22615017, 23500646, 24616004) of JSPS and the Service Science, Solutions and Foundation Integrated Research Program (S3FIRE) from JST.

About the Authors

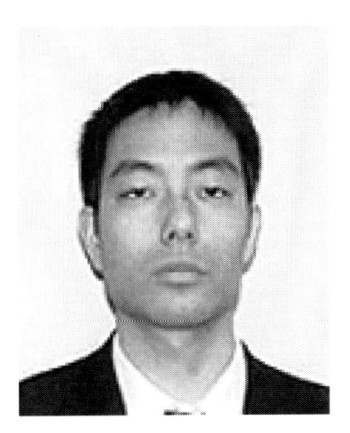

Taro Sugihara is Assistant Professor at School of Knowledge Science, Japan Advanced Institute of Science and Technology (JAIST). He is interest in research of users' behaviour and workplace for human-computer interaction, especially in the fields of caregiving for persons with dementia, university hospital, elementary school and high school. He also conducts resaerch in the area of knowledge management. Taro studied human-computer interaction at Kyoto Institute of Technology and was Doctor of Engineering.

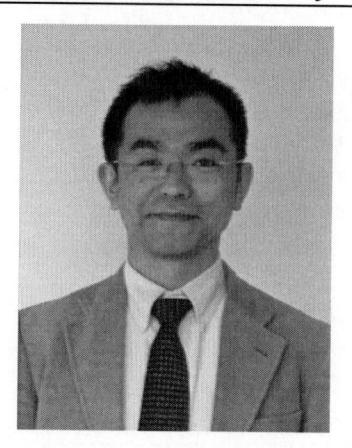

Tsutomu Fujinami is Associate Professor at School of Knowledge Science, Japan Advanced Institute of Science and Technology (JAIST). He is interested in skill acquisition and dementia care. He studied philosophy at Waseda University and was engaged in the research of Artificial Intelligence at Systems Development Laboratory, Hitachi Ltd. He studied Cognitive Science at University of Edinburgh and was awarded his PhD.

References

[1] United Nations Population Division, World Population Prospects: The 2008 Revision Population Database., accessed 30 April, 2011 (2008).
URL http://esa.un.org/unpp/index.asp?panel=2

[2] World Health Organization and Alzheimer's Disease International, *Dementia: a public health priority*, World Health Organization, 2012.

[3] T. Kitwood, *Dementia Reconsidered.*, Open University Press, 1997.

[4] T. Kitwood, K. Bredin, Towards a theory of dementia care: personhood and well-being., *Ageing and society* 12 (1992) 269–287.

[5] K. Hope, H. Waterman, Using multi-sensory environments with older people with dementia, *Journal of Advanced Nursing* 25 (4) (1997) 780–785.

[6] Y. Masuda, T. Yoshimura, K. Nakajima, M. Nambu, T. Hayakawa, T. Tamura, Unconstrained monitoring of prevention of wandering the elderly, in: *Proceedings of the Second Joint EMBS/BMES Conference and the 24th Annual Conference and the Annual Fall Meeting* of the Biomedical Engineering Society, Vol. 3, IEEE, 2002, pp. 1906–1907.

[7] S. Helal, C. Giraldo, Y. Kaddoura, C. Lee, H. El Zabadani, W. Mann, Smart phone based cognitive assistant, in: UbiHealth 2003: *The 2nd International Workshop on Ubiquitous Computing for Pervasive Healthcare Applications*, 2003.

[8] F. Miskelly, A novel system of electronic tagging in patients with dementia and wandering., *Age and ageing* 33 (3) (2004) 304–6.

[9] C.-C. Lin, M.-J. Chiu, C.-C. Hsiao, R.-G. Lee, Y.-S. Tsai, Wireless health care service system for elderly with dementia., *IEEE transactions on information technology in biomedicine* 10 (4) (2006) 696–704.

[10] D. Chen, A. J. Bharucha, H. D. Wactlar, Intelligent video monitoring to improve safety of older persons, in: *Proceedings of 29th Annual International Conference of the IEEE EMBS*, 2007, pp. 3814–7.

[11] A. Arcelus, M. Jones, R. Goubran, F. Knoefel, Integration of smart home technologies in a health monitoring system for the elderly, in: *Proceedings of the 21st International Conference on Advanced Information Networking and Applications Workshops (AINAW'07)*, Vol. 2, IEEE, 2007, pp. 820–825.

[12] D. Zhang, M. Hariz, M. Mokhtari, Assisting Elders with Mild Dementia Staying at Home, *IEEE*, 2008, pp. 692–697.

[13] T. Sugihara, K. Nakagawa, T. Fujinami, R. Takatsuka, Evaluation of a Prototype of the Mimamori-care System for Persons with Dementia, in: *Knowledge-Based Intelligent Information and Engineering Systems*, Springer, 2008, pp. 839–846.

[14] T. Sugihara, T. Fujinami, *Emerging triage support environment of care with camera system for persons with dementia*, Vol. LNCS 6779, 2011, pp. 149–58.

[15] National Institute on Aging, *Glossary, in Alzheimer's Disease: Unraveling the Mystery.*, accessed 19 November, 2012.
URL http://www.nia.nih.gov/alzheimers/publication/alzheimers-disease-unraveling-mystery/glossary

[16] Alzheimer's Associateion, *2011 Alzheimer's disease facts and figures.*, accessed 1 May, 2011.
URL http://www.alz.org/downloads/Facts_Figures_2011.pdf

[17] National Institute of Population and Security Research, *Shakai Hoshou Kyuufu-hi* (Heisei 21-nendo) (Fact sheet 2009: Social Security Benefits)(in Japanese) (2011).

[18] Kaigo Roudou Antei Centre (Care Work Foundation), *Kaigo Roudou Jittai Chousa* (2006 Annual Reports on Care Work Environment in Japan)(in Japanese), accessed 23 September, 2011 (2007).
URL http://www.kaigo-center.or.jp/report/h18_chousa_03.html

[19] Kaigo Roudou Antei Centre (Care Work Foundation), *Kaigo Roudou Jittai Chousa* (2007 Annual Reports on Care Work Environment in Japan)(in Japanese), accessed 23 September, 2011 (2008).
URL http://www.kaigo-center.or.jp/report/h19_chousa_03.html

[20] Kaigo Roudou Antei Centre (Care Work Foundation), *Kaigo Roudou Jittai Chousa* (2008 Annual Reports on Care Work Environment in Japan)(in Japanese), accessed 23 September, 2011 (2009).
URL http://www.kaigo-center.or.jp/report/pdf/h20_chousa_point.pdf

[21] Kaigo Roudou Antei Centre (Care Work Foundation), *Kaigo Roudou Jittai Chousa* (2009 Annual Reports on Care Work Environment in Japan)(in Japanese), accessed 23 September, 2011 (2010).
URL http://www.kaigo-center.or.jp/report/pdf/h21_chousa_point.pdf

[22] Kaigo Roudou Antei Centre (Care Work Foundation), *Kaigo Roudou Jittai Chousa* (2010 Annual Reports on Care Work Environment in Japan)(in Japanese), accessed 23 September, 2011 (2011).
URL http://www.kaigo-center.or.jp/report/pdf/h22_chousa_kekka.pdf

[23] Kaigo Roudou Antei Centre (Care Work Foundation), *Kaigo Roudou Jittai Chousa (2011 Annual Reports on Care Work Environment in Japan)(in Japanese)*, accessed 4 November, 2012 (2012).
URL http://www.kaigo-center.or.jp/report/h23_chousa_01.html

[24] R. L. Kahn, D. M. Wolfe, R. P. Quinn, J. D. Snoek, R. A. Rosenthal, *Organizational stress: Studies in role conflict and ambiguity*, John Wiley, 1964.

[25] J. R. Rizzo, R. J. House, S. I. Lirtzman, Role Conflict and Ambiguity in Complex Organizations, *Administrative Science Quarterly* 15 (2) (1970) 150–163.

[26] C. E. Barber, M. Iwai, Role Conflict and Role Ambiguity as Predictors of Burnout Among Staff Caring for Elderly Dementia Patients., *Journal of Gerontological Social Work* 26 (1996) 101–116.

[27] J. A. Schaefer, R. H. Moos, Effects of work stressors and work climate on long-term care staff's job morale and functioning, *Research in Nursing & Health* 19 (1) (1996) 63–73.

[28] E. Moniz-Cook, D. Clin, D. Millington, M. Silver, Residential care for older people: job satisfaction and psychological health in care staff, *Health & Social Care in the Community* 5 (2) (1997) 124–133.

[29] J. C. Mundt, K. L. Ferber, M. Rizzo, J. H. Greist, Computer-automated dementia screening using a touch-tone telephone., *Archives of internal medicine* 161 (20) (2001) 2481–7.

[30] D. W. Wright, F. C. Goldstein, P. Kilgo, J. R. Brumfield, T. Ravichandran, M. L. Danielson, M. Laplaca, Use of a novel technology for presenting screening measures

to detect mild cognitive impairment in elderly patients., *International journal of clinical practice* 64 (9) (2010) 1190–7.

[31] H. Kim, Y. Cho, E. Do, Computational clock drawing analysis for cognitive impairment screening, in: *Proceedings of the fifth international conference on Tangible, embedded, and embodied interaction*, ACM, 2011, pp. 297–300.

[32] E. Cole, P. Dehdashti, L. Petti, M. Angert, Participatory design for sensitive interface parameters: contributions of traumatic brain injury patients to their prosthetic software, in: *Conference companion on Human factors in computing systems*, ACM, 1994, pp. 115–116.

[33] K. Du, D. Zhang, M. Musa, M. Mokhtari, X. Zhou, Handling Activity Conflicts in Reminding System for Elders with Dementia, in: *Proceedings of the Second International Conference on Future Generation Communication and Networking (FGCN'08).*, IEEE, 2008, pp. 416–421.

[34] Z. Stavros, K. Fotini, T. Magda, Computer based cognitive training for patients with mild cognitive impairment (MCI), in: *Proceedings of the 3rd International Conference on Pervasive Technologies Related to Assistive Environments*, no. Mci, ACM, 2010, pp. 1–3.

[35] M. H. White, S. M. Dorman, Online support for caregivers. Analysis of an Internet Alzheimer mailgroup., *Computers in nursing* 18 (4) (2000) 168–76; quiz 177–9.

[36] E. D. Freeman, L. Clare, N. Savitch, L. Royan, R. Litherland, M. Lindsay, Improving website accessibility for people with early-stage dementia: a preliminary investigation., *Aging & mental health* 9 (5) (2005) 442–8.

[37] S. J. Czaja, M. P. Rubert, Telecommunications technology as an aid to family caregivers of persons with dementia., *Psychosomatic medicine* 64 (3) (2002) 469–76.

[38] D. F. Mahoney, B. J. Tarlow, R. N. Jones, Effects of an automated telephone support system on caregiver burden and anxiety: findings from the REACH for TLC intervention study., *The Gerontologist* 43 (4) (2003) 556–67.

[39] S. Dang, N. Remon, J. Harris, J. Malphurs, L. Sandals, A. L. Cabrera, N. Nedd, Care coordination assisted by technology for multiethnic caregivers of persons with dementia: a pilot clinical demonstration project on caregiver burden and depression., *Journal of telemedicine and telecare* 14 (8) (2008) 443–7.

[40] G. Gowans, J. Campbell, N. Alm, R. Dye, A. Astell, M. Ellis, Designing a multimedia conversation aid for reminiscence therapy in dementia care environments, *Extended abstracts of the 2004 conference on Human factors and computing systems* - CHI '04 (2004) 825–836.

[41] N. Kuwahara, S. Abe, K. Yasuda, K. Kuwabara, *Networked reminiscence therapy for individuals with dementia by using photo and video sharing*, ACM Press, New York, New York, USA, 2006, p. 125.

[42] N. Alm, R. Dye, G. Gowans, J. Campbell, A. Astell, M. Ellis, *Support System for Older People with Dementia*, Computer (May) (2007) 35–41.

[43] C. Marshall, F. Shipman III, Spatial hypertext and the practice of information triage, in: *Proceedings of the eighth ACM conference on Hypertext*, ACM, 1997, pp. 124–133.

[44] R. Badi, S. Bae, J. Moore, K. Meintanis, A. Zacchi, H. Hsieh, F. Shipman, C. Marshall, Recognizing user interest and document value from reading and organizing activities in document triage, in: *Proceedings of the 11th international conference on Intelligent user interfaces*, ACM, 2006, pp. 218–225.

[45] C. Neustaedter, A. Brush, M. Smith, Beyond from and received: exploring the dynamics of email triage, in: *CHI'05 extended abstracts on human factors in computing systems*, ACM, 2005, pp. 1977–1980.

[46] C. Neustaedter, A. Brush, M. Smith, D. Fisher, The social network and relationship finder: Social sorting for email triage, in: *Proceedings of the 2005 Conference on Email and Anti-Spam* (CEAS), 2005.

INDEX

A

abuse, x, 157, 162, 165, 168
academic progress, 100
academic tasks, 30
access, xi, 15, 16, 27, 31, 38, 89, 126, 130, 184
accessibility, 98, 107, 114, 130, 165
accommodations, 13, 26, 32, 34
acupuncture, 44
ADA, 115
adaptability, 52
adaptation, 108, 137, 139, 140, 142, 143, 148, 149, 153, 154, 223
adaptive functioning, 4, 27, 35, 36, 37, 100
ADHD, 3, 4, 24, 25, 50
adjustment, xi, 47, 48, 55, 144, 145, 148, 183, 185, 189, 191, 194
adolescents, 21, 33, 35, 44, 49, 50
adulthood, 2, 10, 36, 37, 38
adults, 12, 20, 22, 24, 32, 33, 37, 38, 42, 49, 54, 178, 198, 200, 205, 216
advancement(s), 90, 99, 138
adverse effects, xi, 158, 184, 203
advocacy, 33, 39, 53
Africa, 128
African-American, 187
age, vii, xi, 2, 3, 4, 7, 10, 11, 19, 21, 24, 25, 26, 27, 29, 30, 32, 35, 38, 42, 47, 56, 58, 61, 79, 127, 130, 141, 142, 145, 148, 149, 159, 160, 161, 184, 185, 186, 187, 191, 195, 198, 200, 201, 219, 222, 223
agencies, 35, 38, 39, 40
age-related diseases, 141
aggression, 9, 13, 121, 155
aggressive behavior, 15, 31, 140
agriculture, 196
algorithm, 115
allied-health workers, xi, 195

ALS, 125, 132, 135
American Psychiatric Association (APA), 4, 24, 48
amniocentesis, 7
amylase, 186
amyotrophic lateral sclerosis, 134, 135
anatomy, 21
anger, 46, 58, 125, 138
ANOVA, 61, 108, 109, 111
anxiety, viii, ix, 7, 13, 21, 24, 25, 30, 42, 52, 57, 58, 59, 60, 61, 62, 63, 71, 72, 74, 75, 126, 127, 134, 137, 138, 140, 143, 148, 149, 150, 151, 152, 159, 179, 185, 200, 203
anxiety disorder, 25, 52, 179
aortic stenosis, 6
apathy, 125
appetite, 172, 185
appraisals, x, 101, 137, 140, 141, 148, 151
aptitude, 216
ARC, 41, 48
arrest, 210
arthritis, 159
articulation, 21
Asia, 166, 204, 206
Asian Americans, 187
assault, 91
assessment, xi, 4, 10, 11, 20, 21, 27, 32, 35, 36, 83, 89, 92, 127, 134, 135, 141, 145, 154, 164, 167, 184, 190, 192, 194, 195, 197, 198, 201, 202, 206, 213, 216, 223
assistive technology, 219
Association of Southeast Asian Nations (ASEAN), 195, 196, 204
ataxia, 219
atmosphere, 38
attachment, 58
attitude measurement, 101
attitudes, ix, 54, 56, 58, 84, 94, 97, 101, 105, 106, 107, 109, 113, 114, 115, 116, 117, 133, 177, 200, 209, 214

attribution, 114
auditory stimuli, 105
authority(ies), 38, 39, 40, 117
autism, 3, 4, 48, 50, 53, 54
autonomy, 70, 71, 83, 128, 130, 202
aversion, 8
avoidance, 172
awareness, 33, 34, 35, 46, 52, 54, 55, 60, 127, 176, 202, 212, 216

B

back pain, 158, 167
background information, 11
banking, 29, 37
barriers, 9, 26, 100, 193
base, 105, 107, 190
batteries, 141
Beck Depression Inventory, vii, 57, 61, 73, 143, 144, 151
bedding, 31
behavioral medicine, 179
behavioral problems, 17, 22, 23, 25, 35, 147, 149, 154, 162, 168, 201, 202
behaviors, 3, 4, 5, 8, 9, 12, 13, 14, 15, 17, 18, 21, 22, 24, 26, 30, 31, 33, 42, 46, 105, 142, 172, 201
benefits, vii, 1, 2, 4, 20, 39, 44, 45, 47, 102, 123, 164, 175
beverages, 221
bioethics, 105
biofeedback, 44
birth rate, 196
birth weight, 6
births, 5, 7
bivariate analysis, 162, 200
blame, 82, 105
blood, 129
bonding, 164
bonds, 58, 69, 81
bottom-up, 65
bowel, 64
brain, 98, 114, 191, 194, 201, 218
brainstorming, 210
Brazil, 217, 218
breast cancer, 133, 187, 192
bridging social networks, 124
bronchitis, 159
bullying, 23, 26
burn, 176
burnout, 140, 153, 172, 173, 174, 175, 176, 177, 178, 179, 180, 181
businesses, 127
buttons, 17

C

Cambodia, 196
cancer, vii, x, xi, 57, 58, 59, 63, 64, 71, 73, 74, 75, 115, 133, 171, 172, 174, 175, 176, 177, 178, 179, 180, 183, 184, 185, 186, 187, 188, 189, 190, 191, 192, 193, 194, 196, 198, 200, 208, 210
cancer care, vii, x, xi, 73, 171, 176, 177, 179, 183, 184, 187, 188, 189, 190, 192, 193, 194
carbohydrates, 218
career development, 86, 212
caregiver burden, vii, x, 125, 126, 135, 154, 157, 158, 159, 160, 161, 162, 163, 165, 167, 189, 192, 193, 196, 197, 198, 199, 200, 202, 203, 204, 241
Caribbean, 128
caries, xii, 217, 218, 219, 220, 222, 223
cartoon, 15
case study, 166
cash, 123
category a, 128
Census, 158, 165, 166, 168
cerebral palsy, vii, 218, 222, 223, 224
cerebrovascular disease, 200
challenges, vii, 1, 2, 3, 4, 5, 8, 21, 23, 32, 33, 34, 42, 43, 45, 46, 47, 54, 57, 79, 88, 98, 123, 124, 158, 160, 162, 163, 165, 166, 173, 177, 185
chaos, 80, 84, 89
charitable organizations, 188
chemical, 121
Chicago, 223
childhood, 2, 8, 23, 31, 32, 47, 59, 68, 218
children, vii, x, xii, 3, 4, 7, 9, 10, 11, 12, 14, 15, 17, 18, 20, 21, 22, 23, 24, 25, 26, 27, 29, 32, 34, 38, 41, 42, 43, 44, 45, 46, 47, 48, 49, 50, 51, 52, 53, 54, 55, 56, 60, 64, 66, 67, 68, 70, 71, 83, 99, 100, 101, 102, 103, 106, 115, 117, 129, 130, 132, 135, 139, 145, 149, 155, 157, 158, 163, 180, 184, 186, 199, 217, 218, 219, 220, 221, 222, 223
China, 133, 139, 157, 195
chorionic villus sampling, 7
chromosome, 5, 6, 7, 49, 55
chronic diseases, 158, 167, 205
chronic fatigue, 172
chronic illness, xi, 128, 129, 139, 159, 195, 196, 197, 198, 199, 200, 202, 203, 204, 205
chronic stress situations, x, 137, 139, 149, 151
circus, 98
civilization, ix, 99, 119, 131
clarity, 175, 178
classes, 22, 113
classification, 3, 48, 88, 115, 117, 222, 223
classroom, 13, 26, 28, 29, 101
cleaning, 218, 220

Index

clients, 163, 172, 211
clinical depression, 201
clinical diagnosis, 50
clinical interventions, 154, 175
clone, 53
close relationships, 59, 154, 164
cluster analysis, 61
clusters, 61, 62, 167
coaches, 34
coding, 133
cognition, 53, 99, 114, 117, 133, 190, 218
cognitive capacity, 39
cognitive deficits, 10
cognitive development, 99
cognitive function, 8, 10, 27, 35, 38, 104
cognitive impairment, 145, 148, 159, 160, 162, 168
cognitive process, 102, 103, 104, 105, 107
cognitive profile, 53
cognitive system, 113
cognitive-behavioral therapy, 163
colic, 9
collaboration, 125, 184, 211
collectivism, 135
college students, 154
color, 19, 116
combined effect, 115
communication, 4, 12, 13, 14, 15, 21, 65, 85, 100, 122, 123, 176, 189, 190, 193, 198, 209, 218
communication abilities, 100
communication skills, 21, 176, 209
communication systems, 21
community(ies), vii, ix, xi, xii, 3, 10, 11, 20, 23, 27, 31, 33, 34, 37, 44, 47, 51, 56, 73, 80, 119, 120, 121, 122, 123, 124, 128, 129, 131, 132, 139, 141, 158, 160, 164, 165, 166, 168, 175, 177, 188, 197, 199, 203, 204, 207, 208, 209, 211, 212, 213, 214, 215, 216, 219, 223
community service, 31, 160, 168
community support, 165
compassion, vii, x, 8, 26, 41, 171, 172, 175, 176, 178, 179, 180, 181, 182
compassion fatigue (CF), vii, x, 171, 172, 173, 174, 175, 176, 177, 178, 179, 180, 181, 182, 214
compensation, xi, 183
competition, 46
complexity, 8, 22, 107, 125, 158, 220
compliance, 123
complications, 6, 7, 184
composition, 130
comprehension, 29
compulsory education, 147
computer, 19, 28
conceptual model, x, 135, 137

conceptualization, 50, 98, 99
confidentiality, 115, 141
conflict, 46, 130, 161, 189, 197, 200
confounders, 161
confrontation, ix, 119, 131
Confucianism, 129
congenital heart disease, 55
Congress, 56, 114, 167, 169
congruence, viii, 57
consciousness, 84, 100, 101
consensus, 106
consent, 39, 40, 65, 141
consolidation, 67
constipation, 7, 9
construction, 64, 73
constructivism, 57
consulting, 31
consumption, 218
content analysis, 74
contour, 116
controversial, 40, 139
conversations, 18, 32, 38, 135
cooking, 18
cooperation, 125, 127
coordination, 4, 9, 10, 20
coping strategies, x, 51, 87, 89, 140, 141, 143, 164, 171, 176, 177, 178, 180, 186, 188, 198, 202, 204
coronary heart disease, 192
correlation, 144, 148, 173, 186
correlations, 144, 145, 148, 161, 173
cortisol, 186
cost, 12, 123, 129, 131, 159, 163, 167, 172, 180, 192, 203
counseling, 36, 42, 44, 161
covering, 142
creative potential, 84
creativity, 6, 215
crises, 138
criticism, 101
cross sectional study
cross-sectional study, 159, 200, 214, 205
cryotherapy, 224
CSS, 142, 143, 144
cues, 24, 33
cultural differences, 130, 187, 188
cultural influence, vii, ix, 119, 127, 128, 130
cultural norms, 58, 187
culture, ix, 67, 113, 119, 121, 128, 130, 133, 174, 187, 190, 200, 203
cure, 128
curriculum, 13, 133, 214
cycles, 9
Cyprus, 128

D

daily care, 160, 186
daily living, 4, 20, 37, 141, 145, 147, 148, 161, 201
danger, 63
data analysis, 112
data set, 61
DEA, 26
deaths, 196, 207
defects, 5, 49
deficiency(ies), 29, 100
deficit, 3, 24, 51, 53, 56, 220
deinstitutionalization, 37
dementia, vii, x, xi, xii, 51, 74, 87, 94, 124, 125, 140, 141, 145, 149, 152, 153, 154, 155, 157, 158, 159, 160, 161, 162, 163, 164, 165, 166, 167, 168, 169, 195, 198, 200, 201, 202, 203, 204, 205, 206, 209, 211, 215
demographic change, 184
denial, 186
dental caries, xii, 217, 218, 220, 222, 223
Department of Education, 3, 56
dependent variable, 110
depression, viii, ix, 7, 57, 58, 59, 60, 61, 62, 63, 72, 74, 125, 126, 127, 134, 137, 138, 140, 143, 148, 149, 150, 151, 152, 159, 162, 164, 167, 185, 186, 187, 189, 190, 192, 193, 198, 201, 203
depressive symptoms, 42, 154, 162, 191, 192
depth, viii, 36, 57, 59, 64, 65
despair, 93
destruction, 9
detachment, 92
detection, xi, 99, 184
developed countries, 184
developmental disorder, 4, 50
diabetes, 196, 200
diagnostic criteria, 3, 4, 24, 25
diagnostic markers, 152
dialysis, 40
diet, 17, 31, 44, 218
diffusion, 139
dignity, 122, 210
dimensionality, 152
dinosaurs, 18
directionality, 150
directives, 33
disability, ix, xi, 3, 4, 5, 6, 7, 8, 23, 24, 26, 34, 35, 42, 45, 46, 48, 50, 53, 54, 55, 97, 98, 100, 106, 107, 108, 109, 110, 111, 112, 113, 114, 115, 116, 117, 119, 120, 121, 122, 128, 129, 130, 131, 141, 161, 195, 200, 202, 218, 220, 222
disclosure, 188, 191, 193
discomfort, 19, 198
discrimination, 34, 98, 101, 115, 122
disease progression, 187
diseases, 125, 130, 159, 165, 196, 209
disorder, 2, 3, 5, 6, 24, 25, 26, 51, 54, 55, 56, 121, 127, 139, 153, 164, 179, 200, 219, 220
dispersion, 59, 75
disposition, 7
distress, 85, 126, 127, 134, 138, 158, 161, 163, 175, 185, 187, 189, 191, 199
distribution, 59, 60, 61, 74, 220
diversity, 115, 193, 196, 199
dizziness, 159
DMF, xii, 217, 219
doctors, 8, 122, 180
DOI, 134, 181
Down syndrome, vii, 1, 2, 4, 5, 7, 22, 41, 44, 46, 49, 50, 51, 53, 54, 98, 108, 116, 117
dream, 69, 88
drugs, 68, 173
DSM-IV-TR, 4, 24
dyslexia, 24
dysthymia, 200

E

early retirement, 159, 174
earnings, 36
East Asia, 129, 167, 204
East Timor, 195
economic development, 203
economic problem, 122, 159
economic resources, 131
economics, 196
editors, 194, 204
education, vii, xii, 8, 24, 25, 26, 27, 33, 36, 39, 101, 103, 106, 107, 109, 112, 113, 115, 116, 117, 127, 128, 129, 132, 145, 160, 161, 163, 175, 176, 200, 205, 207, 208, 209, 212, 213, 214, 215, 216
educational attainment, 26, 187
educational opportunities, 101
educational process, 22
educational programs, 93, 105, 129, 190, 209
educational settings, 25, 51, 73, 107
educational system, vii, 2, 20, 26, 106
educators, 3, 25, 181
elaboration, 121
elastin, 6, 48
elderly population, 158
elders, 74, 95, 128, 166, 167, 168
e-mail, 211, 217
emergency, 51, 172, 179, 209, 210
emotion, 69, 121, 133, 135, 143, 148, 149, 164, 187, 201

emotional distress, x, 140, 164, 183, 192
emotional exhaustion, 176, 179
emotional experience, 94, 135
emotional health, 187
emotional problems, 149, 184
emotional reactions, 6, 128, 174, 180
emotional responses, 58
emotional state, 138, 141, 148, 150
emotional well-being, 13, 30, 185
empathy, x, 6, 23, 41, 171, 173, 177
empirical studies, 82, 175, 179
employees, 173
employers, 34, 35, 101
employment, 34, 50, 51, 55, 115, 186, 200
employment status, 186, 200
empowerment, 113, 122, 132
encouragement, 176
energy, 31, 86, 171
enuresis, 9, 21
environment(s), xii, 11, 12, 14, 15, 17, 19, 20, 23, 26, 29, 34, 38, 47, 51, 103, 107, 108, 109, 110, 111, 112, 121, 122, 125, 133, 172, 177, 202
environmental characteristics, 181
environmental factors, 4, 127
environmental stress, 173
epidemic, 206
equality, ix, 119, 122, 123
equipment, 15, 34
equity, 124
erosion, 196
ethics, ix, 48, 119, 123
ethnic groups, 129, 187
ethnic minority, 187
ethnicity, 187, 193, 200, 202
etiology, 4, 9, 22, 52
Europe, 198
European Commission, 121, 123
everyday life, ix, 65, 66, 71, 119, 120, 138, 179
evidence, viii, x, 4, 13, 41, 72, 77, 105, 106, 129, 130, 153, 157, 158, 171, 172, 175, 178, 185, 189, 201, 204
evil, 129
evolution, 85, 124, 138
examinations, 66
execution, 39
executive functioning, 27, 35
exercise, ix, 31, 39, 44, 97, 177
experimental design, 107, 108
expertise, 8, 44, 88, 100, 125, 181
exposure, 172, 173, 181
extraction, 213
extraversion, 142, 148, 149
eye floaters, 74

F

facial expression, 18
failure to thrive, 9
fairness, 122
faith, 95
families, vii, xi, 2, 4, 5, 8, 9, 10, 11, 20, 21, 25, 32, 35, 39, 46, 48, 51, 65, 94, 95, 122, 124, 125, 126, 128, 129, 132, 158, 160, 167, 168, 180, 191, 193, 199, 201, 207, 208, 209, 210, 216, 223
family functioning, 9, 198
family life, 58, 94, 122
family members, xi, 15, 27, 37, 38, 39, 40, 41, 45, 58, 64, 78, 81, 129, 131, 158, 184, 187, 191, 192, 195, 196, 197, 199, 200, 202, 203, 205
family physician, 184, 193
family support, 108, 164, 196
family system, 42
family violence, 152
fear(s), 8, 49, 58, 89, 122, 185, 212
feelings, 23, 28, 46, 58, 62, 70, 71, 80, 81, 84, 90, 92, 123, 125, 130, 136, 138, 155, 163, 164, 168, 185, 200, 205, 209, 210, 212
fetus, 7
filial piety, x, 129, 157, 158, 165, 166
financial, vii, x, xi, 2, 39, 41, 42, 124, 127, 161, 163, 183, 184, 187, 188, 195, 196, 199, 200, 208, 221
financial records, 39
financial resources, 187
financial support, 161, 188, 208
flexibility, 20, 30, 113, 163
food, 9, 13, 21, 31, 59, 218
football, 68
force, 67, 84, 87, 128
Ford, 141, 153
formal education, 26
formation, 61, 104
fragility, 120
framing, 107
France, v, 116, 119, 128, 190
freedom, viii, 72, 78, 80, 92, 130
funding, 38, 100
funds, xii, 131

G

gait, 202
gastroenterologist, 21
gay men, 151
gender differences, 191
general education, 113
generalized anxiety disorder, 139, 145, 146

genes, 6
genetic disease, 129
genetic disorders, 4, 10, 24, 54
genetic syndromes, 25, 49
genetics, 152
genitourinary tract, 6
genotype, 50
geography, 196
Germany, 100, 124
gerontology, 213
gestures, 12, 71
glioblastoma, 186
globalization, 127, 128
glucose, 6
God, 69, 81
GPS, 20
grants, 222
graph, 103, 105, 108, 110, 112
gravity, 124
Greece, 98
grids, 61, 72
group membership, 106
grouping, 4, 24
growth, xi, 58, 86, 125, 152, 154, 183, 208
guardian, 40, 41, 126
guardianships, vii, 2, 33, 48
guidance, 113, 133
guidelines, 65, 153, 193, 213
guiding principles, 124
guilt, 46, 58, 60, 62, 63, 82, 90, 125, 163, 200
guilty, 70, 82, 83, 221

helplessness, 125
hemiplegia, 219
heredity, 115
heterogeneity, 79, 184
high school, 5, 45, 106, 112, 145
higher education, 160, 161, 165
history, 11, 27, 35, 117, 127, 145, 181, 184, 196
homes, xii, 93, 140, 158, 161, 165, 203
homework, 24, 29
Hong Kong, v, vii, x, 130, 133, 157, 158, 159, 160, 161, 162, 163, 165, 166, 167, 168, 169
hopelessness, 185, 190
hospice, viii, 57, 64, 65, 74, 114, 181, 191, 192
hospital death, 208
hospitalization, 70, 199
hostility, 72
house, 47, 55
housing, 37, 50, 54, 56
human, ix, 34, 52, 97, 98, 99, 100, 102, 120, 121, 124, 130, 151
human dignity, 124
human rights, ix, 97, 98
husband, 67, 69, 70, 71, 81, 83, 187
hybridization, 5
hygiene, 17, 20, 30, 31, 124, 218, 220, 223
hyperactivity, 3, 5, 23, 24, 25, 27, 51, 53, 56
hypercalcemia, 6, 9
hypersomnia, 9
hypertension, 6, 196, 200
hypothesis, 150
hypothyroidism, 6, 49

H

hair, 6, 17, 81
handwriting, 20
harassment, 213
harmony, 130
headache, 159
healing, x, 171, 176
health care, xi, 38, 40, 41, 65, 78, 122, 123, 124, 126, 127, 128, 131, 133, 173, 179, 183, 184, 188, 190, 193, 209, 213, 214, 215
health care professionals, 65, 131, 179, 184
health care system, 124, 126, 127, 184, 188
health condition, 55
health problems, 51, 131, 138, 185
health promotion, 138, 174, 176, 189
health psychology, 44
health services, 215
health status, 148, 150, 186, 190, 198, 200, 203, 223
heart disease, 196
helping behavior, 102

I

ideal, 90, 92, 176
identification, 52, 86, 105, 122, 138
identity, 62, 84
ideology, 128
image, 66, 70, 85
imagery, 176
immersion, 80
immune function, 159
immunity, 167, 196
impairments, 4, 189
implicit association test, 101, 115
improvements, ix, 97, 164
impulsive, 8, 25
impulsivity, 11, 23, 24, 25, 27
in situ hybridization, 5
in transition, 85, 93, 95, 204
inattention, 23, 24, 25, 27
incidence, 7, 58, 184, 185, 190
income, 159, 160, 161, 198, 200

independence, 35, 49, 59, 121, 130, 135, 161
independent living, vii, 2, 4, 17, 37, 38
India, vii, 106, 117, 195, 204
individual characteristics, 148, 149
individual perception, 143
individual students, 176
individual well-being, ix, 47, 119, 123
individuals, vii, ix, 1, 2, 4, 5, 6, 7, 9, 21, 22, 25, 26, 32, 33, 34, 35, 37, 38, 40, 41, 42, 43, 44, 45, 47, 52, 53, 84, 85, 97, 99, 127, 130, 134, 137, 138, 139, 148, 150, 155, 169, 178, 184, 186, 188, 192, 202, 208, 218, 219, 220, 222, 223
Individuals with Disabilities Education Act, 26, 56
Indonesia, 196, 201, 204
industrial chemicals, 51
industry, 196
infancy, 2, 5, 8, 32
infants, 9, 13, 47, 132
inferential processing, 103
influenza, 159, 167
informed consent, 39, 65, 132, 218
infrastructure, 106
inhibition, 132
injury(ies), 9, 10, 14, 120
insecurity, 92
insomnia, 200, 201
institutions, 34, 37, 98, 106, 113, 123, 151, 181, 184
integration, viii, 37, 77, 86, 89, 90, 92, 103, 104, 105, 107, 110, 112, 113, 114, 117, 164
intellectual disability(ies), vii, 4, 48, 50, 51, 52, 55, 98, 101, 107, 111, 115
intelligence, 4, 99, 134, 149
intelligence quotient, 4
intelligence tests, 100
intentionality, 102
interaction effect, 112
interdependence, 125, 127
interference, 192
internal consistency, 142, 143, 144, 198
interpersonal conflict, 85
interpersonal relations, 67, 72, 105, 114, 127, 129
interpersonal relationships, 67, 72, 105, 127, 129
interpersonal skills, 4
intervention, xi, xii, 10, 22, 25, 34, 47, 48, 63, 73, 86, 93, 124, 125, 134, 164, 165, 166, 168, 169, 174, 175, 180, 183, 189, 191, 207, 208, 209, 214, 215, 216
intervention strategies, 48
intimacy, 33, 58
intrinsic motivation, 187
intrinsic rewards, 196
introvert, 70
inversion, 70

investment, 86
Iran, 139
irritability, 9, 125, 172, 201
isolation, xi, 46, 81, 86, 87, 185, 195, 196
issues, ix, 22, 26, 32, 33, 40, 41, 46, 64, 80, 85, 121, 122, 128, 130, 131, 137, 161, 173, 174, 181, 188, 193, 201, 202, 209, 210, 213, 219, 223
Italian family caregivers, vii, 57
Italy, vii, 57, 60, 64, 72, 74, 119, 123, 183

J

Japan, vi, vii, xi, xii, 198, 207, 208, 209, 210, 211, 212, 213, 214, 215, 216, 225
job performance, 173
job satisfaction, 174, 179
junior high school, 45
Jupiter, 120
jurisdiction, 41
juveniles, 73

K

karyotype, 6, 7
kidney, 21
kindergarten, 110, 112
kinship, 145, 148, 149, 200, 201
knots, 91

L

labeling, 16
labor shortage, 34
language acquisition, 9, 16, 21
language development, 8, 9, 10, 12, 53
language proficiency, 103, 104
language skills, 10
languages, 127
lateral sclerosis, 134
laws, 34, 38, 53, 106, 123
lead, x, 7, 9, 17, 22, 24, 28, 33, 42, 58, 60, 63, 81, 82, 85, 88, 93, 99, 102, 103, 113, 125, 129, 157, 162, 165, 172, 184, 196, 200, 203, 212, 218
leadership, 212
learning, 3, 4, 6, 12, 15, 17, 18, 19, 23, 24, 25, 26, 27, 28, 29, 31, 35, 41, 42, 45, 52, 53, 99, 114, 116, 152, 176, 210, 212, 214
learning difficulties, 6
learning disabilities, 24, 52, 114, 116
legislation, 34
legs, 12
leisure, 55, 92, 138

level of education, 44
life cycle, 58
life expectancy, 78, 196
life experiences, 130
life satisfaction, 138
lifestyle behaviors, xi, 184
light, 17, 100, 121, 161, 219
linear function, 109, 112
literacy, 158
living arrangements, 37, 48, 160, 161
living environment, 33
locus, 48, 109
loneliness, 23, 94
longevity, 158, 181, 196, 213
longitudinal study, 168
long-term care facilities, xi, 207, 208, 209, 210, 211, 213, 214, 215
long-term care insurance, 213
love, 8, 22, 41, 44, 45, 62, 68, 69, 71, 88, 105, 114, 129
LTC, 123
lung cancer, 74, 116, 192
Luo, 205

M

magazines, 29
magnets, 19
magnitude, 165, 174
majority, 3, 4, 10, 125, 149, 196, 200, 201
malaise, 127
Malaysia, 196, 201
man, 68, 71, 79, 128
management, xi, 3, 8, 31, 39, 123, 124, 164, 168, 172, 175, 176, 184, 185, 187, 188, 190, 191, 195, 213
marital status, 145, 148, 149, 151, 200
materials, 14, 29
maternal care, 42
mathematics, 24, 28, 37
matter, 17, 78, 81, 87, 93, 105, 120
measurement, 50, 101, 102, 103, 116, 152
mechanical ventilation, 210
media, 49, 127
mediation, 155
Medicaid, 38
medical, vii, 1, 2, 3, 4, 6, 7, 8, 11, 21, 22, 25, 26, 27, 33, 34, 35, 38, 40, 42, 44, 46, 68, 72, 98, 105, 122, 123, 128, 129, 133, 159, 167, 171, 174, 175, 176, 178, 181, 188, 208, 210, 211, 213, 214, 215, 218, 222
medical care, 39, 42, 72, 123, 211
medication, xi, 3, 35, 37, 44, 115, 184, 191

medicine, 128, 132, 181, 214, 216
melatonin, 17
memory, 3, 27, 35, 114, 143, 148, 149, 154, 159, 164, 200, 201
memory function, 164
mental age, 7, 45
mental development, 99
mental disorder, xi, 48, 73, 184
mental health, viii, ix, 32, 35, 44, 51, 78, 83, 92, 126, 137, 140, 141, 149, 153, 175, 176, 185, 186
mental health professionals, 44
mental illness, 114, 134, 148, 197, 199
mental processes, 102, 175
mental retardation, 4, 52, 99, 110, 117
mental states, 101
meta-analysis, 50, 154, 155, 187, 194
methodology, 6, 63, 64, 122, 160
Mexico, 97, 116
migration, 117, 196
Ministry of Education, 208, 210
miscommunication, 193
mission, viii, 77
models, xi, 132, 155, 183
modifications, 3, 13, 17, 113
mood disorder, 187, 190
moral judgment, 102
morality, 68, 216
morbidity, 51, 186, 191
morphology, 10, 49, 55
mortality, 74, 162, 190, 196
mosaic, 7
motivation, 16, 104, 133, 212, 214
motor control, 12, 20
motor skills, 12, 15, 17, 21, 219
multidimensional, 116, 139, 167, 201, 213, 223
multiple sclerosis, 133
muscles, 218, 222
musculoskeletal, 10, 196, 200
music, 6, 7, 14, 17, 30
mutation, 5
mutuality, xi, 184
Myanmar, 196

N

naming, 12
narratives, viii, 65, 77, 80, 82, 90
National Health Service, 124
National Institutes of Health, 43, 44
negative attitudes, 101, 106, 212
negative consequences, 58, 196
negative effects, 140
negative emotions, 46, 130, 135, 160

Index

negative experiences, 58
negative outcomes, 186
negative relation, 186
negotiating, 123, 188
negotiation, 85, 132
neonates, 99
nervous system, 3
Netherlands, 132
networking, 124
neurobiology, 152
neurodevelopmental disorders, vii, 1, 2, 3, 24, 38
neurohormonal, 186
neurological disease, 130
neuromuscular diseases, 125
neurotoxicity, 51
neutral, 58, 84, 106, 198
New England, 54, 222
normal children, 222
normal distribution, 144, 145
North America, 50
Norway, 191
nurses, 69, 95, 171, 172, 173, 175, 176, 177, 179, 180, 181, 182, 209, 215
nursing, 161, 178, 180, 181, 182, 191, 205, 209, 214, 215
nursing home, 161, 209, 215
nutrition, 123, 124

O

obedience, 209
obesity, 31
objective stressors, x, 137
occupational therapy, 11, 49
old age, 7, 135, 158, 161, 162
one dimension, 101
opportunities, x, 16, 19, 26, 29, 33, 34, 49, 98, 101, 117, 171, 177, 212, 214
opportunity costs, 159
oral cavity, 218, 220
oral health, vii, xii, 217, 218, 219, 220, 222, 223
organ, 40, 127
organize, 211
osteoporosis, 159
outpatient(s), 13, 58, 139, 145, 146, 179, 206

P

Pacific, 128, 166, 206
pain, 5, 9, 20, 41, 172, 174, 179, 197, 209, 210, 215, 221
pain management, 209

Pakistan, 106
palate, 218
palliative, vii, xi, xii, 58, 64, 181, 183, 187, 188, 190, 192, 194, 207, 208, 209, 212, 213, 214, 215, 216
pancreatic cancer, 64
parallel, 85, 105, 107, 126, 164, 165
parental control, 132
parenting, 13, 46, 54, 132
parents, ix, 2, 12, 13, 16, 19, 28, 32, 33, 38, 42, 44, 45, 46, 47, 48, 50, 59, 60, 67, 68, 71, 97, 98, 102, 103, 104, 105, 106, 109, 129, 151, 158, 197, 200, 201, 202, 218
participants, ix, 61, 63, 65, 68, 71, 72, 78, 79, 82, 92, 93, 107, 108, 110, 111, 112, 130, 138, 140, 141, 145, 147, 149, 174, 175, 177, 209, 210, 212, 213
pathology, 148
patient care, 126, 174, 178, 188, 197
patient-caregiver dyad, xi, 184
pediatrician, 16, 17, 21, 44
peer relationship, 23, 26, 37, 48
perceived health, 198, 200
peripheral blood, 7
peripheral neuropathy, 5
permission, 19, 20, 39, 88
personal communication, 176
personal hygiene, 123
personal identity, 62
personal life, xi, 82, 85, 185, 195, 196, 197, 200
personal relationship, 58
personal values, 36
personal views, 212
personality, x, 6, 24, 35, 124, 137, 141, 143, 149, 153, 173, 192
personality characteristics, x, 124, 137
personality traits, 141, 143
persons with disabilities, 108, 121
pessimism, 42
phenomenology, 132
phenotype, 50, 52, 56
Philadelphia, 52, 75, 95
Philippines, 196
physical activity, 31, 161
physical health, 42, 121, 154, 155, 159, 162, 173, 185, 186, 187, 192
physical therapist, 10, 31, 32, 175
physical therapy, 11, 20
physical well-being, 162
physicians, 8, 39, 66, 69, 134, 171, 173, 175, 177, 178, 180, 181, 196, 209, 212, 213, 216
physiological mechanisms, 186
pilot study, 107, 159, 164, 209, 224
pitch, 116
placenta, 7

platform, 163
playing, 15, 18, 19, 22, 29, 31, 68, 69, 83, 84, 86
pleasure, 101, 105
policy, xi, 115, 124, 183, 189
policy makers, xi, 37, 124, 183, 189
population, vii, ix, x, xi, 17, 63, 97, 98, 99, 100, 101, 105, 107, 113, 121, 130, 138, 145, 146, 148, 149, 151, 157, 158, 159, 165, 167, 175, 184, 190, 191, 196, 204, 205, 207, 208, 222
Portugal, 77
positive attitudes, 101
positive correlation, 186
positive emotions, 130, 139, 149
positive mental health, 178
positive reinforcement, 18
post-hoc analysis, 61
posttraumatic stress, 139, 153
poverty, 100
prayer, 140, 155
pregnancy, 33
preparation, 79, 115, 184
preschool, 16, 53, 219, 220, 221, 223
preschoolers, 135
presentation skills, 209
preservice teachers, 115
prevalence rate, 159
prevention, 33, 174, 176, 178, 179, 180, 203
primary caregivers, vii, 1, 2, 3, 24, 25, 27, 33, 35, 37, 42, 43, 44, 47, 158, 159
primary degenerative dementia, 154
primary school, 112
priming, 101
principles, 29, 37, 65, 104, 107, 129
private sector, 115
probability, 107, 108, 110, 111, 112, 113, 117, 130
probability judgment, 112
problem behavior, 163, 164, 165
problem-focused coping, 143
problem-solving, 28, 34, 52, 149, 162, 163, 164, 168, 189, 202
problem-solving skills, 149, 163, 189
problem-solving strategies, 34
professional development, 83
professionalism, 178
professionals, viii, ix, xi, 8, 22, 33, 36, 44, 47, 57, 65, 74, 77, 78, 80, 85, 87, 88, 92, 93, 95, 108, 121, 127, 132, 159, 165, 172, 173, 174, 175, 176, 177, 183, 188, 189, 210, 211, 222
prognosis, 47, 64, 188
project, vii, 57, 59, 208, 209, 213
proposition, 86
prostatectomy, 191
protection, 38, 59, 123, 124

protective factors, 139, 148, 159, 160, 161
protective role, 188
psychiatric disorders, 25, 52, 197
psychiatrist, 41, 115
psychological distress, xi, 126, 164, 184, 185, 186, 192
psychological health, 139, 154, 159, 165, 187, 196
psychological problems, 161, 199
psychological stressors, 167
psychological value, 103
psychological well-being, 134, 153, 164
psychologist, 10, 27, 35, 41, 65, 99, 103, 104, 112, 134, 177
psychology, 27, 57, 59, 64, 73, 74, 75, 99, 114, 133, 139
psychometric properties, 143, 152, 153
psychosocial interventions, 95, 188, 194
psychosocial stress, 167
psychosocial support, 8
psychotherapy, 44, 75, 189, 194
PTSD, 139, 145, 146, 148
puberty, 6, 48
public administration, 125
public awareness, 3
public policy, 4
public service, 113
public welfare, 184
punishment, 30, 31, 128

Q

qualitative research, 74, 133
quality of life, vii, xii, 1, 2, 15, 23, 34, 36, 37, 42, 45, 47, 50, 122, 125, 126, 127, 134, 135, 155, 159, 163, 164, 167, 185, 186, 190, 191, 196, 198, 205, 211, 217, 218, 219, 220, 222, 223
quantification, 102
query, 211
questionnaire, xii, 143, 167, 209, 215, 217, 219, 220

R

racing, 18
racism, 117
rationality, 114
reactions, 101
reading, 5, 12, 19, 24, 28, 29, 32, 65, 212
reading disorder, 24
realism, 32
reality, 83, 84, 120, 124, 171, 186
reasoning, 6, 29
recall, 28

Index

recognition, 25, 51, 83, 84, 122, 124, 162, 175, 176
recommendations, vii, 2, 11, 12, 14, 15, 17, 18, 19, 20, 27, 28, 29, 32, 35, 36, 37, 47, 120, 172, 178, 188
reconstruction, 63, 64
recovery, 174, 199
recreational, 55, 163, 177
recruiting, 173, 211
recurrence, 187
redistribution, 126
reflexes, 20, 220, 223
regions of the world, 202
regression, 161
regulations, 39, 101, 123
rehabilitation, 20, 21, 35, 37, 49, 126, 155, 161, 166, 168, 169, 220, 222
Rehabilitation Act, 26
reinforcement, 14, 93
rejection, 48, 53, 71, 123
relapses, 180
relationship quality, 198
relatives, x, 94, 137, 138, 140, 145, 146, 152, 153, 158, 162, 164, 205
relaxation, 176, 189
relevance, 180
reliability, 142, 143, 154, 167, 168, 205
relief, 88, 90, 93
religion, 196
religious beliefs, 177, 186
REM, 9
remorse, 58
renal failure, 200
repetitions, 201
reproduction, 100
reputation, 103
requirements, 131
researchers, 10, 37, 105, 164, 181
resentment, 46, 81, 90
residential, 37, 54
resilience, vii, ix, x, 137, 138, 139, 140, 141, 143, 144, 145, 147, 148, 149, 150, 151, 152, 153, 154, 155
resistance, 9, 88
resolution, 64
resources, vii, x, xi, xii, 1, 2, 5, 11, 12, 20, 27, 32, 34, 35, 36, 43, 46, 47, 59, 61, 66, 80, 88, 90, 92, 98, 117, 128, 131, 137, 138, 140, 141, 148, 149, 150, 151, 164, 171, 172, 173, 184, 186, 189
response, 82, 89, 103, 104, 108, 110, 131, 160, 208
restrictions, 219
retardation, 4, 53, 54, 114, 117
retirement, 177
rewards, 14, 18, 19, 31, 62, 123, 164, 177, 185, 196

rhythm, 7, 116
rights, 26, 41, 98, 100, 115, 121, 188
risk, x, xi, 9, 10, 31, 41, 62, 74, 81, 82, 116, 126, 139, 148, 157, 158, 160, 161, 162, 165, 167, 168, 174, 184, 185, 186, 187, 189, 192, 196, 218, 222
role-playing, 32, 72, 210, 212
romantic relationship, 32, 33, 34, 48
Rosenberg Self-Esteem Scale, 143, 144
routines, 13, 30, 82, 92, 187
rules, 17, 18, 30, 31, 40, 98, 105, 112, 113, 129, 130, 131
rural areas, 211
Russia, 106, 117

S

sadness, 94
safety, 13, 19, 21, 30, 33, 173, 179
saturation, 65
Saturn, 120
savings, 131
scarcity, 131
schema, 104
school, ix, 3, 13, 15, 18, 20, 21, 22, 23, 24, 25, 26, 27, 30, 31, 32, 33, 35, 36, 45, 51, 68, 97, 101, 103, 104, 105, 106, 107, 108, 109, 110, 111, 112, 113, 115, 116, 117, 125, 129, 176, 208, 214, 216, 221
school performance, 30
school work, 31
science, 54
scoliosis, 5
scope, 141
scripts, 18
secondary students, 55
security, 124
segregation, 117
seizure, 5, 218
self-confidence, 30, 35, 59
self-control, 129
self-definition, 85
self-efficacy, x, 58, 142, 148, 149, 154, 157, 159, 162, 164, 165, 166, 198
self-esteem, 19, 23, 34, 58, 59, 148, 149, 152, 172, 176
self-image, 84, 123, 154
self-reflection, 90
self-reports, 191
self-sufficiency, ix, 119, 131
self-worth, 37, 149
seminars, 211, 213
semi-structured interviews, viii, 57
senile dementia, 125

sensation, 218
sensitivity, 5, 100, 168, 188
separateness, 151
sequencing, 19
Serbia, 106
serum, 7, 186
service provider, 39, 124, 163
services, 5, 8, 10, 11, 20, 21, 23, 25, 26, 27, 35, 37, 38, 40, 42, 44, 49, 54, 107, 123, 124, 125, 129, 131, 163, 164, 165, 168, 174, 188, 189, 194, 211
sex, 68, 142, 148, 149, 160, 161, 187, 198, 200, 201, 218
sexual activity, 172
sexual contact, 33, 117
sexual desire, 33
sexual development, 32, 33, 34
sexual intercourse, 114, 116
sexuality, 33, 52, 101, 105, 113, 116
shame, 123, 129, 176
shape, 67, 120
shock, 58
shoot, 133
shortage, xii, 174
shortness of breath, 198
showing, 59, 93, 105, 148, 210
sibling(s), vii, 1, 2, 3, 5, 6, 7, 14, 22, 23, 30, 45, 46, 47, 48, 49, 51, 52, 53, 54, 55
side effects, 172
signaling pathway, 192
signals, 84
significance level, xii, 217, 219
signs, 7, 19, 93, 126, 210
simulation, 211
Singapore, 196, 197, 199, 200, 201, 203, 205
skin, 5, 9
skin picking, 5, 9
sleep deprivation, 185
sleep disturbance, 5, 9, 185, 186
smoking, 115
SMS, 2, 3, 5, 6, 7, 8, 9, 10, 17, 20, 21, 22, 23, 24, 25, 26, 34, 37, 42, 43, 45, 46
sociability, 24
social activities, 23, 89
social care, ix, 119, 123, 131
social cognition, 114
social context, 85, 188
social development, 98, 208
social environment, 101, 107, 108, 109, 112
social events, 100, 172
social impairment, 196
social integration, 129
social interactions, 23, 24, 51, 81, 92
social life, 126, 128

social network, 61, 87
social problems, 46
social relations, 6, 23, 58, 121, 127, 149, 197
social roles, 160
social sciences, 85
Social Security, 39, 213
Social Security Administration, 39
social services, 78, 167
social situations, 19, 24
social skills, 11, 23, 24, 32, 33, 34, 48, 135
social status, 190
social support, x, 42, 48, 50, 75, 88, 98, 127, 131, 137, 140, 147, 148, 149, 154, 155, 162, 163, 165, 168, 180, 186, 187, 192, 198, 200, 202, 203
social welfare, ix, 119, 125, 131, 163
social workers, 8, 92, 164, 171, 175
socialization, 24, 133, 135
societal cost, 167
society, ix, 8, 33, 34, 37, 38, 41, 78, 86, 97, 98, 100, 113, 121, 122, 129, 130, 131, 166, 176, 196, 199, 203, 204
sociocultural contexts, 139
socioeconomic status, 186
solidarity, 124, 131
solitude, 86, 125
solution, 63, 70, 72, 128, 131
South Asia, vii
South Korea, 198
Southeast Asia, vi, xi, 129, 195, 196, 197, 199, 200, 201, 202, 203, 204
Spain, 137
spastic, 219
spasticity, 219, 222, 224
special education, 27, 53, 99, 102, 103, 106, 107, 110, 112, 113, 115, 116
specialists, 22, 32, 190
speech, 3, 5, 8, 9, 10, 15, 20, 21, 22, 27, 32, 47, 53
spending, 131
sphincter, 103, 104
spirituality, 134
spring, 205
sputum, 211, 215
SSA, 39
stability, 83
staff members, 172, 174
standard deviation, 144, 219
state(s), 10, 35, 38, 39, 40, 67, 82, 89, 121, 124, 130, 138, 142, 147, 150, 166, 172, 196
statistics, 144
statutes, 40
stereotypes, 26, 98, 114
stigma, 98, 99, 114
stimulus, 88

stomach, 12, 64
stress, ix, x, 8, 9, 33, 42, 56, 79, 87, 89, 115, 125, 126, 127, 137, 138, 141, 147, 148, 150, 151, 153, 154, 155, 158, 161, 164, 166, 172, 173, 174, 175, 176, 177, 178, 179, 180, 181, 183, 185, 187, 223
stressors, x, xi, 3, 4, 137, 141, 148, 149, 150, 154, 171, 174, 177, 183, 187, 195, 196, 199
stroke, x, xi, 94, 135, 157, 159, 161, 162, 165, 166, 167, 168, 169, 195, 196, 198, 202, 206
structure, 54, 58, 86, 90, 117, 120, 196
style, 17, 58, 132, 152, 187, 209
subjective experience, 59, 65, 121
subjective well-being, 187
succession, 40
suicide, 115
supervision, 30, 35, 99, 141, 218
support programs, viii, 77, 164, 165
support services, 158, 163, 164
support staff, 25
suppression, 131
survival, 58, 59, 71, 120, 128
survivors, 94, 135, 161, 162, 168, 184, 191, 192, 194, 206
sustainability, 131
Sweden, 133, 191
symptoms, ix, x, 24, 42, 60, 124, 125, 127, 129, 137, 138, 140, 143, 148, 149, 150, 159, 160, 162, 165, 166, 169, 171, 172, 174, 175, 176, 177, 178, 188, 202, 204, 209, 210
syndrome, 2, 5, 6, 7, 8, 22, 25, 26, 42, 43, 44, 46, 48, 49, 50, 51, 52, 53, 54, 55, 56, 114, 201
synthesis, 117

T

Taiwan, 128, 198
target, xi, 23, 164, 175, 183, 204, 208
target populations, xi, 183
tax credits, xi, 183
taxonomy, 63
teachers, ix, 8, 23, 25, 26, 28, 97, 98, 101, 103, 104, 106, 107, 112, 114, 116, 117
teaching experience, 106, 111, 112
teams, 8, 25, 174, 203
techniques, ix, 13, 19, 30, 40, 79, 101, 120, 175, 176
technology(ies), vii, xii, 15, 113, 127, 128
teeth, 9, 17, 219, 221
telephone, 164, 165, 169
temperament, 46
tension, 58, 172, 185
terminal patients, 72
terminally ill, 192
territory, 124

testicular cancer, 74
testing, 6, 7, 29
test-retest reliability, 143
textbook, 114
texture, 21
Thailand, 195, 196, 197, 199, 200, 201, 204, 205
theft, viii, 78
therapeutic interventions, 138
therapist, 11, 13, 44, 52
therapy, 11, 13, 17, 20, 21, 22, 32, 44, 47, 125, 152
thoughts, 130, 133, 142, 162, 164, 210
timbre, 116
toddlers, 9, 132
toilet training, 18
tones, 30
toys, 12, 16, 17, 18, 19, 31
trade, 5, 8
traditions, 127
training, x, xi, 25, 27, 34, 36, 44, 45, 79, 99, 106, 117, 122, 128, 129, 131, 132, 134, 157, 161, 162, 163, 164, 175, 176, 181, 183, 184, 188, 189, 202, 203, 209, 211, 214, 215
training programs, x, xi, 99, 157, 176, 183
traits, 7, 53
trajectory, 80, 90, 139, 190, 191, 193
transcendence, 143, 144
transcripts, viii, 57, 65
transformation, 84, 89, 124
transgression, 129
transition to adulthood, 56
translocation, 7
transmission, 173, 213
transport, 127, 164
trauma, 151, 173, 175, 176, 181
traumatic events, 139, 173
treatment, 37, 40, 44, 46, 51, 52, 58, 60, 64, 98, 99, 115, 117, 122, 130, 161, 164, 172, 175, 178, 179, 184, 188, 203, 213, 221, 222
trial, 164, 166, 168, 192, 210, 216
trisomy 21, 7
tumor, 69, 70
turnover, 172, 173, 179
two-dimensional space, 108
Type I error, 145

U

UK, 194
ultrasound, 7
United, 3, 26, 49, 53, 56, 106, 113, 121, 127, 174, 178, 190, 193, 196, 204, 205
United Nations (UN), 121, 127, 190, 196, 204

United States, 3, 26, 49, 53, 56, 121, 174, 178, 193, 205
universe, 127
university education, xii, 207, 208
updating, 27
urban, 132, 196, 201
urbanization, 203
urinary tract, 5, 7, 21
USA, 1, 43, 100, 106, 114, 116

V

validation, xi, 153, 184, 198
valorization, 37, 50, 56
valuation, 103, 104, 105, 107, 112, 113
variables, x, 61, 103, 104, 106, 107, 122, 137, 140, 141, 142, 144, 145, 147, 148, 149, 150, 178, 185, 187, 197, 198, 199, 200
variations, 90, 113
variety of domains, 105
Vatican, 121
ventilation, 138
verbal fluency, 21
victims, 163, 191
video games, 31
videos, 16, 210
violence, 115
vision, ix, 5, 6, 97, 99, 119, 121, 131
visualization, 104
vocational interests, 35, 36
vocational rehabilitation, 35
vote, 121
vulnerability, 42, 92, 100, 120, 173

W

waking, 16, 18
walking, 219
war, 34
Washington, 48, 53, 55, 56, 171, 178
weakness, 10
wear, 15, 19
web, 114, 179
weight gain, 9
weight loss, 25, 159, 172, 185
welfare, 211, 212, 213
well-being, viii, ix, x, xi, 2, 9, 34, 42, 47, 50, 77, 90, 92, 119, 123, 134, 152, 162, 166, 168, 173, 174, 175, 177, 180, 181, 183, 184, 195, 222, 223
wellness, 9, 176, 177, 180, 181
windows, 20
witchcraft, 128
witnesses, 41, 172
work activities, 34
work environment, 34, 172
workers, xi, 36, 52, 101, 115, 174, 175, 176, 177, 179, 181, 195, 197, 202, 209, 215
workforce, 34, 158, 161, 191
workplace, 34, 49, 51, 176, 177, 180, 213
World Bank, 121
World Health Organization (WHO), xii, 4, 56, 100, 106, 115, 117, 121, 122, 135, 204, 205, 217, 223
World War I, 100
worldwide, 5, 6, 7, 167, 184, 190, 209
worry, 197

Y

young adults, 35
young people, 49, 56

Z

zippers, 17